A History of Australia's Early Cosmopolitan Naturopathic Osteopathy

AF875176

Revealing the forgotten ideas and philosophy behind early naturopathic osteopathy, Shirley Murray Strachan presents a reoriented historical view of Thomas Ambrose Bowen and his work, breaking from the prevailing twentieth-century legitimation narrative of mainstream chiropractic and osteopathy and exploring the contributions and practices of Australia's early cosmopolitan naturopathic osteopathy pioneers FG Roberts and Maurice Blackmore.

Viewing Bowen's practice and symbolism through a historical lens, the book examines the forgotten world of early cosmopolitan Australian osteopathy, debunking popular posthumous commercialised claims about Bowen's work and asserts the importance of traditional approaches in naturopathic osteopathy. Though an interrogation of conflicting origin stories and myths about Bowen's work, it highlights the important contributions of naturopathic pioneers FG Roberts and Maurice Blackmore. The background narrative is the struggle of mainstream chiropractic and osteopathy seeking professional recognition and forged from in-fighting between overseas and Australian chiropractic and osteopathic political interests. Counterposed is the posthumous popular interpretations that orphaned Bowen's work from its wellsprings in naturopathic osteopathy.

This is an accessible book for historians and practitioners of early osteopathy, chiropractic and naturopathy, especially to the large, international community of accredited Bowen therapists.

Shirley Murray Strachan is an historian and honorary research associate with the Future Regions Research Centre Federation University, Australia, ND, remedial massage and Bowen Therapist.

A History of Australia's Early Cosmopolitan Naturopathic Osteopathy

The Pioneering Practice and Global Symbolism of Thomas Ambrose Bowen

Shirley Murray Strachan

Routledge
Taylor & Francis Group
LONDON AND NEW YORK

First published 2025
by Routledge
4 Park Square, Milton Park, Abingdon, Oxon OX14 4RN

and by Routledge
605 Third Avenue, New York, NY 10158

Routledge is an imprint of the Taylor & Francis Group, an informa business

British Library Cataloguing-in-Publication Data
A catalogue record for this book is available from the British Library

ISBN: 978-1-032-99067-5 (hbk)
ISBN: 978-1-032-99068-2 (pbk)
ISBN: 978-1-003-60212-5 (ebk)

DOI: 10.4324/9781003602125

Typeset in Galliard
by Apex CoVantage, LLC

Contents

Figures

Tables

Acknowledgements

I thank colleagues Professor Keir Reeves and Dr Brad Duncan for their review of the manuscript and helpful suggestions, Romney Smeeton DC, Ron Phelan, Lynn Wilson and Maryann Cosic for kindly allowing the use of their images, Robert Ryder and Ron Phelan for access to and use of their video and sound recordings, and all the contributors too many to name who provided their valuable memories with Tom Bowen for the centennial *Healing Hands* anthology and afterwards. I also thank A/Prof Hans Baer for his suggestion of the Medical Pluralism theme.

Introduction

How did an uneducated blue-collar worker and football masseur who assumed the title of osteopath become the subject of a book?

Today Bowen's name is attached to an international modality called Bowen Technique or Bowen Therapy, taught around the world as part of complementary and alternative medicine (CAM) with practitioners accredited in major jurisdictions of Australia, Britain, Europe, America and Canada with an influence in India, Malaysia, Japan, South Africa and Alaska.

Bowen in the late 1970s (see Figure 0.1) did not leave any memoirs or writings about his work, nor did he call what he did Bowen Technique or Therapy. Any clinic records were destroyed. Surviving documentary records are limited to his 1973 transcript of an interview at the *Victorian Government Inquiry into Chiropractic, Osteopathy and Naturopathy*; records by first-hand observers in training manuals, presentations and articles; and over fifty oral histories compiled by the author as a 2016 celebratory centennial anthology of unsung voices that included accounts from his college-trained clinic associates, former patients, family and friends.

Bowen's language preserved in transcripts, oral and media accounts provides valuable clues about the origins of his work alongside what is remembered of his techniques – interpreted in global teachings and perfected in clinical practice by the few college-trained observers who had the privilege of watching him treat his patients. This book is an exploration into the historical landscape around Bowen to understand his journey from genius to victim of regulation to the posthumous figurehead of a global modality taking its unique place among other CAM bodywork forms.

The popularised global portrayal of Bowen is untrained and a divinely inspired originator of his methods. However, Bowen's language and what has survived the delivery of his work in memory and practice resonates with early and traditional osteopathic sources. This has allowed comparable practice and ideas to be found in a long-forgotten form of early osteopathy called neuropathy. Neuropathy was brought to Australian shores from America – not via graduates of modernised osteopathy colleges but via the nature cure route and disseminated by Australia's founding naturopathic pioneers – FG Roberts

DOI: 10.4324/9781003602125-1

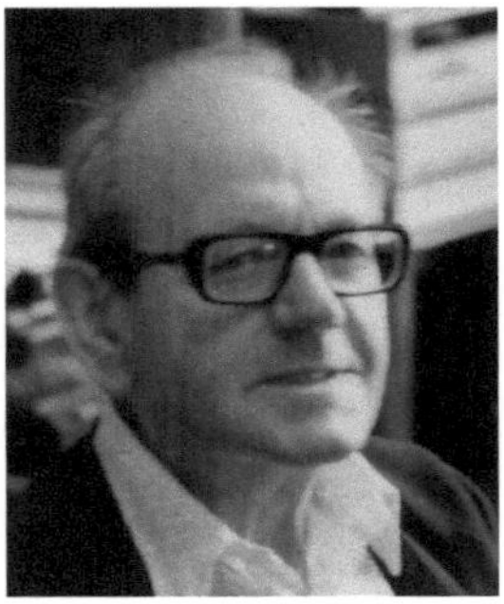

Figure 0.1 Bowen on a social visit to Smeeton Home in Colac, late 1970s.

Source: Image Courtesy of Romney Smeeton.

principally and Maurice Blackmore. Attention to Bowen's language and clinic style also correlate with traditional and original moves of osteopathy's pioneer Dr A T Still MD, DO, preserved by his disciples who formed a roundtable in 1924, five years after his death due to concern that the heart of Still's work was becoming lost to developments in education.

Some will repel any suggestion that Bowen's work has a historical source and prefer to continue to portray him as a lone soul, orphaned in space and time from osteopathy and operating apart from formal knowledge and interaction with like-minded osteopathic peers; others may remain attached to the view that a legendary football masseur called Saunders imparted Japanese acupressure techniques to Bowen and that Saunders is Bowen's mentor despite the lack of congruence in his style. Others may see that reappraising him in a historical context and viewing him as a representative of early naturopathic osteopathy allows his genius to stand out. Finding a home for the historical origins of Bowen's work does not detract from his pioneering innovation in developing an approach that embodies a consummate mastery of Dr Still MD, DO's dictum, 'Find it. Fix it. Leave it Alone' sometimes extended to 'and Nature will do the rest.' Bowen was not a learned man in the academic sense and his pioneering status has nothing to do with expounding a new theory, but simply with his brilliance and in developing a system of sequential minimalist techniques that expertly achieved Dr Still MD, DO's objectives to use minimal interventions. Bowen applied a unique sensory giftedness and remarkable intuition to the creative delivery of highly nuanced minimalist techniques applied with finely honed tactile finesse. In doing so, Bowen developed something altogether different, posthumously called Bowen Therapy or Technique that is practised globally today. His system is so versatile that even simplistic renditions in good hands give therapeutic benefit but to quote

Romney Smeeton DC writing in 1992, there is unfinished work and depths to plumb to fully honour his legacy:

> While working with Mr Bowen, we were given the basis of his approach. Unfortunately, many of his 'secrets' he took with him when he died ten years ago. It is up to us to further the technique to gain the maximum potential of this work. The scope of the progression is limited only by the practitioner's inability to understand the basis of his approach and thereby failing to utilise the immense potential.[1]

Note

1 Romney Smeeton. "The Bowen Approach to Manipulative Therapy," 1992 (see full statement in Chapter 1).

1 Bowen's World

Under American Pressure, Legitimation of Osteopathy and the Sidelining of Naturopathic Osteopathy

> It is clear that so long as a man is to practise medicine, the public is equally concerned in his right preparation for that profession, whatever he call himself, – allopath, homeopath, eclectic, osteopath or whatnot. It is equally clear he should be grounded in the fundamental sciences upon which medicine rests, whether he practices under one name or under another.
>
> Henry S Pritchett, President Carnegie Foundation[1]

Introduction: Bowen Biography

Who was Thomas Ambrose Bowen (1916–1982) and how does he relate to these chapter themes? Despite his immense talent and after two decades of successful practice under the self-chosen title of osteopath, Bowen became a victim of regulation and was stripped of any right to use this professional designation. He represents not only the untold story of those cast aside as the grand narrative of the legitimation of chiropractic and osteopathy played out with its own battles towards a successful conclusion but also that his work resonates with a forgotten practice in early osteopathy called neuropathy brought to Australian shores by naturopathic pioneers; namely FG Roberts and Maurice Blackmore. Bowen's individual genius allowed him to develop these early techniques and hone them into a unique system now posthumously called Bowen Technique or Therapy and taught the world over. Along the way, he incorporated other traditional ideas of Dr Still MD, DO osteopathy's pioneer and his disciples.

The Bowen story is one of rise from humble beginnings to posthumous international fame. He was born in Melbourne, the third child of an immigrant family from Wolverhampton, UK, whose early home in Brunswick, Victoria, became a 'sacred place' after his parents' religious conversion within the Salvation Army around 1920.[2] Avidly pursuing their calling, his parents William and Norah became a devout driving force in the founding of Geelong's early citadels. Before her retirement some years ago, Bowen's eldest daughter Pamela Trigg (1943–2024) held the high rank of Lieutenant Colonel of the Australian Southern Territory. With education not valued by his father, the teenage Bowen became a milk carter and assisted his carpenter-father in the

DOI: 10.4324/9781003602125-2

building trade, before holding various menial jobs on the floors of Geelong's blue-collar industries. According to his sister Agnes, her brother had always wanted to be a medical doctor but during the Depression years (1930–1939 in Australia) and their father facing bankruptcy, to her brother's great disappointment, his ambitions were thwarted.[3]

With a passion for football and associated enjoyment of beer and cigarettes that led his angered father to discipline his son, Bowen satisfied his calling by rising through the ranks of football masseurs and gave early attention to victims of polio. He said he found his gift in the war and oral history evidence begins in the mid-1950s with him treating people in the homes of workmates. In 1959, the year his father died, Bowen moved to discard his dungarees from his cement works' employment as locomotive cleaner to become a white-collar professional carrying the title of osteopath (see Figure 1.1). Though an unregulated profession at the time, the tides of change were underway with the Royal Commission in Western Australia 1958–1964; set up to investigate natural therapies. This resulted in the *Chiropractors Registration Act 1964* and heralded developments on the eastern seaboard. Osteopathy had not fared well and it is interesting, given this negative profile that Bowen chose this profession, rather than chiropractic. It seems from the outset that Bowen was clear in his chosen vocation and this surfaces again in Chapter 7 with his remarks to the Ward Inquiry and his membership of the Victorian Society of Specialist Osteopaths (VSSO). Until 1961, during his part-time transition to test the waters and ensure he could financially support his family, others appreciated Bowen's abilities. The Hazeltons stepped in to help and gave Bowen work driving their truck to protect his hands.[4] In the lead-up, the pressures were great and Bowen reportedly had a health episode of some kind leading to a short stay at the Ballarat Asylum. Scandalously for his religious family's strictures, his business ally was another woman, the formidable Irene (Rene) Horwood, recently widowed to Stan Horwood, Bowen's friend and workmate

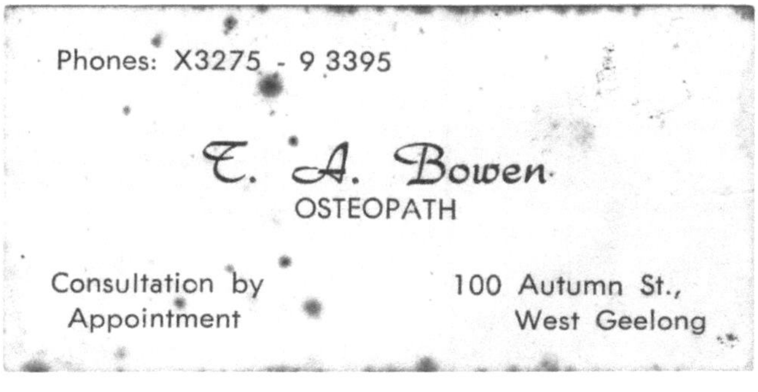

Figure 1.1 Bowen's first business card denoting 'Osteopath' 100 Autumn Street, Geelong West.

Source: Image courtesy Ron Phelan, Custodian Rene Horwood Collection.

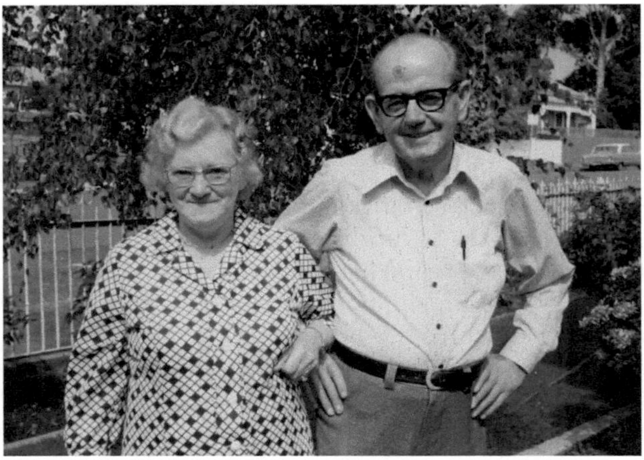

Figure 1.2 Bowen and Horwood at 30 Villamanta Street, late 1970s.
Source: Image courtesy Ron Phelan, Custodian Rene Horwood Collection.

at the Portland Cement Plant (see Figure 1.2).[5] As First Aid Officer at the plant, Bowen had helped Stan injured in a fall, and by 1958, the Horwoods were supporting Bowen's talent by offering him the stability of a treatment room and study space at their home at 100 Autumn Street, Geelong West (see Figure 1.3 where the property is in the background across the street from the Tom Bowen *Healing Hands* memorial).[6] Rene brought homely cheer and an iron will for order over the incessant traffic at all of Bowen's clinics that followed establishing a professional presence: at the main thoroughfare of Latrobe Terrace; at no. 99 (1958–1963) and no. 283 (1963–1976/77) followed by Villamanta Street, Geelong West at no. 30 (1976/77–1980) then lastly, no. 26 (1980–1982). Bowen's first clinic was in high demand, cars parked in Autumn Street blocked the fire brigade's access to the station across the street.[7] He attracted jealousies and derision from local competitors who held either prestigious overseas degrees or Australian credentials. Other than doctors and physiotherapists (including registered masseurs) who enjoyed legal protection and status, all practitioners were viewed as quacks.

Bowen's choice of vocation and regulation in Victoria is set against the historical context of the new forms of drugless systems of medicine that had their debut in America during the last quarter of the nineteenth century. These new medicines emerged alongside each other and appeared concurrently as osteopathy, chiropractic and naturopathy. The latter in its original form was an umbrella concept that embraced all forms of drugless healing, whether ingestive, manual medicine or lifestyle interventions. Osteopathy was pioneered by Andrew Taylor Still (Dr Still MD, DO) as a new drugless system of medicine in 1874 and taught at his college the American School of Osteopathy (ASO) founded in Kirksville, Missouri, in 1892. By 1902, Daniel David Palmer

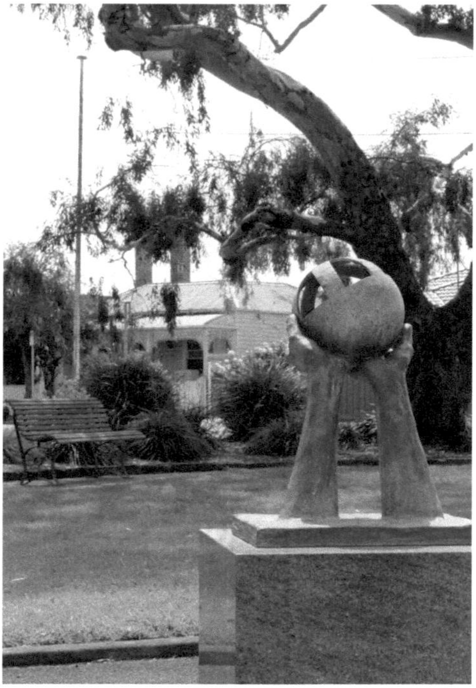

Figure 1.3 The Bowen *Healing Hands* memorial showing Bowen's hands holding a globe representing the international reach of his work and facing 100 Autumn Street where his professional career began.

Source: Image courtesy of Lynn Wilson, Bowen Therapist, New Zealand.

had pioneered a chiropractic school in Davenport, Ohio. There is evidence of early contact between Still and Palmer whose ideas overlapped, though techniques and philosophy differed. In modern terms, their holistic concepts were person-centred and founded on the holistic wellbeing philosophy that the body had innate powers of self-regulation and healing. This outlook was in opposition to the reductionist approach of mainstream allopathic medicine that involved the application of sometimes dangerous drugs and surgery in Still's time.

Osteopaths and chiropractors alike were concerned with the structural integrity of the body and the optimal functioning of its systems. Both rectified bony misalignments of the spine, with a view to optimal innervation of the body; however, osteopaths also attended to the appendicular joints and the limbs, though some chiropractic approaches such as 'diversified' did too. Alignment of the spine restored nerve flows. Osteopaths were also concerned with blood and lymph flow and later, for those who adopted craniosacral therapy, cerebrospinal fluid flow. While chiropractic relied on robust thrusts commonly described as bone-cracking to bring alignment to the spine and free impingements to nerve flow, osteopaths influenced tissue tensions that allowed bones to gently roll back to alignment to optimise healthy circulatory flow of blood, lymph and nerve activity. Osteopaths uniquely developed a strong palpatory awareness of changes in tissue and nervous system tone and detected blockages or 'lesions' that represented somatic dysfunction. Chiropractors instead embraced the old concept of spinal 'subluxations' as misalignments that affected nerve flow. Osteopaths and chiropractors both used limbs as levers to bring about tension/structural changes to the pelvis and spine. Both regarded their professions as complete systems of medicine but during the twentieth century, boundaries were blurred due to practitioners subsuming each other's techniques.

The teaching of these new drugless forms of therapy in the USA irked the medical mainstream because of the proliferation of doctor titles by those without medical degrees. However, many of the leaders of these new systems were also medically trained and carried the titles of medical doctor (MD) alongside Doctor of Naturopathy, Chiropractic or Osteopathy (ND, DC and DO), respectively. Tensions erupted in the USA and subsequently spread overseas. Aimed at educational reform, the American 1910 Flexner Report was written during a time when there was no licensing of medical doctors or therapists of any kind in the USA. Abraham Flexner, a reformist and expert in education, was strongly influenced by the 'German pedagogic style of medical education' founded on laboratory work and the 'hyper rationale system of German science'.[8] Flexner divided institutions he visited into three tiers and was scathing of those USA medical institutions which fell under tier three, to which he added those schools flourishing around the new and increasingly popular modalities of osteopathy, chiropractic and naturopathy. The Flexner Report also hit a nerve highlighting tensions within osteopathic teaching, where among those medically trained, were those who upset Dr Still MD, DO and advocated the integration of their allopathic medicine with osteopathic training. The Flexner Report heralded curricula development in the USA that imposed scientific standards on university training aligned to the biomedical sciences. From this, uniquely in America, osteopathic training evolved to allow practitioners who pursued these pathways to graduate with the same status and practising rights as a medical doctor and today can also practise surgery and prescribe drugs. Elsewhere Flexner's reform agenda influenced curricula development in the early prestigious osteopathy colleges in the UK. These included the British School of Osteopathy (BSO – founded in 1917) and the London School of Osteopathy (LSO – established in 1949). Both aspired to the more stringent standards but strong medical opposition prevented their credentials receiving equivalent equal standing like the USA by medical doctors. Vested medical interests in Europe strenuously debarred osteopaths from the right to practise. Consequently, the European School of Osteopathy (ESO) founded in Paris in 1950 was forced to relocate to the UK in 1965. Dr Still MD, DO resisted a medicalised direction for his ASO.

As the fight for professional legitimation progressed in America, Canada, and Europe, common themes that affected overseas jurisdictions were likewise reflected in Australia. There were issues and different theories defining professionalisation, strategies adopted by mainstream osteopaths against organised medical resistance – by setting up training schools, forming nationalised associations, redefining the scope of practice and monopolistic strategies and lobbying political and economic elites.[9] These themes appeared in a journal article that explored the unique USA's situation where the legacy of the Flexner Report of 1910 resulted in co-optation of osteopathy by organised medicine.[10] Katherine Miller identified issues around co-optation and the tensions between Still's articulation of identity counterposed against practice adopted within the medical model. Miller pursued the phenomenological approach which regards professions as a folk category which relies upon how people in society determine who is a professional and who is not, how the professionals define themselves by their activities and what the consequences are for the way in which they see themselves and perform their work.[11] In 1998, Miller concluded by saying, 'It may be impossible for osteopathy to craft an identity that justifies a distinctive and separate profession in the coming century'.[12]

Osteopathy Graduates in Australia: Still's College and the Nature Cure Route

The early graduates of Still's ASO entered the Australian scene early in the twentieth century against the backdrop of tensions flowing from the Flexner Report. Coincidentally their arrival was when massage was undergoing regulation – effected in Victoria with the *Masseurs Act 1922* (Vic). The histories of Still's disciples across the Atlantic have been researched by other authors who covered the UK, Europe and Australia.[13] This professional stratum was first addressed by Hawkins and O'Neill who traced the first eighty years of osteopathy introduced to Australian shores by the first wave of graduates of Andrew Still's pioneering college in Kirksville, Missouri.[14] Their practices soon attracted the attentions of the Australian medical establishment resulting in legal actions against their use of doctor titles.[15] An important point is that these individuals never taught osteopathy and were superseded by graduates from derivative USA colleges and the prestigious mainstream UK establishments who formed their own exclusive Australian Osteopathy Association (AOA) and set about attempting to disenfranchise graduates of the leading Australian colleges of rights to be registered. Hawkins and O'Neill recognised the dearth of records of Australian home-grown students and a lack of accounts.[16]

An important distinction for the research in this book is that the teachings of osteopathy in the early period came via the naturopathic route and not directly from graduates of Still's ASO or any of the Flexner-compliant institutions. The naturopathic practitioners who pioneered early osteopathic and chiropractic education in Australia did so initially under a naturopathic umbrella and include the Tasmanian FG Roberts who established the Institute of Naturopathy, ca

1929, Englishman Maurice Blackmore who formed the Blackmores Australian College of Naturopathy, ca 1940 and the later entrant, the Australian of Bavarian descent, Alfred Kaufmann who formed the Sydney College of Osteopathy in 1959 by which time the naturopathy phase was starting to be supplanted by chiropractic. All were initially educated at UK naturopathic colleges – the London School of Natural Therapeutics (Roberts and Kaufmann), the London College of Biotherapy (Kauffman) and the British College of Naturopathy (understood to be Stanley Lief's College) (Blackmore). Roberts also undertook additional correspondence studies with USA nature cure schools and formed a strong connection with America's naturopathic pioneer, Benedict Lust MD and carried credentials of ND, DO and DC, among others. Although the Scot James Edward Boyle established the Ballarat-based Pax Osteopathic College of Australasia around 1937 and is said to have started off apprenticed to a Canadian osteopath, new evidence indicates he practised herbalism and Jean Doyle said he trained with Roberts in Australia while setting up Pax College.[17] The naturopathic colleges above eventually evolved away from these beginnings and ended up focusing on chiropractic and osteopathy, chiropractic mainly, to satisfy regulatory requirements for the registration of their graduates. In Australia, the long-term effects of the Flexner Report made their influence felt in State and Commonwealth Government Inquiries of the 1970s and dominated considerations of desirable education standards, now benchmarked against biomedical sciences in college curricula. The colleges of FG Roberts in Melbourne and Alfred Kaufmann in Sydney evolved to become government-recognised and produce prescribed qualifications when regulation arrived in Victoria and New South Wales in 1978. Along the way, Roberts' Institute of Naturopathy changed to the British and Australian Institute of Naturopathy (BAIN) then became the Chiropractic and Osteopathic College of Australasia (COCA) in 1959 and by the late 1970s the Chiropractic College of Australasia. Kaufmann's college started in 1959 as the Sydney College of Osteopathy and became the Sydney College of Chiropractic in 1973. This politically-driven name change and trajectory had a huge influence on the college offerings. Chapter 7 will reveal that the Roberts' college came to neglect osteopathy in its teachings whereas the Sydney College gave attention to both. The naturopathic wellsprings of Roberts' college fell by the wayside in favour of evolving Americanised standards and philosophy and the colleges became dedicated to chiropractic. These were all landmark changes on the journey to legitimation which were done under a chiropractic umbrella and osteopathy was a secondary consideration. Bowen became a member of the VSSO and Chapter 7 captures the voices and misgivings of those who studied osteopathy with Roberts' college as it started to prioritise chiropractic.

Naturopathic Pioneers FG Roberts and Maurice Blackmore

This research is concerned not only with teachings of osteopathy before Roberts' college pursued a chiropractic tangent but also what Roberts disseminated in the period before 1945, when alongside his college presence, he had a strong national public profile promoting naturopathy and all the other systems of healing it entailed. In addition to traditional apprentice models of learning for formally enrolled students, those with a calling could also access Roberts' ideas through his generous early dissemination of content in his magazine, *Natures Path to Health*, distance learning and his widespread speaking engagements, demonstrations and radio segments. He was also accessible through shops nationally and likewise, plus clinics in Victoria. In the early period, others imitated Roberts and set up their own schools and are discussed in Chapter 2. Maurice Blackmore was based in Queensland and had an organised association-school complex operating in Queensland, New South Wales and Victoria under the National Association of Naturopaths (NAN) formed in 1946, becoming NANOC in 1970 and returning later to NAN again.[18] The early Roberts' outreach phase that lasted until the mid-1940s has not been given detailed consideration, but new research of early advertising activities of both Roberts and Blackmore has unearthed information about the practice of neuropathy that illustrates styles of work that resonate with Bowen's language and practice. This new material is explored in Chapter 3. The early Roberts' outreach phase came to an end, he focused on his soy foods business and gradually handed the reins of his college onto others, but this book demonstrates that aspects of early work brought to Australia through the naturopathic route have survived, advanced and perfected in Bowen's practice.

Towards Regulation in Australia

Tensions over regulation had early beginnings in Australia. In 1935, FG Roberts established the United Practitioners Association of Australasia (UPAA) to represent naturopaths, chiropractors and osteopaths and during his time as president was an advocate to the government seeking recognition of these modalities.[19] In New South Wales, the Australian Chiropractors, Osteopaths and Naturopathic Physicians Association Limited (ACONPAL) was established in 1936 a year after the threat of legislation in NSW, 'preventing nature healers, chiropractors, osteopaths, herbalists and the like' from practising.[20] Gerritt Janssen was instrumental in this, he too was educated at the British College of Naturopathy and started practice in 1933.[21] By 1971, ACONPAL directors formed a Victorian Branch and the South Pacific Federation of Natural Therapeutists (SPFNT) as an umbrella organisation for all colleges and associations until a name change in 1975 to council. In 1975, under the influence of the national United Chiropractors Association of Australasia (UCAA), a body formed from the United Chiropractors Association (UCA) that was synonymous with Roberts' Melbourne college, an exodus took place from the SPFNT. The exodus included the Roberts' College of Chiropractic and Osteopathy Australia (COCA), the Sydney College of Chiropractic (SCC) and the South Australian College of Chiropractic and Osteopathy (SACO). These colleges were all influenced by pressure from the inter-related American and British offshoot mainstream models and their graduates increasingly oriented to a chiropractic identity and curriculum standards of leading overseas specialised schools. The UCAA became the successful vehicle to register leading Australian-school graduates in the face of opposition of those with overseas credentials and the medical mainstream. This South Pacific and UCAA space are explored in Chapter 6 and brought to life through Bowen as an actor whose work was in demand in both domains.

The SPFNT (renamed a council post exodus) and ACONPAL left a small record. Analysis in Chapter 6 draws on formal company papers, available rare publications, correspondence and submissions to the government along with government inquiry transcripts of organisational representatives. This research is aimed to better understand Bowen's exposure to a wider culture of ideas including Eastern themes and his own increasing professional profile that led to others adopting his osteopathic approach even though he was fated to be stripped of his professional identity. Other than mentions and a table of membership numbers in the Ward Inquiry Report, a useful appendix in the Webb Inquiry Report and coverage in Baer, there are no detailed histories about these organisations or the individual personalities involved.[22] The focus is on a microhistory of Bowen and his connections in this sphere and allows new insights to emerge about his influence when he is viewed as an involved actor in this domain with his contemporaries.

After the formation of the first branch of ACONPAL in 1936, South Australia proclaimed its *Chiropractic Act* (1949); in 1958, the Western Australian parliament responded to pressure to draft a Natural Therapists Bill to register osteopaths, chiropractors and naturopaths and the ripples of pending change began in earnest. In Western Australia, only the chiropractors got satisfaction with the *Chiropractors Registration Act 1964* and this paved the way for intensified chiropractic-led pressure on the eastern seaboard. The Royal Commission 1958–1964 was the first to grapple with difficulties that beset all future inquiries in Australia, around questions of education standards, adequacy of training establishments and definition of individual therapies (given the overlaps in philosophy and practice). In the west, the Commission dealt with chiropractors who strenuously objected to being aligned with natural therapists in the proposed legislation. Future inquiries faced the dual problem of strong opposition of the medical lobby and physiotherapists towards any legitimation of chiropractic and osteopathy, compounded by professional associations in Australia that represented overseas-trained chiropractors and osteopaths, equally opposed to recognition of their Australian-trained counterparts whose training they regarded as inferior to their own. The elite mainstream schools became specialised with curricula following a biomedical sciences model. Other colleges were mixers and regarded as 'second stream'. Writing in 1957, Parnell Bradbury who was educated in America and worked in England said that though there had been clear demarcation between the two systems of chiropractic and osteopathy when he was a student, 'more recently the exponents of both schools have borrowed freely from each other'.[23]

Osteopathy had not fared well in the West Australian Commission process and the United Osteopaths Association formed by FG Roberts in 1961 folded afterwards.[24] During the progress of the Western Australian Commission's deliberations towards registration of chiropractors, the American-led Victorian Chiropractors Association aspired to registration in 1962 and was met with strong opposition from physiotherapists.[25] By the early 1970s, pressure was increasing which led to the Victorian branch of ACONPAL in 1971. Soon after, in 1972, the New South Wales government initiated an 'Inquiry into the question of registration of chiropractic' (Teece Inquiry) and in 1973, the Victorian government followed suit by appointing a joint select committee into chiropractic, osteopathy and naturopathy (Ward Inquiry). The federal government then followed with the Chiropractic, Osteopathy, Homeopathy and Naturopathy Committee of Inquiry (Webb Inquiry). Each of these recommended registration of chiropractors and osteopaths, but not naturopaths, eventually resulting in state legislation in NSW and Victoria in 1978 and followed by Queensland in 1979. This outcome represents the victor narrative of the hard-won fight for the legitimation of chiropractic and osteopathy, albeit the latter swept in under the chiropractic umbrella.

Clinician and Lay Observers at Bowen's Clinic in the 1970s

While all these developments were happening and before regulation in Victoria in 1978 and after Bowen had responded to the Ward Inquiry in 1973, four qualified clinician chiropractors became associated with Bowen's clinic as observers from 1974–1982, two dually qualified as naturopaths (Keith Davis DC/ND and Nigel Love DC/ND who trained at FG Roberts' early BAIN qualifying in 1958) and two were awarded student of the year (Kevin Neave DC and Romney Smeeton DC). Neave and Smeeton overtly qualified as 'straight' chiropractors in 1976 during the later iteration of the Roberts' college as the COCA – soon to become the Chiropractic College of Australasia (CCA). Later on after the proclamation of the *Chiropractors and Osteopaths Act 1978 (Vic)*, Kevin Ryan DO, then a student-in-training in osteopathy at the Southern School of Natural Therapies (SSNT) joined as an observer from 1979 to 1982. Ryan was registered shortly before Bowen's death. The chiropractors and osteopath were long-term observers with a presence on individual days covering the period from 1974 until Bowen's death in 1982. Smeeton enjoyed the longest continuous contact from 1977 to 1982. Also starting in 1974 and finishing in 1976, Oswald Rentsch, a young lay-taught masseur and aspiring natural therapist from the rural far west of Victoria made visits to Bowen's clinic too. ACONPAL appears to have played a role in bringing Bowen's observers together. Both Davis DC from Frankston on the Mornington Peninsula and Rentsch described meeting Bowen at a conference of therapists. The organisation was never named but deduced from research to be either ACONPAL or possibly Blackmores National Association of Naturopaths, Osteopaths and Chiropractors (NANOC). NANOC was a derivative of the original NAN association-school founded in 1946 and focused on chiropractic teaching and remedies. Davis DC/ND was a confirmed member of both but had left NANOC by 1973 meaning an ACONPAL event as most likely where he met Bowen as Bowen formally joined ACONPAL in 1972. The ACONPAL membership structure was tiered to accommodate those qualified and those attending as guests. Bowen's initial status is not known but he was a registered member on a surviving business card (shown later in Chapter 7). Chapter 6 describes the leadership of this professional environment as part of the South Pacific, along with membership characteristics and qualifications for full membership and how Bowen was perceived in this domain.

The college-trained observers appreciated Bowen's flair in obtaining faster and better results for their patients; the chiropractic clinicians were intrigued by the outcomes of Bowen's methods without the use of any bony adjustments. All, including the osteopath, recognised that Bowen worked with an understanding of the relationship between structure and function and applied the discipline of a trained professional in arriving at a working diagnosis before proceeding to treat and would follow up with post-treatment checks to ensure a change had occurred. Bowen was not a communicator and expected his observers to learn by watching him work. All assumed he had no formal training of any kind, but this is reappraised in Chapter 2 using oral history evidence. Oswald Rentsch and other masseurs who attended Bowen's clinics were intrigued by Bowen's formidable reputation and seemingly miraculous results compared to massage. Rentsch decided to build a business around Bowen's methods and was keen to teach them while Bowen was alive, but Bowen insisted that those interested do so by personally attending his clinic. Bowen was particular about who he would impart his techniques and quickly rejected anyone who he felt did not have the hands for the work or who did not grasp what he was doing. Others enjoyed brief associations with Bowen's clinics born of Bowen's later invitation to therapists at the new Australian Natural Therapists Association (ANTA), one of the associations formed after the demise of ACONPAL. Neil Skilbeck DC/DO (SSNT) took up the offer of travelling from Gippsland involving several hours drive from the east of Victoria and developed a teaching module in the late 1970s called the Bowen Way.

Regulatory Tensions Escalate

While Bowen was hosting observers at his clinics throughout the 1970s, regulatory tensions were escalating. The Webb Inquiry had cast an international net over the UK and USA training institutions and commissioned specific research. Professor Webb did not visit Dr Still MD, DO's ASO (better known by the 1970s as the Kirksville College of Osteopathic Medicine – (KCOM) – now the Andrew Taylor Still University (ATSU)). The Webb Inquiry was focused on the leading north American chiropractic institutions. In the UK, the Bournemouth College of Chiropractic was visited and found to be substandard to the American colleges and only the London School of Osteopathy (LSO) was inspected, undoubtedly because a prerequisite for enrolment was medical credentials.[26] Professor Webb identified that the British School of Osteopathy

(BSO) was of interest.[27] There was no mention of either the European School of Osteopathy (ESO) or the BCNO (now the British College of Osteopathic Medicine) in the Webb Inquiry Report.

In Victoria, regulation began with the *Chiropractor and Osteopaths Act 1978*. In the same year in New South Wales, the *Chiropractic Registration Act* 1978 was proclaimed, followed in 1979 with the *Chiropractic Manipulative Therapy Act* (Qld). South Australia had already enacted chiropractic legislation in 1949. The Victorian legislation registered and protected suitably qualified chiropractors and osteopaths who held prescribed credentials from the three key schools, namely the Sydney College of Chiropractic, Melbourne's Preston Institute (today's Royal Melbourne Institute of Technology (RMIT)) and Adelaide's College of Chiropractic. Successful automatic registration was achieved for those Australia-trained who had joined the UCAA. With regulation, ACONPAL folded and under the leadership of Alfred Jacka – a former leader of Blackmores' NANOC association-school in Victoria, and successor dean and owner of the SSNT, the Australian Natural Therapists Association (ANTA) was formed. ANTA accommodated members from the demise of NANOC, ACONPAL and the South Pacific and of necessity became the only professional refuge for Bowen and his elder talented osteopathic colleagues who had formed the VSSO. The VSSO members were marooned from registration either because they were credentialled and had refused to join the UCAA or lacked formal credentials but enjoyed successful careers and community standing. ANTA continued to advocate for those marginalised.

Disparate Implementation of the Grandfather Clause for Uncredentialled but Talented Practitioners

As Chapter 7 will show, with the unfolding of regulation in Victoria, long-standing practitioners like Bowen were supposed to have been grandfathered into registration, via a special provision in May 1981 inserted into the *Chiropractors and Osteopaths Act 1978*. However, the Registration Board established under the Act was dominated by medical interests along with representatives of mainstream chiropractic and osteopathy and forced these eligible practitioners to attend examinations (later found to be illegal); and criticised as designed to make it impossible for them to pass. There was no parallel like the flexibility afforded to Kirsté Martinovich, registered in Western Australia under the *Chiropractors Registration Act 1964* following pressure from community, business and political champions who had advocated for his talent.[28] Nor was there a repeat of the respect extended to the Saunders' father and son duo in 1935 and 1957, respectively, and registered under the *Masseurs Act 1928* (Vic) without credentials but possessing remarkable talent. The New South Wales *Chiropractic Registration Act* provided a grandfather clause from the outset, and although then parliamentarians Tom Roper and Rod Mackenzie OAM attempted to rectify this in Victoria with the May 1981 amendment, the Board requested those who applied to present for examination even though there was no head of power in the Act to allow them to do so.

One of the effects of the 1978 legislation was that massage, regulated since the early 1920s, lapsed as a protected profession and was superseded with the *Physiotherapy Act 1978*. As a result, lay therapists, chiropractors and osteopaths holding unrecognised qualifications that previously denied them registration could continue their remunerated work as massage if they wished, without fear of retribution and were able to join ANTA in Victoria and the Australian Traditional Medicine (ATMS) in New South Wales. Some like Bowen as an ANTA member elected to call himself a natural therapist.

Victor Narrative of Legitimation and the Sidelined Narrative of Marginalisation and Victims of Regulation

Accounts and research of this era of regulation and legitimation are focused on the victor narrative and overcoming forces of marginalisation from the medical mainstream, physiotherapists and those holding qualifications from elite overseas schools with curricula founded on biomedical sciences. The history of the legitimation of mainstream chiropractic and osteopathy and natural therapies in Australia was prominently covered by Hans Baer in several journal articles and the coverage of Australian organisations drawn from government and official inquiry reports; Baer also addressed the international ground and described complexities in different jurisdictions that impacted the professionalisation and legitimation of osteopathy and naturopathy.[29] The overall Australian story of the marginalised is reflected in similar tensions in the late nineteenth century in America between the medical hierarchies and those described as village bonesetters culminating in the introduction of osteopathy and chiropractic. These are described by Erland Pettman's historical overview.[30] In the UK, Sir Herbert Barker wrote his own biography and journey through similar initial discrimination as a bonesetter.[31] The ethnography of Welsh bonesetter Leyshen resonated strongly with that of Bowen.[32] Unlike the various articles on native bone setting in India and histories of British families, no body of literature has been found to exist on Australian bone setting traditions. Common themes that prevail in accounts of these grassroots traditions are the shared experience of accusations of quackery offset with community trust and demand for bonesetters' services. These practitioners shared a commitment to service, being accessible, providing caring expertise and only charging modest fees, or none.

With legitimation secured, Australian chiropractic and osteopathy research theses and journal articles tend to focus on the history of education, philosophy and practice or themes related to legitimation that impacted the professions.[33] The Sydney-based chiropractic history group's recent work provided a person-focused history of the Sydney College of Chiropractic (SCC) set against historical and legislative developments.[34] Covered are identities involved in establishing the college, successful navigation of government enquiries and the strategies adopted to win against both an entrenched medical mainstream and the powerful overseas lobbies vehemently opposed to recognition of any graduates of Australian institutions. Compared to Hawkins and O'Neill, more information appears on FG Roberts, Doyle and Kaufman, presented in the context of the development of the SCC.[35] The SCC taught chiropractic and osteopathy concurrently with graduates emerging with dual diplomas for the same course.[36] For this reason, the NSW *Chiropractic Registration Act* provided for three categories of registration: osteopath, chiropractor or dual. The UCAA campaign fostered a chiropractic identity for registration and there are Roberts' college BAIN period graduates who identified as osteopaths in the electoral rolls but held out to be DCs when registered – one example being Bowen observer, Nigel Love DC. In the lead-up to regulation, the VSSO described in Chapter 7 wished to identify solely as osteopaths but had no recourse to a similar registration mechanism championed for chiropractors.[37]

Against this victor narrative backdrop that succeeded in the face of American pressure and the Australian colleges that fought against marginalisation by overseas-trained elites, another stratum of marginalisation exists below these surface currents. The role of Bowen and the voices of others who individually and collectively collaborated to hold out for a sole osteopathic identity and preserve their kind of osteopathic practice are heard individually in Chapter 7 through their presentations to the Victorian Ward Inquiry. As members of the VSSO, they distinguished themselves from chiropractors by reliance on tactile ability alone, more nuanced manipulations and no use of x-rays. They were not a homogenous group with respect to the formal knowledge they called upon for their professional development and it becomes evident some were attempting to keep up with literature in mainstream schools in America while members like Bowen continued to develop his own work and remained cued to the original tenets of Dr Still MD, DO.

In Australia, those who established large health retreats or teaching schools (or both) have received disparate attention. Australia's naturopathic pioneers, the Tasmanian-born FG Roberts and the English-born Maurice Blackmore have not received any in-depth attention by historians. To date, no individual dedicated biographies have been produced of either of these major naturopathic pioneers of manual medicine in the naturopathic sphere. FG Roberts was referenced often in a history of soy foods and receives attention in Devereaux et al., but Maurice Blackmore who is represented in the National Library of Australia is reflected there in only one newspaper cutting.[38] Other famous figures of the time were more fortunate and include the Swedish-born Ernst Kjellberg, who, unusually, was the subject of several dedicated monographs.[39] Kjellberg's clinic at Millaa Millaa, located in the far north of Queensland featured a philanthropic *modus operandi* similar to Bowen, Saunders and others. Not all early college-educated Australian leaders have left a trail lit by historians either. Individuals who became connected with Bowen and established their own colleges or were leading spokesmen for the naturopathic voice such as Robert Lucy and his associate Gerritt Janssen were men of vision whose pre-regulation endeavours have become lost to regulation and history. In addition to Lucy, other leaders in the networks to which Bowen belonged include Alfred Jacka ND and Peter Derig DC/DO/ND and all established and headed up the new professional organisations of ANTA and ATMS respectively for natural therapists (still existing today) when regulation obliterated the landscape of older networks in 1978 introduced here and described in Chapter 6.

This trend is also true for the history of Australia's talented masseurs. Bentley and Dunstan recently wrote a history of Australian physiotherapy.[40] No mention was made of the roles of the talented non-college educated masseurs such as the Melbourne-based Saunders men – neither the senior Ernest Saunders' profile in the Victorian Football League (VFL renamed Australian from 1990) and as honorary masseur to the Australian Olympics team for Berlin in 1936 nor his son George Saunders as Physiotherapy Director to Olympic and most Empire Games' teams between 1950 and 1982. In Bentley and Dunstan, the formal history of Australian physiotherapy at the Olympics begins in 1976 when a physiotherapist first attended the Montreal Olympiad. Likewise, an entire history of talented masseurs who were not registered with a massage association has been overlooked for the period before then. A recent paper by Strachan and Reeves aimed to address this oversight and highlight the selection of men of talent to the Olympics team who can be demonstrated to have connections with formal knowledge, which belied the amateur ethos.[41] Lisa Casanelia and David Stelfox provided a paragraph on Bowen's contemporaries in VFL football, namely healer-masseurs William (Billy) Mitchell and Keith Cleaver, a Mitchell apprentice.[42] Those who worked in the culture of football and who like Bowen had reputations as community healers are covered in Chapter 8. Many lacked education and the press of the day were arbiters of their legacy. Ernest Saunders was regaled while alive, yet apart from a couple of brief press mentions, he was forgotten in death. His legacy endured through media coverage of his son. Bowen and his well-known other contemporaries such as Albert (Bert) Donald and Bill Mitchell generally avoided publicity and left no personal memoirs.[43] Many VFL and local football team masseurs have been forgotten and their biographical details remain largely unknown. This pattern is reflected elsewhere and replicated overseas. Bovine's paper on William Rae the famous Blantyre Bonesetter confirms how uneducated healers were unable to leave their own record. Rae was feted by the press, but within seven months of his death, he was forgotten and quickly replaced by another assigned the role of curing community ills. Available literature reflects that it is the more educated and wealthy pioneers that have been given attention than those pejoratively disparaged as 'quacks'. However, Bowen's story did not die with his death. Chapter 6 covers his connections in the South Pacific organisation and its subsidiary ACONPAL and how he was welcomed in the UCAA environment. The contrasting tangents of popularised teachings and professional advancement in the clinical practice of his work ensures his work has survived.

Retracing the Origins of Bowen's Methods Through His Practice and Symbolism

The task of claiming Bowen to osteopathic identity, specifically one with naturopathic origins and how Bowen's techniques are remembered and practised posthumously, is set against this historical backdrop. However, the greater historical focus is on language and methods used that trace Bowen's work in particular to earlier forgotten forms of osteopathy that came to Australia through the naturopathic route – through early naturopathic colleges, and via Roberts in particular who operated both a college and a wide outreach program for the public and aspiring lay therapists. These outreach activities died away by the mid-1940s and by 1959, Roberts' college left behind its naturopathic wellsprings to become the COCA then CCA with a chiropractic pathway prioritised under new leadership increasingly influenced by overseas and political developments. Roberts moved out of the spotlight to focus on his soy food business and private practice and did not participate in the government inquiries of the 1970s; he died in 1977, the year the federal Webb Inquiry report was released. There is a lack of historical documentation on the practice and development of early Australian osteopathy disseminated by naturopathic pioneers. The work and language of Thomas Ambrose Bowen, his like-minded colleagues in the VSSO and others who responded to the Ward Inquiry are echoes that fill an important gap in understanding this topic. This research highlights that Bowen's style of work was a throwback to more original and much older forms of osteopathy he encountered when younger, either directly or indirectly through a naturopathic source in his learning period in the 1940s and 1950s. Geographically, through Roberts directly, or indirectly via a practitioner of his techniques is more likely as Roberts lived in Victoria and had shops and clinics where Bowen lived and worked. Bowen retained this older style of working and refined and pioneered a highly minimalist and systematised approach that was richly creative depending on patient presentation and effective in addressing musculoskeletal and other bodily ills.

Bowen was victimised because he was not formally educated and his approach was a relic of a bygone era. Though more authentically aligned to Still's original teachings, the pressure movements of neuropathy were not a style of working recognised or in vogue by 1970. Ironically, Bowen may not have known the name of the origins of his practice as he acquired and held up a book on Namikoshi's shiatsu to explain the basis of his work to Smeeton DC in the late 1970s. The research identifies that Bowen's ideas, symbolism and practice had their origins in neuropathy, a forgotten and different name for osteopathy taught at various American naturopathic colleges early last century and brought to Australia by naturopathic pioneers. Both FG Roberts and Maurice Blackmore advertised neuropathy in the early period and Roberts identified as a neuropath on electoral rolls until 1945.[44]

Bowen's Posthumous Legacy

Posthumously, and referring to the 1960s, at least one Bowen patient, Cec Capon noted similarities of Bowen's style to Michael Chadwick, a UK BSO osteopath who worked in Geelong at the time, 'None of them were chiropractic like, more myotherapist by comparison, it was just different'.[45] The posthumous representations of Bowen's approach are understood differently in the world of successful clinical practice of his college-trained observers who drew upon the formal knowledge system of chiropractic and osteopathy and who, over several decades of practice, have treated many thousands of patients over their five respective clinic careers, compared to how it was successfully presented for wide international public consumption by the masseur Rentsch who orphaned his teachings from osteopathy. After launching his interpretation in the late 1980s, Bowen's legacy was spread globally and offshoot schools formed within a decade leading to widespread popularity of Bowen's methods. In the midst of these developments, a decade after Bowen's death, Smeeton wrote a piece about Bowen, reproduced with permission (see Table 1.1).[46]

Table 1.1 Romney Smeeton, 'The Bowen Approach to Manipulative Therapy'

The Bowen approach as practised by the late Tom Bowen of Geelong is a gentle soft tissue technique, involving the combination of muscle and connective tissue manipulations, which restore balance to the body's structure, thereby stimulating the corrective flow of the body's energy allowing for nature's own correction of spinal (structural) imbalances.
The approach does not involve any osseous adjusting at all and can be used safely at any age for a vast range of conditions – particularly useful for treating babies and the aged.
A series of carefully planned manoeuvres begin the process of structural correction using gentle finger pressure only. Its scope of effectiveness ranges from purely orthopaedic (spinal and joint problems – and other musculoskeletal troubles) to a range of visceral complaints such as digestive disorders, infertility, colic and gastric reflux in babies.
All disorders that can be helped by conventional chiropractic and osteopathic care can likewise benefit from this approach with the advantage it is much less invasive on the body and therefore more easily tolerated.
Tom Bowen practised in Geelong and he only passed on in any detail the basis of his approach to a limited number of people. Of those who were given exposure to this amazing man, only three are still practising full-time. Two in Geelong (one DC and one DO) and a chiropractor in Frankston.
While not necessary, conventional chiropractic and osteopathic techniques can be incorporated into the general case management, where applicable.
While working with Mr Bowen, we were given the basis of his approach. Unfortunately, many of his 'secrets' he took with him when he died ten years ago. It is up to us to further the technique to gain the maximum potential of this work.
The scope of the progression is limited only by the practitioner's inability to understand the basis of the approach and thereby failing to utilise the immense potential.

During Bowen's lifetime, Davis DC/ND and Neave DC demonstrated Bowen's work on his behalf and with his approval at the SCC in 1979 and Neave continued to show chiropractic associates in Melbourne and Brisbane and posthumously. Chiropractors Davis and Smeeton had no aspirations to teach, but in the last two decades, Smeeton has been in demand internationally to impart a deeper appreciation of Bowen's work. Ryan DO received Bowen's blessings to teach before he died and taught Bowen's techniques to professionals in Melbourne and the Gold Coast in 1984 then later for nine years to fifth-year osteopathy students at the RMIT – the modern successor to Roberts' CCA. Ryan has since developed a system that combines Traditional Chinese Medicine (TCM) with Bowen methods and teaches this currently at workshops and online.

These two tangents were forged from different knowledge systems and worldviews. Those college-trained viewed Bowen through the chiropractic/osteopathy perspective of their training and in the case of Ryan DO, incorporated a TCM lens from his acupuncture qualifications, whereas the initial popularised teachings orphaned Bowen from osteopathy in the belief Bowen only assumed this unregulated title, so he could set up in business. In a culture that falls within the definition of a New Religious Movement (NRM), the focus was on creating a simplified teachable format to a mass audience imbued with Bowen's mystique and successes and what the techniques could achieve if delivered in the set way taught. The challenge for everyone was that Bowen did not document his work nor leave any memoir to explain his thinking. The offshoot schools were secular and many strived to interpret Bowen's techniques based on formal knowledge drawn from fascia science emerging in the massage/physical therapy field and the growing influence of Eastern medicine and anatomy. One school was influenced by the work of Major Bertrand de Jarnette DC and his work on sacro-occipital technique.[47] A critical mass of Bowen therapists came into being leading to the need to establish professional associations. This laid the groundwork for Bowen Therapy or Bowen Technique to become subject to government quality control and accreditation in Australia and through official bodies overseas. Internationally, the Bowtech school has the largest footprint, in 2014 outnumbering other schools by a ratio of three to one, with overall figures of certifications issued then reaching 40,000 overall.[48] A decade later, the Bowtech school figures alone are stated to be 50,000 trained.[49]

However, Bowen did not arrive at mastery in a vacuum. His symbolism is captured in expressions and explanations at the Ward Inquiry, oral history and in the media. These together with his techniques and how he applied them provide important clues to trace the origins of the approach he pioneered and perfected into a skilled system that brought highly effective results in his hands. Accordingly, the next chapter begins by exploring uncharted territory to reveal more about the nature of early training opportunities in the new systems of manual medicine that would have been potentially accessible to a lay person like Bowen. There is evidence that Bowen was active for several years treating co-workers, the community and footballers long before he made the decision to become professional and formally set up a business as an osteopath in 1959. Ultimately, this book is about historically restoring the legacy of Bowen to his chosen vocation of osteopathy and recognising the heritage of his work to Still's original ideas and the work of his close disciples early last century that aimed to preserve them. With historical research, Bowen emerges out of the posthumous vacuum that masked his osteopathic stature and reinstates his legacy as representative of early osteopathy introduced by Australia's early naturopathic pioneers from overseas training beginning in America, hence the term *naturopathic osteopathy*. As a pioneer, he developed the neuropathy branch of this work within the discipline of osteopathic rules to not overtreat to minimise hyper reflexes. As such, he developed an astounding consummate mastery in minimalism. This honours Andrew Taylor Still's famous dictum of 'Find it, Fix it and Leave it alone', often extended to 'and Nature do the Rest.'[50]

Notes

1 Henry S. Pritchett, "Introduction," in Abraham Flexner, *Medical Education in the United States and Canada, A Report to the Carnegie foundation with an introduction by Henry Pritchett, President, Bulletin No. 4* (Fifth Avenue, New York City: D. B. Updike, Merrymount Press, 1910), viii.

2 "In the Ranks of the Reservists," *The Musician*, Salvation Army National Headquarters Melbourne, July 1948, 165.

3 Agnes Shaw, interview by Ron Phelan 2003, in Shirley Strachan, *Healing Hands, Unsung Voices* (London: Cloister House Press, 2016), 56.

4 Rosemary Hazelton interview by author, June 3, 2018.

5 Bowen and Horwood outside 30 Villamanta Street, late 1970s. Image Courtesy Ron Phelan, Custodian, Rene Horwood Collection.

6 Image courtesy Lynn Wilson. The *Healing Hands* monument in the foreground was erected by Phelan to commemorate Bowen in 2002; the hands stretch out towards 100 Autumn Street (sold for development in 2024) and the globe represents the international reach of his work.

7 Rene Horwood interview by Ron Phelan 1998, transcribed by author.

8 Thomas P. Duffy, "The Flexner Report – 100 Years Later," *The Yale Journal of Biology and Medicine* 84, no. 3 (2011): 269–76.

9 Hans A. Baer, "The Drive for Professionalization in British Osteopathy," *Social Science and Medicine* 19, no. 7 (1984): 717–72.

10 Hans A. Baer, "The Organizational Rejuvenation of Osteopathy: A Reflection of the Decline of Professional Dominance in Medicine," *Social Science and Medicine* 15, no. 5 (1981): 701–11.

11 Katherine Miller, "The Evolution of Professional Identity: The Case of Osteopathic Medicine," *Social Science and Medicine* 47, no. 11 (1998): 1739 referencing E. Freidson "The Theory of the Professions: State of the Art," in *The Sociology of the Professions: Lawyers, Doctors and Others*, ed. R. Dingwall (London: Macmillan, 1983), 27.

12 Miller, "The Evolution of Professional Identity: The Case of Osteopathic Medicine," 1747.

13 Peter Hawkins and Arthur O'Neill, *Osteopathy in Australia* (Bundoora, Australia: Phillip Institute of Technology Press, 1990), 19–26; Edwin Devereaux, Brian O'Reilly, and John Cice, *History of the Sydney College of Chiropractic* (Sydney: Macquarie Lighthouse Press, 2012).

14 Hawkins and O'Neill, *Osteopathy in Australia*, 19–16.
15 Hawkins and O'Neill, *Osteopathy in Australia*, 19.
16 Hawkins and O'Neill, *Osteopathy in Australia*, 2.
17 Herbalist in Caulfield West, 29 Glenhuntly Road, 1937 *Australia, Electoral Rolls, 1903–1980;* PROV, VPRS 3253/P1/, Unit 47, Doyle transcript, 463.
18 Ward Inquiry Report, 263.
19 Devereaux et al., *History of the Sydney College of Chiropractic*, 4–5.
20 "Our Country as I See It," *and Settler (Sydney)*, September 5, 1935: 1.
21 PROV, VPRS 241/P/ Unit 14, South Pacific Federation transcript (Janssen), 890.
22 Ward Enquiry Report, 9; Webb Inquiry Report, appendix 3, Brief History of Organisations, 261–75.
23 Parnell Bradbury, *Healing by Hand* (Harvill Press: London 1957), 35.
24 Steven A. Campbell, "The Rise and Legitimation of Chiropractic, A Study of Professionalisation" (Masters with Honours thesis, University of New England, 1985), 200.
25 PROV, Chiropractic Treatment and Reports, VPRS 6345/P/, Unit 155, General Correspondence Files, Letter Leigh Wedlick, Masseurs Registration Board to Mack, Minister for Health, January 23, 1962.
26 Webb Inquiry Report, Appendix 14, 747–55 and 756–62.
27 Webb Inquiry Report, Appendix 14, 760.
28 E. Jaggard, "Kristé Martinovich (1903–1966)," National Centre of Biography, Australian National University, accessed December 3, 2018, published first in hardcopy 2000; the Saunders story is covered in Chapter 4.
29 Hans Baer, "Osteopathy in Australasia: From Marginality to a Fully Professionalised System of Health Care," *International Journal of Osteopathic Medicine* 12 (2009): 25–31; Hans Baer, "The Drive for Legitimation in Australian Naturopathy: Successes and Dilemmas," *Social Science and Medicine* 63 (2006): 1771–73; Hans Baer, *The History of Complementary Medicine in Australia and New Zealand: Its Popularisation Legitimation and Dilemmas* (London and New York: Routledge, Taylor and Francis, 2009).
30 Erland Pettman, "A History of Manipulative Therapy," *Journal of Manipulative Therapy* 15, no. 3 (2007): 165–74.
31 Herbert Barker, *Leaves from my Life* (London: Hutchinson & Co, 1927).
32 Simon Leyson, "A Man of his People, a Concise Ethnography of a Welsh Bonesetter," in *Healing by Hand*, eds. Kathryn Oths and Servando S. Hinojosa (Walnut Creek, CA: Alta Mira Press, Rowan and Littlefield, 2004), 237–64.
33 Melanie Cameron, "An International Study of Osteopathic Practice" (Masters thesis, Victoria University of Technology, Melbourne, 1999), 38; Keith J. Simpson, "The Five Eras of Chiropractic and the Future of Chiropractic as seen through the Eyes of a Participant Observer," *Journal of Chiropractic and Manual Therapies* 20, no. 1 (2012): 1–8.
34 Devereaux et al., *History of the Sydney College of Chiropractic.*
35 Devereaux et al., *History of the Sydney College of Chiropractic*, chapters 1, 2 and 3.
36 Devereaux et al., *History of the Sydney College of Chiropractic*, 119; Hawkins and O'Neill, *Osteopathy in Australia*, 27–28.
37 Devereaux et al., *History of the Sydney College of Chiropractic*, 132–33.
38 William Shurtleff and Akiko Aoyagi, *Soyinfo Center, History of Soybeans and Soyfoods in Australia, New Zealand and Oceania 1770–2010, extensively annotated bibliography and Sourcebook (*Lafayette, CA: SoyInfo Center, 2010): Biographical cuttings on Maurice Blackmore, businessman, containing one or more cuttings from newspapers or journals, National Library of Australia.
39 Kathleen Rock, *Kjellberg, The Man and the Healer* (Bowen Hills Brisbane: Boolarong Publications, 1991); Kevin Sommerfeld, *E. E. J. Kjellberg, Healing Hands, A Review of the Life and Times of a Master* (Brisbane: Boolarong Press, 2001);

Henry and Elaine Tranter, *Ernst Kjellberg, Swedish Chiropractor* (Millaa Millaa: Eacham Historical Society, n.d.).

40 Philip Bentley with David Dunstan, *The Path to Professionalism, Physiotherapy in Australia to the 1980s* (Melbourne, Victoria: Australian Physiotherapy Association, 2006).

41 Shirley Strachan and Keir Reeves, "Through the Lens of the Trainer-Masseurs: Australia's Incongruous Engagement with the Olympic Amateur Ethos," *International Journal of the History of Sport* 39, no. 6 (2022): 631–52.

42 Lisa Casanelia and David Stelfox, *Foundations of Massage* (Chatswood, New South Wales: Churchill Livingstone, Elsevier Australia, 2010), 16–17.

43 Libby Gordon and Brian Smart, *Tom Bowen Personal Reflections* (Australia: BTAV and BTSA, 1999).

44 *Australia, Electoral Rolls 1903–1980*, available on *Ancestry.com.*

45 Cec Capon interview by author, in Shirley Strachan, *Healing Hands, Unsung Voices, Thomas Ambrose Bowen Osteopath (1916–1982)* (United Kingdom: Cloister House Press, 2016), 86.

46 Smeeton, "The Bowen Approach to Manipulative Therapy," reproduced with permission.

47 This is the school for NeuroStructural Integration Technique (NST); *NST Development*, NST Website.

48 Shirley Strachan, "Bowen Therapy Today, A 2014 Overview," 23–24, accessed November 17, 2024, https://www.bowentherapy.org.uk/docs/articles/shirley--strachan-report-on-tom-bowen-18Apr14.pdf.

49 "Bowtech, The Original Bowen Technique," Bowtech Website.

50 The image 'Andrew Taylor Still Caricature Postcard with Phrase "Find it, Fix it, and Leave it Alone" is in the collection of the Museum of Osteopathic Medicine, Kirksville, MO [1975.67.02.02 cropped].

Bibliography

Newspapers

"Our Country as I See It." *Farmer and Settler (Sydney)*, September 5, 1935: 1. (col.5). Accessed November 17, 2024. http://nla.gov.au/nla.news-article117208654.

Primary Sources

Ancestry.com [database on-line]. Provo, UT, USA: Ancestry.com Operations, Inc. *Australia Electoral Rolls 1903–1980.*

Barker, Herbert Atkinson. *Leaves from My Life*. London: Hutchinson & Co, 1927.

Biographical cuttings on Maurice Blackmore, businessman, containing one or more cuttings from newspapers or journals. National Library of Australia. Accessed November 17, 2024. http://nla.gov.au/nla.cat-vn219268.

Cameron, Melanie. "An International Study of Osteopathic Practice." Masters thesis, Victoria University of Technology, Melbourne, 1999, 38. Accessed November 17, 2024. http://vuir.vu.edu.au/17921/1/CAMERON_1999compressed.pdf.

Campbell, Stephen A. "The Rise and Legitimation of Chiropractic. A Study of Professionalisation." Masters with Honours thesis, University of New England, 1985, 201–2. Accessed November 17, 2024. https://hdl.handle.net/1959.11/12799.

Capon, Cec. Interview by author, August 4, 2015, transcript in Strachan, Shirley. *Healing Hands, Unsung Voices, Thomas Ambrose Bowen Osteopath (1916–1982)*. London: Cloister House Press, 2016.

Flexner, Abraham. *Medical Education in the United States and Canada, A Report to the Carnegie foundation with an introduction by Henry Pritchett, President, Bulletin No.*

4. Fifth Avenue, New York City: D. B. Updike, Merrymount Press, 1910. Accessed November 17, 2024. https://archive.org/details/medicaleducation04flexuoft/medicaleducation04flexuoft.

Hazelton, Rosemary. Interview by author, June 3, 2016.

Horwood, Rene, Interview by Ron Phelan, July–October, 1998. Transcript excerpts in Strachan, Shirley. *Healing Hands, Unsung Voices, Thomas Ambrose Bowen 1916–1982, Osteopath.* London: Cloister House Press, 2016.

PROV. Chiropractic Treatment and Reports, VPRS 6345/P/, Unit 155. General Correspondence Files. Letter Leigh Wedlick, Masseurs Registration Board to Mack, Minister for Health, January 23, 1962.

PROV. Osteopathy, Chiropractic and Naturopath Joint Select Committee pp. 783–938, VPRS 241/P/, Unit 14, Transcripts of Committee, South Pacific Federation of Natural Therapeutics represented by Janssen, Lucy and Goulson, transcript: 890–914.

PROV. Report and evidence Osteopathy Committee (Pt.1–4), 27/11/975 (Pt. 2) 2261, VPRS 3253/P1/, Unit 47. Original papers tabled in the Legislative Assembly, transcripts of proceedings, Bowen transcript: 672–78.

PROV. Report and evidence Osteopathy Committee (Pt.1–4), 27/11/975 (Pt. 2) 2261, VPRS 3253/P1/, Unit 47. Original papers tabled in the Legislative Assembly, transcripts of proceedings, Doyle transcript: 463–68.

PROV. Report and evidence Osteopathy Committee (Pt.1–4), 27/11/975 (Pt. 2) 2261, VPRS 3253/P1/, Unit 50, Original papers tabled in the Legislative Assembly, transcripts of proceedings, McAlister transcript: 3424–60.

Shaw, Agnes. Interview by Ron Phelan, n.d. 2003. Transcript by Phelan in Strachan, Shirley. *Healing Hands, Unsung Voices, Thomas Ambrose Bowen 1916–1982, Osteopath.* United Kingdom: Cloister House Press, 2016.

Smeeton, Romney. "The Bowen Approach to Manipulative Therapy." 1992.

Ward Inquiry Report. Full title: Victoria Parliament, Osteopathy, Chiropractic and Naturopathy Committee, et al. *Report from the Osteopathy, Chiropractic and Naturopathy Committee: Together with Appendices.* Melbourne: C. H. Rixon, Government Printer, 1975. Accessed November 17, 2024. http://www6.austlii.edu.au/au/other/vic/VicLASelCPubInq/1975/1.pdf.

Secondary Sources

Baer, Hans A. "The Organizational Rejuvenation of Osteopathy: A Reflection of the Decline of Professional Dominance in Medicine." *Social Science and Medicine* 15, no. 5 (1981): 701–11. Accessed November 18, 2024. https://doi.org/10.1016/0271-7123(81)90093-6.

Baer, Hans A. "The Drive for Professionalisation in British Osteopathy." *Social Science and Medicine* 19, no. 7 (1984): 717–25. Accessed November 18, 2024. http://doi.org/10.1016/0277-9536(84)902442.

Baer, Hans A. "The Drive for Legitimation by Osteopathy and Chiropractic in Australia: Between Heterodoxy and Orthodoxy." *Journal of Evidence Based Integrative Medicine* (April 1, 2006): 77–94. Accessed November 17, 2024. https://journals.sagepub.com/doi/pdf/10.1177/1533210106292467.

Baer, Hans A. "The Drive for Legitimation in Australian Naturopathy: Successes and Dilemmas." *Social Science and Medicine* 63 (2006): 1771–73.

Baer, Hans A. *Complementary Medicine in Australia and New Zealand: Its Popularisation Legitimation and Dilemmas.* London and New York: Routledge, Taylor and Francis, 2009.

Baer, Hans A. "Osteopathy in Australasia: From Marginality to a Fully Professionalised System of Health Care." *International Journal of Osteopathic Medicine* 12, no. 1 (2009): 25–31. Accessed November 18, 2024. https://doi.org/10.1016/j.ijosm.2008.05.002.

Bentley, Philip with Dunstan, David. *The Path to Professionalism, Physiotherapy in Australia to the 1980s.* Melbourne, Victoria: Australian Physiotherapy Association, 2006.
Bradbury, Parnell. *Healing by Hand.* London: The Harvill Press, 1957.
Casanelia, Lisa, and David Stelfox. *Foundations of Massage.* 3rd ed. Sydney: Churchill Elsevier, 2010.
Devereaux, Edwin, Brian O'Reilly, and John Cice. *History of the Sydney College of Chiropractic.* Sydney: Macquarie Lighthouse Press, 2012.
Duffy, Thomas P. "The Flexner Report – 100 Years Later." *The Yale Journal of Biology and Medicine* 84, no. 3 (2011): 269–76. Accessed November 17, 2024. http://www.ncbi.nlm.nih.gov/pmc/articles/PMC3178858.
Gordon, Libby, and Brian Smart. *Tom Bowen Personal Reflections.* Australia: BTAV and BTSA, 1999.
Hawkins, Peter, and Arthur O'Neill. *Osteopathy in Australia.* Bundoora, Australia: Phillip Institute of Technology Press, 1990.
Leyson, Simon. "A Man of His People, a Concise Ethnography of Welsh Bonesetter." In *Healing by Hand: Manual Medicine and Bonesetting in the Global Perspective*, edited by Kathryn Oths and Servando Z. Hinojosa, 237–64. Walnut Creek, CA: Alta Mira Press, Rowan and Littlefield, 2004.
Miller, Katherine. "The Evolution of Professional Identity: The Case of Osteopathic Medicine." *Social Science and Medicine* 47, no. 11 (1998): 1739–48. Accessed November 17, 2024. https://doi.org/10.1016/S0277-9536(98)00247-0.
Oths, Kathryn, and Servando S. Hinojosa, eds. *Healing by Hand.* Walnut Creek, CA: Alta Mira Press, Rowan and Littlefield, 2004.
Pettman, Erland. "A History of Manipulative Therapy." *Journal of Manipulative Therapy* 15, no. 3 (2007): 165–74.
Rock, Kathleen. *Kjellberg, the Man and the Healer.* Bowen Hills, Brisbane: Boolarong Publications, 1991.
Salvation Army National Headquarters Melbourne, "In the Ranks of the Reservists." *The Musician*, July 1948, 165.
Shurtleff, William, and Akiko Aoyagi. *Soyinfo Center, History of Soybeans and Soyfoods in Australia, New Zealand and Oceania 1770–2010, Extensively Annotated Bibliography and Sourcebook,* Lafayette, CA: SoyInfo Center, 2010. Accessed November 17, 2024. www.soyinfocenter.com/pdf/138/Ocea2.pdf.
Sommerfeld, Kevin. *E. E. J.* Kjellberg, *Healing Hands, A Review of the Life and Times of a Master.* Brisbane: Boolarong Press, 2001.
Strachan, Shirley. "Bowen Therapy Today an April 18, 2014 Overview." Accessed November 17, 2024. https://www.bowentherapy.org.uk/docs/articles/shirley-strachan-report-on-tom-bowen-18Apr14.pdf.
Strachan, Shirley, and Keir Reeves. "Through the Lens of the Trainer-Masseurs: Australia's Incongruous Engagement with the Olympic Amateur Ethos." *The International Journal of the History of Sport* 39, no. 6 (2022): 631–52. https://doi.org/10.1080/09523367.2022.2095369.

Websites

"Bowtech, The Original Bowen Technique." Accessed November 17, 2024. http://www.bowtech.com/WebsiteProj/Pages/About/Welcome.aspx
Jaggard, E. "Kristé Martinovich (1903–1966)." *National Centre of Biography, Australian National University.* Accessed November 17, 2024. http://adb.anu.edu.au/biography/martinovich-kriste-11075/text19713. Published first in hardcopy 2000.
Nixon-Livy, Michael. "NST Development." Accessed November 17, 2024. https://nsthealth.com/development/.

2 Through Bowen's World, Early Educational Opportunities in Osteopathy

He must have somehow got onto this osteopathy from England and this is where he started. He'd done all this study from England – actually through correspondence – and he even got to the stage that in the finish he could have became [*sic*] so clever with it he could have gone to England for two years and become a Doctor of Osteopath[y], but he told me, 'That people here in Australia needed him more than he needed to be a doctor'.

Walter (Wal) Hayward, long-term friend[1]

Introduction

Thomas Ambrose Bowen is posthumously regarded as having intuitively invented the sequential set of procedures now promoted and taught globally as Bowen Therapy/Technique, with Bowen originally portrayed in hagiographic, saintly terms. Bowen's blue-collar, cement plant worker period 1955–1961 has been romanticised with views of him polarised between mystical healer who suddenly discovered he had a gift to those who saw him as 'just one of the cementies, a regular bloke'.[2] Rising out of this ground is the emergent professional who discarded his greasy dungarees for shirt and tie with business cards declaring the title of osteopath operating his business registered with the Department of Health from 1959 at the Horwood home at 101 Autumn Street. In 1963, early in his career, Bowen was already poised to competently address complex problems and treated Brian Anderson who faced the medical advice of being wheelchair-bound after a spinal injury from football and was suffering painful nerve reactions, 'Thank God for Tom Bowen! That's all I can say'.[3]

Bowen's Schooling

Bowen's transcript to the Victorian Government Ward Inquiry on October 8, 1973, revealed he went to Geelong's Ashby and Flinders State Schools leaving at fourteen in 1930.[4] Before employment at the cement works in 1955 and his additional important role there as First Aid Officer, Bowen's sources of employment included as a milk carter for Whistler Lee, working for his

DOI: 10.4324/9781003602125-3

carpenter-father in the building trade in Melbourne and later included the industries of North Geelong: the Harbour Trust, International Harvesters Company, Pilkington Glass and Fords Motor Plant, all of which, especially the latter, offered great networking opportunities with men involved in sport. This theme is developed further in Chapter 4 to explore influences around Bowen as a participant among sports' trainer-masseurs and the overlap in Bowen's world there with in-training and qualified osteopaths. Former employees at International Harvesters and Pilkington Glass remembered Bowen as a masseur and treating people then.[5] Several other accounts exist of Bowen, while connected to football trainer-masseurs, treating the public and gaining a strong reputation. All of this suggests a practitioner gaining wide experience and confidence in his work before the romanticised cement works period of 1955–1961 and setting up in business in 1959, full-time from 1961. Stanley (Stan) William Horwood (1904–1957) was an older workmate employed as a boilermaker's assistant at the cement works since 1944.[6] After the death of his first wife in 1952, Stan remarried in 1956 to Emily (Rene) Horwood who was to play a significant role in Bowen's future as his clinic manager.[7] Stan Horwood's sudden death in November 1957 was a blow to Bowen but Rene honoured Stan's dying wish for Bowen to be looked after and remained a staunch ally and supporter until his death. Bowen said of demand for his services 'It got that big I went to Melbourne to the Health Department for permission to practice'.[8]

Bowen's friends just assumed his work was an expression of something he 'just had in him' or 'something just out of his spirit'.[9] Family friend Barry Tattersall remembered first seeing Bowen in 1956 for a football injury to his back:

> I remember Autumn Street really well. I think it must have been early in his career because he would often ring me and say, 'I haven't seen you for a while, I've got some new ideas come in, I want someone to try them on'. He was good, but he also used me as a guinea pig during his earlier learning period.[10]

Association with Practitioners Connected to Naturopathic Pioneers

Bowen described himself as 'self-taught' in 1973 at the Victorian government inquiry into chiropractic, osteopathy and naturopathy.[11] However, the historical evidence questions the view that the inspiration for his treatment approach was entirely original and unique to him and provides clues of attempts at formal (but not completed) training at an English college, along with evidence of ongoing study of formal sources and interacting with peers on master-apprentice lines. Bowen had contact with other practitioners in professional circles sharing ideas and practice – in particular, students and graduates connected to early naturopathic pioneers, notably FG Roberts and Maurice Blackmore. Both pioneers set up teaching schools in Australia and brought to Australia early ideas about osteopathy and chiropractic as promulgated in British nature cure colleges they had attended in London. Roberts had attended the London School of Natural Therapeutics (LSNT) and he obtained further doctorates awarded from studies with Benedict Lust MD in the USA. Maurice Blackmore was educated on-campus at the British Naturopathic College of London graduating in 1925 and the British Chiropractic College and held a membership of the British Naturopathic Association in 1935.[12]

The use of 'college' rather than 'school' supports the college attended by Blackmore to be Stanley Lief's British College of Naturopathy (BCN) located in London – a college that enjoyed a positive relationship with LSNT. Others in Bowen's networks are found to be connected to Lief's establishment too, among them another Geelong man Percy Alfred (Alf) Jacka (1920–1988), a key figure in the Blackmores Victorian school-association network NAN/NANOC (National Association of Naturopaths – later separately adding osteopathy and chiropractic), though naturopathy at the time encompassed all the healing arts. Jacka also undertook his correspondence studies at Lief's BCN. This is confirmed by the fact that Jacka remembered in his sworn transcript to the Ward Inquiry in 1973 that he had undertaken theoretical studies in the early 1940s with the 'British Naturopathic College'.[13] When asked about the address, he responded in slight error, instead of stating correctly Netherhall Gardens, he said, 'I think it is Wetherley Gardens'.[14] Jacka's practical hands-on training in Australia was with consultant USA chiropractors Hansen and Feeley.[15] Jacka became the president of the newly founded Australian Natural Therapists Association (ANTA) to which Bowen belonged after the advent of regulation in 1978 destroyed the naturopathic association networks that existed prior that were primarily established around Roberts and Blackmore and others heading up their suborganisations and schools. Gerritt Janssen introduced later in Chapter 6 also completed studies at the BCN in 1933 and played a major role in Australia establishing leading organisations for naturopaths. Chapter 6 also finds Janssen connected to Thomas Dummer (principal of the European School of Osteopathy (ESO)) and Dummer's dual role as honorary secretary of the International Federation of Practitioners of Natural Therapeutics (IFPNT) in accrediting teaching schools internationally, including Australia in line with the Federation's standards. Today, the ESO continues to maintain a strong relationship with the modern college, the British College of Osteopathic Medicine (BCOM) that evolved from Lief's BCN.[16]

Oral History Evidence of Bowens' Uncompleted Attempts at Formal Studies

There is no documentary proof of Bowen's involvement in formal studies; any study records and correspondence that might have existed have perished along with just about all of his clinic records reportedly burned after his death. However, there is a rich enough tapestry of oral history recollections and lore that indicate Bowen was engaged in formal studies by correspondence overseas, an English establishment the strongest prospect. Research indicates correspondence pathways can be narrowed to Lief's BCN. However, Bowen did not complete the formal educational journey. Entwined, there is lore that Bowen actually travelled overseas, though the family deny Bowen ever travelled outside of Australia. Bowen's youngest sister Agnes Shaw (born in 1924) remembered her brother undertaking correspondence studies during the Great Depression and the study materials were on display (recollected by Agnes to be medically related), but that her brother had dropped out of formal studies to be a doctor as his father couldn't pay the fees.[17] In Australia, the effects of the Great Depression started in the late 1920s and formalised with the Wall Street crash of 1929, with effects continuing for a decade.[18] Agnes Shaw lived in Melbourne between 1937 and 1943 and returned to Geelong between then and 1949. Talking of the Bowen home at 31 McDougall Street, as 'a kid' and reference to the Great Depression period, Agnes said:

> We had a very big bathroom and he had a table in there and my memory of him was – papers all over the table and he was doing correspondence courses. But what they were, me being a kid I sort of didn't cotton on to what they were. All I knew was that he was studying something but it would be medical. It would have been medical, because that was his ambition actually, to be a doctor.[19]

According to Shaw, ambitions were thwarted when facing bankruptcy, their father William focused on clearing his debts:

> Well, that was the Depression and dad had a building business and he lost all his money then and he could have gone bankrupt but he wouldn't go bankrupt. He paid all his debtors and he said at least he could walk with his head high. That was important to him and therefore there wasn't the money to put Tom through [his studies]. So, but I don't know whether Tom actually got over that. That was a big, big disappointment. He [Tom] was aware of the circumstances, but deep down I don't know whether, he didn't hold it against my father, deep down the disappointment was there and I think he sort of felt it.[20]

Although training opportunities existed for soldiers in the 1940s under the Commonwealth Reconstruction Training Scheme (CRTS) 1944–1950, these can be discounted for Bowen as the CRTS allowed only returned soldiers the benefit of tertiary education, but Bowen was not eligible as he did not see active service, only the Civil Militia Force (CMF).[21]

Bowen's friend Walter (Wal) Hayward quoted at chapter's epigraph shows he understood from what Bowen told him personally that he had undertaken correspondence studies with an English institution. In support of this, clinic observer Dr Romney Smeeton DC was also personally told by Bowen between 1976 and 1982 that he had sent a manuscript to England but had not heard back and surmised it was forgotten in a bottom drawer somewhere. The existence of the manuscript was later validated posthumously to Smeeton through a patient connected to the friend of Bowen who had typed the manuscript for him. Unfortunately, other than Smeeton, the individuals involved in the manuscript account are now deceased. If Bowen retained a copy, the mystery manuscript has perished. Later, in Bowen's career (also in the 1970s), Anne Mortelliti recounted the following exchange with Bowen and got the impression his treatment style was learned from overseas:

> Anyway, so one day while we were talking, I said to Mr Bowen . . . . 'What do you call what you do? 'Well' he said, 'I work on pressure points'. Right? 'On pressure points'. I said, 'Yes, well where did you learn that?' He told me, 'overseas'.[22]

Other oral histories such as Peter Scott's account also carried the impression of Bowen and overseas connections:

> No, no, the impression was – and get this, this is only the story, he'd been somewhere and they taught him how to do it and then he'd come back and he had that ability himself, I always believed that.[23]

The several oral history sources and Bowen's personal remark to Smeeton take priority over other possible domestic explanations of association with a British college. Robert Lucy's transcript made reference to a British School which related to the correspondence course in chiropractic offered in Australia by Blackmore based on a British curriculum.[24] Blackmore had attended the London Chiropractic College.[25] It was considered that Hayward's association with Britain perhaps came from the early title of FG Roberts' College, the 'British and Australian Institute of Naturopathy' (BAIN) which existed before the name-change in 1959 to Chiropractic and Osteopathy College of Australia (COCA). However, given oral history evidence directly linked to Bowen from friend Hayward and long-standing clinic associate Smeeton, these domestic explanations are weak to explain the overseas theme. Lief's English BCN emerges as the strongest possibility for the college Bowen enrolled in but had to withdraw – the college is represented in the backgrounds of others in Bowen's networks and was evidently a popular choice among key Australians leading naturopathic education last century.

Despite the unfinished formal studies, from her association with Bowen from the mid-1950s, Rene Horwood confirmed Bowen also did a lot of reading and self-education.[26] With a family keen on music, Bowen set up at 100 Autumn Street to study there with quiet. Other oral history evidence reveals Bowen next engaged in studies in 1959, the year he registered his business. Tensions between Bowen and his father William Bowen were not uncommon as Bowen senior thought to thwart any ambitions of his son unrelated to salvationist culture and aspirations. William Arthur Bowen was experiencing frustrations of his own – he suffered the ongoing discomfort of a hernia that had permanently precluded military service including the Great War.[27]

In 1948, William had relinquished his position of Lieutenant Major of the Geelong West Salvation Army brass band corps on account of failing eyesight and was assigned to the band's reserves as a soldier.[28] Tensions escalated in 1959 within the Bowen family and a stressful standoff saw Tom admitted to the Ballarat Mental Hospital for a month in March 1959.[29] In September 1959, Bowen's father died 'passed to glory'.[30] This year too, Bowen was working with the gifted masseur Ron Garner at the Horwood home in Autumn Street.[31] This provided the impetus for Bowen to formally register his business and capitalise on the opportunity provided by ongoing use of the treatment space provided by Rene Horwood. Bowen's study efforts intensified at this time.

In 1959, the same tumultuous year that Bowen formally registered his business, the FG Roberts' BAIN overtly realigned itself to engage in chiropractic-dominated registration politics and was renamed COCA. Bowen was treating long-term patient Thérèse Vahland at the time. Then in her early teens, Vahland said her father worked at the Elephant and Castle Hotel 1954–1961 and Bowen spoke with him often.[32] The father brought the conversations home to the family dinner table and she stated:

> I had the impression that other chiropractors or osteopaths in Geelong were upset with him [Bowen] because he was seeing lots of people and taking their business away. There was talk he had to become registered or closed down. Well, he didn't have time for study as he was always treating people. He trained in osteopathy. I remember hearing from dad that he found it [the study] difficult mentally.[33]

Vahland's recollection is when her father was 45 years old, which confirmed 1959. Tensions in the political scene may well have propelled Bowen to intensify study effort with a view again to formal credentials as he activated his professional aspirations in 1959. Masseur Doug Sells who often helped Bowen in the evenings at the Latrobe Terrace clinic in the 1960s remembered textbooks on the shelves there too.

Anti-quack legislation first proposed in NSW in 1937 was followed up in Victoria in 1954.[34] In 1959, Western Australia initiated a Royal Commission completed in 1964 into the registration of naturopaths, encompassing chiropractic and osteopathy. Osteopathy had not fared well and the United Osteopaths Association formed by FG Roberts in 1961 folded afterwards.[35] That year, Alfred Jacka as Honorary Secretary of the former Australian National Naturopathic Association wrote to the minister for health responding to lobbying for registration by the Victorian Branch of the Australian Chiropractors Association (ACA) which catered to American graduates.[36] The official reply denied plans for legislation.[37] In this climate, Bowen operated his business full-time from 1961 as an osteopath with the indomitable Rene Horwood who provided encouragement, managerial skills, financial support and assets towards this and future clinics which she regarded as much hers as his.[38] In 1964, further controversy followed as the ACA reacted negatively to the formal Australian qualifications offered through Roberts' COCA.[39]

Bowen is also connected at home in networks with graduates of early Australian schools teaching osteopathy under the naturopathic umbrella whose knowledge originally hailed from overseas, notably both FG Roberts whose education spanned the UK and the USA and Maurice Blackmore with Lief in the UK. FG Roberts was accessible to Bowen at physical sites in Melbourne near where Bowen worked for his father in the 1930s and lived for a period during the war in the Dandenong area to the East. Through FG Roberts' communications and touring presence, access to early local osteopathy study opportunities were available to a working-class labourer like Bowen as well as others sharing these interests who were engaged as masseurs and looking after VFL footballers. Roberts gave lectures on nature cure during the depression at the Young Men's Christian Association (YMCA).[40] Roberts started a clinic in Latrobe Street Melbourne in 1929 and was prosecuted for practising as a medical practitioner.[41] The court case is enlightening as it described new information that Roberts undertook additional training with American institutions after his early LSNT period in the UK and acquired additional doctorates by correspondence.[42] This helps explain Roberts' strong alliance with Dr Benedict Lust, the USA Father of Naturopathy. Of the pioneers, Roberts was earliest on the scene in a significant way and handled by far the largest number of trainees and graduates. Roberts 'loved to travel, and at all these places he lectured, taught and treated people'.[43] For those who could afford formal studies, Roberts offered low-cost study, flexibly delivered through correspondence pathways and direct clinic contact. Very importantly, he accepted men like Bowen who had not matriculated. Cecil Wells who lectured for Roberts in the 1930s was interviewed by Campbell in 1980 and stated his objection to Roberts training people who were not educated.[44] Roberts had an extensive presence on the eastern seaboard and wide public engagement with radio work and free lectures and consultations ensured he was well known.[45] The accessibility and affordability to the untrained was part of his deeper mission spread from the 'Home of the Nature Cure Movement' at 430 St Kilda Road Melbourne.[46] Roberts had a street presence first as a health food store then as dietician services at 284 Post Office place in Melbourne from 1937.[47] Roberts' school was soon renamed the BAIN, first in the press in 1935 and shortened to Roberts Institute of Naturopathy in his magazine *Natures Path to Health* (NPH) and using the full title for course advertising in 1941.[48] Roberts established a presence in the far north beginning in 1930 in Rockhampton and Mackay extending south to Melbourne and the regional centres of Ballarat and Geelong by 1937. This was complemented by the multi-location Roberts Health Service and clinics around Australia. Prospective students would have been aware of his courses in NPH or attending his lectures where more information and practical demonstrations were available.

Roberts published NPH between 1928 and 1952. A complete set of Roberts' journals does not exist in one institution and only the holdings at Deakin Library were inspected which include items from 1934 to 1950.[49] Readers of NPH enjoyed a privileged connection to a prime knowledge network of ideas and practice of leading overseas pioneers and teachers. Roberts made the naturopathic world accessible to all and extended to profiling manual therapies, including osteopathy and chiropractic. Many of the invitees to Roberts' first Australian Health Congress in Melbourne in 1939 included contributors to his magazine, including Dr Benedict Lust (USA), Herbert Shelton (USA), Dr George Starr White (USA), William F Lucas (his UK contributor) and Dr Uliric Williams (NZ).[50] Much of the content was republished from Dr Benedict Lust's *The Naturopath and Herald of Health* from 1902–1927 and from 1924 entitled *Nature's Path*. Lust was a contributing editor to NPH. Among the reprinted Lust articles were twenty-three lessons on Osteopathy, Chiropractic and Mental Therapeutics. Lust's 1918 *Universal Naturopathic Dictionary* contained an international directory of like-minded professionals and numerous articles.[51] Through Lust, Roberts remained abreast of the thinking and development of osteopathy and chiropractic from the pioneers; Andrew Taylor Still (osteopathy) and David D Palmer (chiropractic) with his college 'joining in force'.[52] Roberts advertised a lecture circuit in the press and his magazine, the earliest newspaper advertisement dating to 1928 at the Victorian Hardware Club, 386 Bourke Street.[53] By mid-1930 Roberts lectured at the new Hardware Club at 386 Post Office Place, near his future clinic at number 284.[54] Coinciding with the outbreak of the war and the end of the Great Depression, Roberts' home study course ceased and he developed other offerings.

Roberts' home study offerings would have been convenient as an introduction for any would-be osteopath or chiropractor. Roberts had a shop in Geelong, Bowen's hometown and later professional base and shop in nearby Ballarat.[55] One of Roberts' earliest students was Agnes Marie Cogan of Ballarat dating to 1933.[56] Cogan started her practice before 1942 and used language at the Ward Inquiry about leveraging pressure off nerves and pinched nerves to describe her work which matches that of Bowen at the same inquiry.[57] It is not known what sources Roberts used to teach osteopathy, though evidence in Chapter 3 points to neuropathy as a key orientation.

By 1939, Roberts started to promote 'courses for the layman and practitioner' on the 'practice and theory of chiropractic adjustments and soft tissue therapy'. Running for almost a year, it cost £1.00 per week and included a free-of-charge textbook.[58] In 1940, the average yearly wages of a factory worker was £248 5s 8d, amounting to less than £5.00 a week, resulting in an investment of one-fifth of earnings.[59] Throughout the 1940s, Roberts' Institute continued to conduct courses in chiropractic and osteopathy with direct classroom lectures.[60] Examples of others known to have completed correspondence training with Roberts in the 1940s are Alan Goldby of Ballarat and William Pruss of Sydney. Goldby was Director of Physical Education with the YMCA and studied for eighteen months to two years with Roberts involving correspondence studies, lectures and practical application before graduating at BAIN in 1948.[61] William Pruss was later observed at Bowen's clinics and taught a similar technique as Bowen called Pruss Alignment Techniques. Pruss had also studied in Sydney with Roberts' brother William in the 1930s and 1940s. From there Pruss headed to Melbourne in the 1940s to study by correspondence alongside practical time in Roberts' clinics.[62] Pruss received his naturopathic diploma from FG Roberts in 1949 and later in 1964 completed studies at the Sydney College of Osteopathy (SCO) qualifying simultaneously as DO/DC.[63] Costly training was outside of Bowen's purview, but the boundaries between those trained and sharing ideas to interested others was not a stringent at the time as they are now.

Roberts had an influence on another Geelong man who established a teaching presence in Queensland but does not emerge as a notable avenue for correspondence studies by Bowen and those in his networks. For a brief period starting in 1927, courses on osteopathy, chiropractic and medical electricity were advertised to be held in Brisbane.[64] These were offered by Claude Alfred Beales (1888–1963) from Geelong. Beales was an associate of Roberts and had escaped north to evade persecution. Beales described himself a professor and 'pioneer of chiropractic in Australia'.[65] He supported a Roberts' lecture in Rockhampton in 1930.[66] Although Beales' offerings were not advertised as correspondence studies, a 1947 story on Gilbert Richard Wheeler reveals he obtained a degree of Doctor of Osteopathy 'by correspondence' through the Australian Hygeian Institute operated by Beales in Fortitude Valley, Brisbane.[67] Beales was not high profile and he became connected to Maurice Blackmore who was also associated with Roberts' activities in the north. The possibilities for osteopathy studies within Australia from the 1930s are otherwise extremely narrow with constancy of opportunity limited to the fledgling FG Roberts' school already established in Melbourne in 1929 and operating initially as the Australian College of Naturopathy (ACN) and also described as the Australian School of Mutual Therapeutics in 1930.[68] Apprenticeships were also available through Blackmores Queensland-based association-college that had branches elsewhere and began as National Association of Naturopaths (NAN). Alister McAlister who was known to Bowen taught apprentices for Blackmore before he qualified with Roberts as a DO in 1958 and provided placements for his students too. This is determined from the role he played as mentor to Andrew Fraser DO who settled in Geelong in the 1970s and whose training was with Blackmore.[69] McAlister also offered placements to Roberts' students too in the 1960s.[70] The presence of FG Roberts in Geelong and Melbourne surely cannot have escaped Bowen's notice, given his interests in manual therapy, nor the presence of Blackmores school given McAlister's connection with it.

Another local college is dismissed as a training route for Bowen. Pax College was set up in Ballarat by a Scot, James Edward Doyle. Chiropractic historians accept Pax College commenced in 1937.[71] However, according to Campbell who quoted the Webb Inquiry Report, it was when Pax moved to Ballarat in

1947 that teaching really began by Doyle.[72] Research confirms Doyle's second wife Jean Doyle (married in 1949) said the Ballarat move was that year.[73] Cameron's thesis indicated Doyle trained in Canada under an apprenticeship of some kind.[74] Jean Doyle also said her husband had also trained with FG Roberts.[75] A James Edward Doyle is listed as 'herbalist' on the electoral rolls in Melbourne in 1937.[76] At the end of his first doomed two-year marriage in 1944, Doyle was described an osteopath with a flourishing practice in the city.[77] No proof of teaching activities pre-1947 has been found. Though closer to Geelong, Doyle's College is not a likely drawcard for Bowen; Pax offered training later than Roberts and was more selective, producing only three graduates in 1953.[78] Pax courses were three years initially in apprentice-style teaching then later four and six months full-time with a substantial investment outlay which precludes Bowen affording his training.[79] However, James Doyle and FG Roberts enjoyed a positive relationship and both men, Doyle in particular, was close to Alfred Kaufmann who established the forerunner to the Sydney College of Chiropractic (SCC), initially an osteopathy college in 1959.[80] The strength of the ties is revealed by Doyle bequeathing Pax to Kaufmann when Doyle died in 1965.[81] All were members of Roberts' United Practitioners' Association of Australasia in 1941.[82]

John Garner, son of Ron Garner, Bowen's early 1950s business associate at Autumn Street, said 'Bowen always told me he "found his gift in the war"'.[83] During the war, Bowen was enlisted in the CMF with the 21/23rd Battalion (the Geelong Regiment/Victorian Rangers) and for a period was engaged in tactical training at Balcombe/Mount Martha on the East side of Port Phillip Bay.[84] Mount Martha was a large camp catering to thousands of soldiers including the second Australian Infantry Force (AIF) and the CMF, which provided a great opportunity for Bowen to connect and share interests with many others, including those involved with the YMCA and the Red Cross Units that had a presence there.[85] Alister (Lal) McAlister was a champion foot runner and won a race in soldier sport at Mount Martha in November 1940 and developed a reputation for massaging other soldiers.[86] McAlister – later DO, is certainly connected to Bowen after the war and afterwards in the regulatory 1970s as a member to the small eleven-member Victorian Society of Specialist Osteopaths (VSSO). The war period could be when these two men first met and Bowen discovered he too had a yen for manual therapies. Among the VSSO men, McAlister is the closest link found to Bowen. From a Scottish emigrant family, hailing first from Smeaton, Victoria, the McAlister family was working class with the father a waterside worker. Alister was born in 1915 in West Melbourne.[87] Melbourne addresses for the McAlister family are on the west side including 103 Stanley Street in Maribyrnong from 1937 an address that is a short distance from the Footscray Football Club which becomes topical.[88] From 1962 to 1966, McAlister was engaged as an osteopath to the Footscray Football Club and was also treating the public from there. His earlier work included factory-hand then foreman graduating to an AMP insurance salesman before turning osteopath; his brother Graham became a Labor MP.

Later when married, Alister was located at 105 Market Street, Essendon from around 1954. McAlister was self-learning osteopathy in the 1950s and had a practice in Collingwood before later completing a Diploma with the Roberts College in 1958.[89] McAlister achieved this over two years part-time and three nights a week.[90] Through his protégé Fraser DO, in the early period, McAlister was also involved with the Blackmores network and provided apprenticeships to Blackmores students members to the NAN (later NANC to reflect chiropractic, established in 1946). NANC evolved to incorporate osteopathy in 1970. NANOC is the forerunner of today's Southern School of Natural Therapies formed in 1971 and led by Jacka who trained at Lief's BCN like Blackmore did.

There are oral history accounts from Bowen's daughters that place Bowen associated with a group of men for a two-year period in the 1950s at the Footscray and Moonee Ponds area of Melbourne. The famous name of VFL trainer-masseur Ernest Saunders was recalled in connection with these Melbourne meetings, but Saunders is definitely not a match for the chronology, as he died in February 1951 and was ill in the months prior. Instead, Footscray and Moonee Ponds venues closely point to Alister (Lal) McAlister as the connection to the suburbs recalled. As described earlier, he lived on the west side of Melbourne when younger; he served as an osteopath at Footscray Football Club in the 1960s and afterwards operated his osteopathy practice at 151 Pascoe Vale Road, Moonee Ponds.[91] As well as the documented VSSO connection, oral accounts from an apprentice of McAlister confirmed that the men were personally known to each other.[92] The reasonable conclusion is McAlister and Bowen were meeting up with others in Footscray and Moonee Ponds in the 1950s/1960s to share ideas about treatments and participate in this master-apprentice form of learning. A protégé of McAlister, Andrew Fraser set up his practice in Geelong was educated at Blackmores school and credits McAlister as his mentor.[93] The recalled contact with Saunders on the west side of Melbourne would have to relate to an earlier period. Neither Footscray nor Moonee Ponds are convenient to Saunders' clinic located further eastward in Victoria Street, Richmond. As a Victorian Football League (VFL) trainer until 1935, the members of the trainers' association may well have met at various clubs around the city. Bowen's connections in the football sphere are explored in Chapter 4 which reveals that Footscray Football Club was a drawcard to manual therapists, given its advanced facilities for treating VFL players. Bowen's contact with Saunders is of unknown timing pre-1951 and considered in that context.

In Bowen's day, the professional demarcations that later separately defined osteopath and chiropractor as protected professional titles (similar to that enjoyed by physiotherapists since the 1950s) were yet to happen. At the time, many of the college graduates held joint titles of DC/DO revealing the closeness and overlapping of the two modalities in the lead-up to regulation. Among the men who formed the VSSO in 1975, several had been formally enrolled in Roberts' Melbourne college before it took off strategically on a chiropractic bent by 1959 in response to survival politics and pressures of the day. Some had a connection to Blackmores school too and this is covered in Chapter 7. The VSSO men include Bowen, McAlister, Alan Wilkie, Robin Gardini and Richard Bennett, among others. The VSSO men were a minority of eleven men and held out for their osteopathic identity and refused to be legitimised under the chiropractic umbrella that subsumed osteopathy at the time. Their critical views of the chiropractic direction of Roberts' college are also captured in Chapter 7.

Both FG Roberts and Maurice Blackmore identified as neuropaths earlier in their careers. In Chapter 3, the historical evidence of what the practice of neuropathy entailed becomes useful as a reference point for Bowens' symbolism and practice and that of his college-educated peers interviewed at the Ward Inquiry. This demonstrates neuropathy to be a foundational home of Bowen's approach and further reinforces Bowen's connection with leaders of nature cure osteopathy in Australia. Already in existence in osteopathic and nature cure circles was the Universal Natural Tonic Treatment Tonic (UNTT) developed by Dr FW Collins and a roundtable of leaders and students of Still such as Dr Charles F Haverin, Drs Andrew Victory, EK Stretch and Jacob Lang to restore Still's principles to osteopathy.[94] The roundtable was concerned that the general osteopathic treatments contained too many moves and stimulated hyper reflexes. The work of several practitioners was reviewed by the roundtable, including Still, Barber, Murray, McFadden and German texts on manual therapies to develop the UNTT. The UNTT involved a minimalist sequence of moves that effected comprehensive therapeutic benefit.[95] Leon Chaitow DO also stated the UNTT or General Naturopathic Tonic Treatment (GNTT) was represented in a few manual therapy movements, including Bowen Technique, Reflexology and NMT, all of which he also considered to be 'constitutional therapies'.[96]

Chaitow described that as well as correcting specific lesions found, the manner of delivery of a treatment in the UNTT provided simultaneous diagnosis.[97] As observed by Smeeton, this was an element that challenged observers of Bowen; differentiating whether a hand movement was a therapeutic intervention or whether Bowen was just simply assessing and diagnosing tissue states. Bowen's work was so subtle and he worked so swiftly it was difficult to follow without close attention to what he was doing.[98] Bowen's minimalist style and sequential approach and use of only fingers and thumbs to influence specific levels of tissue structure are echoed in UNTT.

Bowen's Connections to Liefs' British College of Naturopathy and Opportunities for Correspondence Studies

It is proposed from available oral history that Bowen had a fleeting association with Stanley Lief's college based on evidence from friend Hayward and clinic-associate Smeeton DC. Unfortunately, enquires to BCOM have failed to unearth any early archive about any possible Australian enrolments and training by correspondence for the 1930–1960 period. Both Blackmore and Jacka obtained their education at Lief's British College of Naturopathy. The following maps out the slim overseas landscape of training by correspondence opportunities in the UK and the USA. The mainstream colleges in the UK and the USA did not provide correspondence pathways and can be safely eliminated. These included the British School of Osteopathy (BSO) and the London School of Osteopathy (LSO) and the ESO each established in the UK in 1917, 1949 and 1965 respectively. In the 1930s, the UK climate was tense with bonesetter [Sir] Herbert Barker in the news and calls for registration of osteopathy and training to fall under the scrutiny of Parliament.[99] The mainstream schools in America can also be eliminated; in the early 1900s, osteopathy had become a specialism and separated in the mainstream from naturopathic manual medicine, and an association drive had stamped out correspondence training by the leading institutions.[100] Some opportunities existed in non-mainstream nature cure colleges. A home study osteopathy course was published by The Psychic Research Company and Columbia College of Osteopathy but not referred to in Australian circles.[101] In the 1920s, correspondence studies were available via the Manchester School of Natural Therapeutics (MSNT), originally established by Dr William Looker in 1921, as the Manchester School of Bloodless Surgery.[102] By the late 1920s, the college was under J Allen Pattreiouex who continued to offer training by home study.[103] The well-known Parnell Bradbury enrolled in full-time study around 1920, as MSNT was becoming affiliated with the Wellington School of Chiropractic at Stockport, led by a graduate of the National College of Chiropractic in Chicago.[104] It was renamed to the Manchester College of Osteopathy and Chiropractic and apparently eventually relocated to London.[105] These colleges are not specifically named by respondents to the Australian government enquiries and did not attract the attention of Australian followers of naturopathic modalities. FG Roberts had attended on-campus training at the LSNT suggesting the school did not have correspondence training.[106] The LSNT later incorporated osteopathy and Dr Milton Powell taught the subject in the 1940s while his brother Eric Powell ran the London School of Biotherapy, primarily a homeopathy school where Alfred Kaufmann of the SCO enrolled on-campus in 1940.[107] By 1934, the LSNT had moved to a four-year fulltime course with matriculation entry requirements which eliminates it as a college Bowen could have accessed directly in the Great Depression period.[108]

Opportunities are narrowed to Stanley Lief's BCN in England (retitled BNCO in the 1950s).[109] The college still exists today (renamed again in 2002 as the BCOM), though its website now reverts to the BCNO group with ESO as a subsidiary.[110] Correspondence study was available at BCN in its early period. The Latvian and nature cure leader, Stanley Lief, is said to have founded the BCN in 1936.[111] However, a reference in the British Newspaper Archive referred to court action against a graduate and the details indicate BCN was offering naturopathy and osteopathy earlier from 1926 via correspondence and other study before the building was destroyed in the war.[112] Additional information confirmed the original site was at Wyndham Place, before relocating and establishing at Netherhall Gardens, evolving to become the BCNO in 1953.[113] Lief and cousin Boris Chaitow developed Neuromuscular Technique (NMT) in the lead-up to and during the Second World War.[114] Lief had originally studied in the USA with Bernarr McFadden's School of Physcultopathy and founded Champney's Nature Cure Home in 1914 offering dietetics, alongside hydrotherapy, osteopathy, chiropractic and massage.[115] McFadden and Dr Lust were also close friends.[116]

FG Roberts' enjoyed a strong relationship with Benedict Lust and it is evident that correspondence studies were available to Roberts through the USA nature cure route, in addition to his on-campus training at the LSNT. Stanley Lief had also pursued direct training in America with Bernarr McFadden. Overall, the USA is not topical among Australian practitioners in Bowen's time as a training source of osteopathy, other than Roberts' education with Lust and Jacka's training with USA chiropractors who visited Australia after he completed studies at BCN. England remains the drawcard for those in networks in which Bowen participated and Stanley Lief's London college of naturopathy, soon to include osteopathy emerged as the predominant college. Lief also advertised his *Health for All* publication advertised extensively in Australian newspapers between 1926 and the early 1950s. Given his educational and financial circumstances, any formal pathway to a qualification for Bowen can only have been achieved through a naturopathic college route. His thwarted attempt at formal study did not deter Bowen from pursuing ongoing self-directed study and seeking out personal interaction with others who shared his osteopathic interests. He interacted with others trained with Roberts' in Australia and Roberts was an accessible presence to men like Bowen. There are also personal and professional linkages to Blackmores school through McAlister and Jacka.

The popularised posthumous view of Bowen is that he adopted the title of osteopath simply as a convenience so he could register a business and legally practise. It was certainly easier than setting up as a masseur – a profession regulated in Victoria since the introduction of the *Masseurs Registration Act* in 1922. In 1957, the tensions and control over masseurs and growing power of physiotherapists were evidenced by special legislation enacted to solely register George Saunders, son of Ernie Saunders and these men are covered in Chapter 4.[117] The Physiotherapy and Massage Association and the Massage Registration Board formally objected wishing to limit registration to those qualified.[118] The Board supplied documentation detailing the three years of training required to be registered as a masseur.[119] As a result, the proposed Bill was amended to prohibit Saunders from using varying titles including physiotherapist. Given the tensions surrounding masseurs and those around nationally with osteopathy, it is unlikely that Bowen was not aware of these. Bowen was aware of George Saunders' registration at the Ward Inquiry.[120] Rene Horwood indicated that Bowen was always careful to have no black marks against him.[121] Equally, the decision to identify himself as an osteopath in 1961 was a brave one given how Roberts wound down the osteopathy association he had established that same year and then focused on chiropractic as a result of the outcomes of the Western Australian Commission process.

Connections to Practitioners Trained with the Naturopathic Pioneers, FG Roberts and Blackmore

By October 1961, Bowen had a huge patient load. Throughout the 1960s, qualification pathways were available with Roberts' COCA via clinic placements with a qualified osteopath undertaken in conjunction with other non-osteopathic training.[122] McAlister was self-taught in osteopathy practising for years before he studied at the FG Roberts College (BAIN), qualifying as DO in late 1958 after two years part-time involving three nights a week.[123] McAlister was also connected through NANC/NANOC with Blackmores trainees: an example being his protégé Andrew Fraser DO, and Fraser too originally worked as head football trainer for an undisclosed Melbourne football club.[124] Fraser started his osteopathic training in 1937 – determined from research to be with Blackmores/NANC (later NANOC) and dedicated a book to McAlister, assisted by Paul Schmidt.[125] This logically leads to the conclusion that Fraser received early apprenticeship training under Blackmores school with McAlister before completing his studies with Jacka who ran Blackmores NANOC association school in Victoria until 1971 when it became his own college, the Southern School of Natural Therapies (SSNT). Fraser also set up practice in Geelong. He had a big personality and a competitive view of Bowen giving others the impression that Bowen referred difficult cases to him.[126] McAlister was also a member of NANOC and later the Australian Chiropractors Osteopaths and Naturopathic Practitioners Association Ltd. (ACONPAL), an organisation that Bowen also joined by the time of his interview with the Victorian government inquiry in 1973.[127] Professor Murtagh was a teenage patient of McAlister in the 1960s.[128] Murtagh (unaware that McAlister was credentialed as DO at the time) acknowledged McAlister's ability as a masseur in his retrospective in musculoskeletal medicine.[129]

When the VSSO was formed in 1975 involving a small group of eleven men with decades of experience, Bowen and McAlister were among them.[130] These members were joined by invitation only and would have been well known to each other by long reputation and acquaintance.[131] The VSSO is discussed further in Chapter 7. Fraser is expected to be a member too. Later on, after the Victorian regulation was in force, Bowen, McAlister and Fraser became members of the newly formed ANTA with Jacka as president.[132]

Sometime before 1951 Bowen also had contact with the Melbourne-based VFL trainer-masseur, Ernest (Ernie) Saunders (1878–1951) a 'legend' in football, sports and other circles and a renowned 'manipulator'.[133] This contact with hearsay described in Chapters 4 and 5 has been popularly inflated to suggest Saunders was Bowen's mentor and introduced him to Japanese acupoints learned on a trip to America between the wars. This claim is analysed in

Chapter 4 which describes Saunders' quite different style from Bowen and the lack of evidence to support the hearsay.

Bowen never gave a clear picture of the origins of his work though he clearly had strong connections with others associated with FG Roberts and Maurice Blackmore and their training. After joining Bowen's clinic as an observer in 1976, Dr Kevin Neave DC on was one of the very few who thought to ask Bowen outright 'so, where did all this start Tommy? I'd like to know'. Bowen replied enigmatically with words recalled as 'an old fellow from Gove'. When Neave said, 'I'd like to meet with him', Bowen replied, 'he'll have nothing to do with you' and was reluctant to discuss further.[134] It cannot be guaranteed that Neave heard Bowen correctly as there exists the expression 'cove', which is old-fashioned British and Australian meaning 'a fellow' or 'chap'.[135] Bowen may just have been repeating two similar expressions. Either way, Neave respected this and let it be, but formed the impression that this related to someone now quite old and still alive who came from the far north of Australia as Gove is in Arnhem Land. This disclosure was subsequently published in a Bowen Association newsletter and gave rise to rumours that Bowen's inspiration came from an Indigenous source.[136] A more realistic possibility for Bowen's elusive response to the mystery identity is FG Roberts. Apart from Roberts' geographical proximity to Bowen's life and influence on others in Bowen's circle, Roberts fits the mystery identity – born in 1882, he was an old man in his eighties and still living in 1976, the year Neave started observing Bowen. Roberts was semi-retired after an accident in 1960 but still operating a clinic in the 1970s at Prahran. By 1973, he was not well enough to present to the Ward Inquiry and was not described in a particularly flattering light. An explanation for Bowen's ideas about Roberts' negative attitude to Neave, a straight chiropractor may lie in the following:

> There was also a major philosophical difference between F. G. Roberts who was a 'mixer' making use of various techniques (naturopathy, osteopathy, chiropractic, herbalism) and the second generation of chiropractors – the 'straights' who wanted to practice the discipline exclusively.[137]

Roberts was a holistic 'nature cure' adept and may have been disenchanted about this and how his own legacy as a phenomenal and indefatigable naturopathic entrepreneur had played out. Roberts was included as a 'notable citizen' of Sydney in 1940.[138] Only one biographical piece has been written of him, an unpublished manuscript by Paul Smith, who owned Roberts Health foods (now taken over as Gluten Free World) and assisted Shurtleff and Aoyagi in their history of soy production in Australia that also extensively utilised NPH references.[139] Campbell conducted rare interviews of family and others associated with Roberts' college.[140] Roberts died in Nunawading, Victoria, in March 1977 before the Federal Webb Inquiry released its report. Maurice Blackmore (1906–1977) was also living at the time of this exchange but was Queensland-based and his presence in Victoria was through intermediaries such as Jacka leading his association-school NAN/NANOC. Blackmore was a respondent to the Ward Inquiry but carries a much lower profile than Roberts in the discussion and Blackmore retained his identity as naturopathic. By then, Roberts' college was poised to become a prescribed college under the forthcoming legislation whereas Blackmores NAN/NANOC in Victoria morphed into the Southern School of Natural Therapies under Jacka's ownership. If either of these two men is the mystery mentor, Roberts is a more likely contender than Blackmore and given his public appearances in Victoria and early philosophy, personally more accessible to Bowen.

Summary

In conclusion, self-taught does not mean that Bowen invented his techniques; he clearly informed himself with ideas from formal osteopathic studies most likely overseas-based with Lief's BCN/BCNO in England the initial wellspring but failed to complete. It is reported he 'constantly studied a variety of medical and osteopathic texts' and in 1981 Bowen himself said he supported a 'knack' he had 'by studying books containing information relevant to osteopathic [*sic*]'.[141] He pursued ongoing self-study and participated in get-togethers with others who shared ideas in osteopathic practice and his acquaintance with Alister McAlister is key as McAlister bridges the world between Blackmores and Roberts' training. Like Bowen, McAlister evolved from football masseur status and was initially self-taught. Unlike Bowen, he proceeded to formally qualify as DO in 1958 through the Roberts' school and his readings disclosed at the Ward Inquiry reveal how his interests were more transitional and consulted more mainstream college texts such as Stoddard and Cyriax. Chapter 3 will consider Bowen's style of working and terminology against early styles of osteopathy espoused by Roberts and Blackmore called neuropathy which involved lifting pressure off nerves. Both FG Roberts and Blackmore identified as neuropaths and neuropathy emerges as foundational and a sound alignment for the language and approach adopted by Bowen in his own practice. This is also shared by other early Roberts' trained graduates who were interviewed at the Ward Inquiry. Chapter 3 will explore neuropathy as the origins of Bowen's practice, a preferred title for osteopathy in various USA nature cure colleges and brought to Australia by FG Roberts and Blackmore.

Notes

1 Walter (Wal) Hayward interview (excerpt) by Robert Ryder, Geelong, October n.d., 2003, extract of transcript in Shirley Strachan, *Healing Hands, Unsung Voices, Thomas Ambrose Bowen Osteopath (1916–1982)* (United Kingdom: Cloister House Press, 2016), 265.
2 Paul and Sandy Forman, interview by author, June 18, 2018.
3 Brian Anderson, interview by author, transcript in Shirley Strachan, *Healing Hands*, 101.
4 PROV, VPRS 3253/P1/, Unit 47, Bowen transcript, 673.

5 John Reid personal communication to author November 20. 2015; Keith Cowland email to author in Strachan, *Healing Hands*, 193.
6 Stanley William Horwood Registration Birth, 26008/1904, Registration Death 24499/1957 Births Deaths and Marriages Victoria; Horwood's position at the Portland Cement plant was recorded on his employment card when accessible at the former cement works museum, the collection is now lodged with the Geelong Heritage Records Centre and not yet catalogued.
7 Stanley William Horwood and Emily Rene Hansen (nee Wood) Registration Marriage 19552/1956, Births Deaths and Marriages Victoria.
8 PROV, Report and evidence Osteopathy Committee, Pt.1–4 27/11/975 (Pt. 2) 2261, VPRS 3253/P1, Unit 47 Original papers tabled in the legislative assembly, transcripts of proceedings, Bowen transcript: 672–78, 672.
9 Barry Tattersall interview by author January 9, 2015, transcript in Strachan, *Healing Hands*, 8.
10 Tattersall interview by author, 6.
11 PROV, Report and evidence Osteopathy Committee, Bowen transcript: 672–78, 672.
12 "Advertising," *Daily Mercury (Mackay)*, November 14, 1935: 13.
13 PROV, Report and evidence Osteopathy Committee, Pt.1–4 27/11/975 (Pt. 2) 2261, VPRS 3253/P1/, Unit 47, Original papers tabled in the Legislative Assembly, transcripts of proceedings, Jacka transcript: 16.
14 PROV, Report and evidence Osteopathy Committee, Jacka transcript: 16.; No colleges have been found to be listed at Wetherley Gardens.
15 PROV, Report and evidence Osteopathy Committee, Jacka transcript: 16.
16 Refer to website https://bcnogroup.ac.uk/ which shows the logos of both organizations together.
17 Agnes Shaw interview by Ron Phelan, 2003, transcribed by Phelan in Strachan, *Healing Hands*, 6.
18 "Defining Moments, Great Depression," National Museum of Australia, accessed November 19, 2024, http://www.nma.gov.au/defining-moments/resources/great-depression.
19 Agnes Shaw interview by Ron Phelan, 2003, transcribed by Phelan in Strachan, *Healing Hands*, 6.
20 Agnes Shaw interview by Ron Phelan, 2003, transcribed by Phelan in Strachan, *Healing Hands*, 6.
21 "Commonwealth Reconstruction Training Scheme."
22 Ann Mortelliti, interview by author June 26, 2018.
23 Peter Scott interview by author, transcript in Strachan, *Healing Hands*, 208.
24 PROV, Osteopathy, Chiropractic and Naturopath Joint Select Committee pp. 783–938, VPRS 241/P/, Unit 14, Transcripts of Committee, South Pacific Federation of Natural Therapeutics represented by Janssen, Lucy and Goulson, transcript: 890–914, 897.
25 "Advertising," *Daily Mercury (Mackay)*, November 14, 1935: 13.
26 Rene Horwood interview by Ron Phelan, September 11, 1998, transcript extract by Phelan in Strachan, *Healing Hands*, 32.
27 NAA MT1486/1, William Arthur Bowen.
28 "In the Ranks of the Reservists," *The Musician*, Salvation Army, July 1948, 165.
29 Murray, *In Search*, 101.
30 Archivist Lindsay Cox Salvation Army Heritage Centre personal communication, July 30, 2018.
31 John Garner, interview by author June 22, 2015, transcript in Strachan, *Healing Hands*, 37.
32 Therese Vahland, interview by author, transcript in Strachan, *Healing Hands*, 80.

33 Therese Vahland, interview by author, transcript in Strachan, *Healing Hands*, 83.
34 *Natures Path to Health*, November–December 1937, editorial; Edwin Devereaux, Brian O'Reilly, and John Cice, *History of the Sydney College of Chiropractic* (Sydney: Macquarie Lighthouse Press, 2012), 25.
35 Steven A. Campbell, "The Rise and Legitimation of Chiropractic, A Study of Professionalisation" (Masters with Honours thesis, University of New England, 1985), 200.
36 PROV, Chiropractic Treatment – Letters and Reports Pt 1, VPRS 6345/P/, Unit 155, General Correspondence Files, Letter Jacka to Mack Minister for Health, August 25, 1961.
37 PROV, Chiropractic Treatment – Letters and Reports Pt 1, VPRS 6345/P/, Unit 155, General Correspondence Files, Letter Minister for Health to Jacka, August 29, 1961.
38 Rene Horwood interview by Ron Phelan, October 8, 1998, transcribed by author, September 30, 2018.
39 "Vic. Riddled with Scoundrelly Quacks," *Advertiser (Adelaide),* June 15, 1954: 3, accessed February 14, 2018, http://nla.gov.au/nla.news-article48110658; Devereaux et al., *History of the Sydney College of Chiropractic,* 25 (quoting *Sun* (Melbourne), March 25, 1964).
40 Campbell, "The Rise," 197.
41 "Practitioner Fined," *Weekly Times,* January 5, 1929: 12.
42 "Practitioner Fined."
43 William Shurtleff and Akiko Ayoyagi, *Soyinfo Center, History of Soybeans and Soyfoods in Australia, New Zealand and Oceania 1770–2010, Extensively Annotated Bibliography and Sourcebook* (Lafayette, CA: SoyInfo Center, 2010), 373.
44 Campbell, "The Rise," 201.
45 *Natures Path to Health*, November 1939, 25.
46 *Natures Path to Health*, January/February 1937, 25.
47 The lease was advertised in February. "Advertising," "Factories &c to Let," *Argus,* February 11, 1937: 2 (col.7); A smart girl was wanted for the health food store was sought in October. "Advertising," "Wanted Smart Girl," *Argus,* October 25, 1937: 20 (col.2), Roberts' dietician services were offered in November, "Advertising," "Medical- Roberts Health Academy," *Herald,* November 30, 1937: 23 (col.4).
48 "Social," *Maryborough Chronicle, Wide Bay and Burnett Advertiser*, October 1, 1935: 8; *Natures Path to Health*, October 1939, 36 and January–February 1941: 18.
49 "Social," *Maryborough Chronicle, Wide Bay and Burnett Advertiser*, October 1, 1935: 8; *Natures Path to Health* October 1939, 36 and January–February 1941: 18, various editions January/February 1937–February/March 1949, Alfred Deakin Prime Ministerial Library, Deakin University, Geelong.
50 *Natures Path to Health*, December 1939, 4.
51 Benedict Lust, ed., *Universal Naturopathic Encyclopaedia and Buyers Guide 1918–1919* (Butler, NJ: Benedict Lust MD, ND, 1918), 84 and 1149.
52 *Natures Path to Health,* November–December, 1937: 27.
53 "Advertising," "Meetings and Lectures – Natural Health Society," *Age*, November 13, 1928: 16 (col. 5)
54 "Advertising" "Meetings and Lectures – Natural Health Society," 16 (col. 5).
55 *Natures Path to Health*, May–June 1937: 20–21.
56 PROV, Osteopathy, Chiropractic and Naturopathy Committee, VPRS 16439/P1/, Unit 13, Committee Records, Cogan transcript: 428–35, 431–32.
57 PROV, VPRS 16439/P1, Unit 13, Cogan transcript, 429–30.
58 The free of charge textbook was the hot-off-the-press first edition of Janse, Hauser and Wells, *Chiropractic Principles and Technic* (Wheaton Illinois, 1939)

an indication of how closely in touch Roberts was with developments overseas. Though the text and anatomical terminology would have been difficult for a lay person to follow, it is illustrated with numerous diagrams and clear photographs of procedures.

59 "Wages in Victoria, Average Yearly Wages Factory Workers," *State Library of Victoria*, accessed August 12, 2024, http://guides.slv.vic.gov.au/whatitcost/earnings.

60 Devereaux et al., *History of the Sydney College of Chiropractic*, 9.

61 PROV, Osteopathy, Chiropractic and Naturopathy Committee, 16439/P1 Committee Records, Unit 13, Goldby transcript: 447–54, 447–48.

62 Devereaux et al., *History of the Sydney College of Chiropractic*, 51.

63 Devereaux et al., *History of the Sydney College of Chiropractic*, 51; W. Pruss, "Natural Therapies from the 1890s to the 1950s," *Journal of the Australian Natural Therapists Association* 21, no. 1 (2006): 31–33.

64 "Advertising," *Daily Standard (Brisbane)*, September 19, 1927, 3.

65 "Advertising," "When Others Fail See Claude Beales," *Queensland Times (Ipswich)*, May 28, 1929: 3.

66 "Visit of Mr. F.G. Roberts," *Morning Bulletin (Rockhampton)*, July 26, 1930: 8.

67 "Whacko! Wheeler the Healer!" *Truth (Sydney)*, March 16, 1947: 29; "Exchange and Mart," *World's News*, March 17, 1951: 29.

68 "Visit of Mr. F.G. Roberts."

69 Fraser's own book and correspondence to the Minister for Health confirm his connection to Blackmores school: Andrew Fraser, *Osteopathic Natural Treatments* (Drysdale: Dr A Fraser, 1994), 121–69; PROV, Chiropractic Treatments – Letters and Reports, Pt.1, VPRS 6345/P/, Unit 155, Andrew Fraser letter to Sir (Minister for Health), November 22, 1972.

70 Michael Quinlivan personal communication.

71 Devereaux et al., *History of the Sydney College of Chiropractic*, 21.

72 Steven A. Campbell, "The Rise and Legitimation of Chiropractic, A Study of Professionalisation" (Masters with Honours thesis, University of New England, 1985), 201–2.

73 PROV, Report and evidence Osteopathy Committee, Pt.1–4 27/11/975 (Pt. 2) 2261, VPRS 3253/P1/, Unit 47, Original papers tabled in the Legislative Assembly, Transcripts of Proceedings, Doyle transcript: 463–68, 463.

74 Cameron, "An International Study of Osteopathic Practice" (Master's thesis, Victoria University of Technology, Melbourne, 1999), 38.

75 PROV, VPRS 3253/P1/, Unit 47, Doyle transcript, 463.

76 Herbalist in Caulfield West, 29 Glenhuntly Road, 1937 *Australia, Electoral Rolls, 1903–1980.*

77 "Xmas Wedding Was Far from Merry," *Mirror*, December 30, 1944: 15.

78 Campbell, "The Rise," 202.

79 Campbell, "The Rise"; Devereaux et al., *History of the Sydney College of Chiropractic*, 22. Devereaux et al. utilise excerpts from the Pax Submission to the WA Commission of Inquiry into chiropractic in 1959 and describe Doyle's Pax course as 4.5 years full-time, fees as £525 plus textbooks and other miscellaneous overheads.

80 Devereaux et al., *History of the Sydney College of Chiropractic*, 40.

81 Devereaux et al., *History of the Sydney College of Chiropractic*, 32.

82 Devereaux et al., *History of the Sydney College of Chiropractic*, 5.

83 John Garner personal communication to author and Romney Smeeton, June 24, 2016.

84 "Routine Orders," Australian War Memorial, AWM 52 8/3/61; "Training Camp," *Camperdown Chronicle (VIC)*, November 19, 1940: 3.

85 "Militia Training," *Riverine Herald*, August 30, 1940: 1; "Y.M.C.A. Work for Soldiers," *Wodonga and Towong Sentinel*, January 5, 1940: 2.

86 "Soldiers' Sports McAlister wins at Mt Martha," *Argus (Melbourne)*, November 21, 1940: 14; Heather Hay personal communication to the author February 9, 2019.
87 Alistair Graham McAlister, Registration Birth 23714/1915, Births Deaths and Marriages Victoria.
88 Australia Electoral Roles, 1903–1980 available on *Ancestry.com.*
89 PROV, VPRS 3253/P1/, Unit 50, McAlister transcript: 3425
90 PROV, VPRS 3253/P1/, Unit 50, McAlister transcript: 3425, 3426.
91 PROV, VPRS 3253/P1/, Unit 50, McAlister transcript: 3427.
92 Heather Hay personal communication to author July 29, 2018 and February 9, 2019.
93 Andrew Fraser, *Osteopathic Treatments* (Geelong: Deakin University Press, 1994), frontispiece.
94 Leon Chaitow, ed., *Naturopathic Physical Medicine* (Edinburgh: Churchill Livingstone, 2008), 70.
95 Chaitow, *Naturopathic Physical Medicine.*
96 Chaitow, *Naturopathic Physical Medicine*, 70.
97 Chaitow, *Naturopathic Physical Medicine*, 71.
98 Chaitow, *Naturopathic Physical Medicine*, 71.
99 Martin Collins, *The British School of Osteopathy, the First Hundred Years* (United Kingdom: XLibrispublishing.co.uk, 2016), 29–30; John O'Brien, "The First Steps on the Road to State Regulation of British Osteopaths," in John O'Brien, *Bonesetters: A History of British Osteopathy* (Tunbridge Wells, Kent: Anshan Ltd, 2013), 35–46.
100 Emmons Rutledge Booth, *History of Osteopathy and Twentieth Century Medical Practice* (Cincinnati, USA: Caxton Press, 1924), 261, 273.
101 *Osteopathy, Massage and Manual Therapeutics,* Psychic Research Company (London: Temple Chambers, 1900).
102 Hans Baer, "The Drive for Professionalisation in British Osteopathy," *Social Science and Medicine* 19, no. 7 (1984): 718.
103 Tom Dummer, "The History and Development of Osteopathy in the UK," in Dummer, *Textbook of Osteopathy* (Berrington Press, UK, JoTom Publications, 1999), 45–47.
104 Parnell Bradbury, *Healing by Hand* (London: The Harvill Press, 1957), xiv.
105 Baer, "The Drive for Professionalisation"; Bradbury, *Healing by Hand.*
106 Ward Inquiry Report, 5.
107 *Natures Path to Health,* Christmas, 1937: 15; Devereaux et al., *History of the Sydney College of Chiropractic*, 38.
108 Jane Adams, "Developing Naturopathy in Interwar Britain," in *Routledge Handbook of Complementary Medicine*, eds. Nicola K. Gale and Jean V. McHale (Abingdon, Oxon: Routledge, 2019), 68.
109 Hayward interview by Robert Ryder, in Strachan, *Healing Hands*, 265.
110 "History of the British College of Osteopathic Medicine," *BCOM Website*, accessed November 17, 2024, https://www.bcom.ac.uk/about-bcom/history-of-bcom/.
111 Leon Chaitow with Judith DeLany, *Modern Neuromuscular Techniques* (New York: Churchill Livingstone, 1996), 19–21.
112 "Osteopath's use of Physician as Title," *Eastbourne Herald*, September 27, 1950: 3.
113 "British College of Osteopathic Medicine," *Telegraph*, July 28, 2016. (Note, Wyndham Place is in Marylebone, City of Westminster, London).
114 Chaitow and DeLany, *Modern Neuromuscular Techniques*, 19–21.
115 "Local News, Burnley Valley," *Todmorden* and *District News*, November 25, 1927: 5.

116 Joseph E. Pizzorno, Michael T. Murray, and George W. Cody, "History of Natural Medicine," in *A Textbook of Natural Medicine,* by Joseph E. Pizzorno and Michael T. Murray (Seattle, WA: John Bastyr College Publications, 1985), I: HistNM-17.
117 *An Act to provide for the Registration of a Certain Person as a Masseur under the Masseurs Acts*, No 6078, June 4, 1957.
118 PROV, Masseurs Registration Bill – G. E Saunders VPRS6345/P/, Unit 64, General Correspondence Files 1094/4, Letter from the Victorian Massage and Physiotherapy Association to the Hon. H. Bolte, Premier April 14, 1957 and letter Massage Registration Board – Victoria to the Hon. E. P Cameron, Minister for Health, April 19, 1957.
119 PROV, Masseurs Registration Bill VPRS6345/P/Unit 64, Pamphlet, Training in Massage, Masseurs' Registration Board.
120 PROV, VPRS 3253/P1/, Unit 47, Bowen transcript 676.
121 Rene Horwood interview by Ron Phelan, September 11, 1998, transcribed by Phelan in Strachan, *Healing Hands,* 27.
122 Michael Quinlivan personal communication to author, June 9 and 22, 2017.
123 PROV. Report and evidence Osteopathy Committee (Pt.1–4), 27/11/975 (Pt. 2) 2261, VPRS 3253/P1/, Unit 50, Original papers tabled in the Legislative Assembly, transcripts of proceedings, McAlister transcript: 3425.
124 Andrew Fraser, *Osteopathic Natural Treatments* (Geelong: Dr A. Fraser, Deakin University, 1994), 'About the Author'.
125 Fraser, *Osteopathic Natural Treatments.*
126 Paul Schmidt personal communication to author, n.d., 2015.
127 PROV, Report and evidence Osteopathy Committee, Pt.1–4 27/11/975 (Pt. 2) 2261 VPRS 3253/P1/, Unit 50 Original papers tabled in the legislative assembly, transcripts of proceedings, McAlister, 3424–60: 3428; McAlister states, 'National Association of Osteopaths, Chiropractors and Naturopaths'. NANOC is assumed as McAlister provided clinic placements for NANOC trainees.
128 Professor John Murtagh personal communication to author, October 13, 2015.
129 John Murtagh, "Musculoskeletal Medicine in Australia: A 50 Year Journey and Perspective," Australasian Musculoskeletal Medicine 18, no. 1 (2013): 8–9.
130 VIC, Parliamentary Debates, Legislative Council, Vol. 362, December 9, 1981, 4493–506: 4497.
131 PROV, Chiropractors and Osteopaths Board, VPRS 6345/P/, Unit 556, General Correspondence, letter Alan Wilkie of VSSO to Minister Houghton, April 5, 1978.
132 Kevin Ryan personal communication to author, February 13, 2019.
133 Gordon and Smart, *Tom Bowen Personal Reflections*, 7 and 14; "What Goes on? Ernie's Hands Put Athletes Back on Map," *Argus* February 21, 1951.
134 Kevin Neave letter to Ron Phelan, May 9, 2002.
135 *Collins English Dictionary* (Sydney, Auckland, Glasgow: Collins, 1979), 345.
136 Ron Phelan, "Tom Bowen – the Technique Where Did It Come from?" *Bowen News Australia*, December, 2009: 29.
137 Ward Inquiry Report, 7.
138 *Notable Citizens of Sydney* (Sydney: Notable publications of Australia, 1940), 240–41.
139 Shurtleff and Ayoyagi, *Soyinfo Center, History of Soybeans,* numerous references throughout.
140 Campbell, "The Rise," 201–2 and "B4. Persons Interviewed," 362–63.
141 Jan Breen, "Red Tape Ties Healing Man's Hands," *Geelong Advertiser*, March 31, 1982.

Bibliography

Newspapers

"Advertising." *Daily Standard (Brisbane),* September 19, 1927: 3 (col.5, bottom). Accessed November 17, 2024. http://nla.gov.au/nla.news-article184914232.
"Advertising." *Daily Mercury (Mackay),* November 14, 1935: 13 (col.1). Accessed November 17, 2024. http://nla.gov.au/nla.news-article173339866.
"Advertising." "Medical – Roberts Health Academy." *Herald,* November 30, 1937: 23 (col.4),AccessedNovember17,2024.http://nla.gov.au/nla.news-article244543063.
"Advertising." "Meetings and Lectures." *Age (Melbourne)*, November 13, 1928: 16 (col.5, middle). Accessed November 17, 2024. http://nla.gov.au/nla.news-article204254489.
"Advertising." "Meetings and Lectures." *Age (Melbourne)*, June 14, 1930: 16 (col.1). Accessed November 17, 2024. http://nla.gov.au/nla.news-article203083733.
"Advertising." "Meetings and Lectures-Natural Health society." *Age* November 13, 1928: 16 (col.5). Accessed November 17, 2024, http://nla.gov.au/nla.news-article204254489.
"Advertising." "Shops, Factories &c, To Let." *Argus*, February 11, 1937: 2 (col.7). Accessed November 17, 2024. http://nla.gov.au/nla.news-article11967941.
"Advertising." "When Others Fail, See Claude Beales." *Queensland Times (Ipswich),* May 28, 1929: 3. Accessed November 17, 2024. (col.2). http://trove.nla.gov.au/newspaper/article/118481600#
Breen, Jan. "Red Tape Ties Healing Man's Hands." *Geelong Advertiser*, March 31, 1982: 22.
"Exchange and Mart." "All Skin Diseases Treated." *World's News*, March 17, 1951: 29 (col.2). Accessed November 17, 2024. http://nla.gov.au/nla.news-article139910275.
"Local News, Burnley Valley." *Todmorden* and *District News*, November 25, 1927: 5.
"Militia Training." *Riverine Herald*, August 30, 1940: 1. Accessed November 17, 2024. http://nla.gov.au/nla.news-article116295985.
"Practitioner Fined." *Weekly Times*, January 5, 1929: 12. Accessed November 17, 2024. http://nla.gov.au/nla.news-article223821867.
"Social." *Maryborough Chronicle, Wide Bay and Burnett Advertiser,* October 1, 1935: 8. Accessed November 17, 2024. http://nla.gov.au/nla.news-article149950624.
"Soldiers' Sports McAlister Wins at Mt. Martha." *Argus (Melbourne),* November 21, 1940: 14. Accessed November 17, 2024. http://nla.gov.au/nla.news-article11319833.
"Training Camp." *Camperdown Chronicle (VIC)*, November 19, 1940: 3. Accessed November 17, 2024. http://nla.gov.au/nla.news-article26544437.
"Vic. Riddled with Scoundrelly Quacks." *Advertiser Adelaide,* June 15, 1954: 3. Accessed November 17, 2024. http://nla.gov.au/nla.news-article48110658.
"Visit of Mr. F.G. Roberts." *Morning Bulletin Rockhampton*, July 26, 1930: 8. Accessed November 17, 2024. http://nla.gov.au/nla.news-article55375684.
"Wanted Smart Girl." *Argus*, October 25, 1937: 20 (col.2). Accessed November 17, 2024. http://nla.gov.au/nla.news-article11103119.
"Whacko! Wheeler the Healer!" *Truth Sydney, NSW: 1894 – 1954*, March 16, 1947: 29. Accessed November 17, 2024. http://nla.gov.au/nla.news-article169366106.
"What Goes on? Ernie's Hands Put Athletes Back on Map." *Argus*, February 21, 1951: 6. Accessed November 17, 2024. http://nla.gov.au/nla.news-article23035440.
"Xmas Wedding Was Far from Merry." *Mirror*, December 30, 1944: 15. Accessed November 17, 2024. http://nla.gov.au/nla.news-article76007921.
"Y.M.C.A. Work for Soldiers." *Wodonga and Towong Sentinel*, January 5, 1940: 2. Accessed November 17, 2024. http://nla.gov.au/nla.news-article69639462.

Primary Sources

An Act to Provide for the Registration of a certain Person as a Masseur under the Masseurs Acts, No 6078, June 4, 1957. Accessed November 17, 2024. www.austlii.edu.au/au/legis/vic/hist_act/ma1957271.pdf.

Ancestry.com [database on-line]. Provo, UT, USA: Ancestry.com Operations, Inc. *Australia Electoral Rolls 1903–1980.*

Cameron, Melanie. "An International Study of Osteopathic Practice." Masters thesis, Victoria University of Technology, Melbourne, 1999, 38. Accessed November 17, 2024. http://vuir.vu.edu.au/17921/1/CAMERON_1999compressed.pdf.

Campbell, Stephen A. "The Rise and Legitimation of Chiropractic. A Study of Professionalisation." Masters with Honours thesis, University of New England, 1985. Accessed November 17, 2024. https://hdl.handle.net/1959.11/12799.

Forman, Paul and Sandy. Interview by the author, June 18, 2018.

Garner, John. Interview by author June 22, 2015, Transcript in Strachan, Shirley. *Healing Hands, Unsung Voices, Thomas Ambrose Bowen 1916–1982 Osteopath.* London: Cloister House Press, 2016.

Hayward, Walter (Wal). Interview by Robert Ryder October n.d., 2003. Transcribed by author, *Healing Hands, Unsung Voices, Thomas Ambrose Bowen 1916–1982 Osteopath.* United Kingdom: Cloister House Press, 2016.

Horwood, Rene. Interview by Ron Phelan. Transcript extract in *Healing Hands, Unsung Voices, Thomas Ambrose Bowen 1916–1982 Osteopath.* United Kingdom: Cloister House Press, 2016.

Horwood, Rene. Interview by Ron Phelan, October 8, 1998, transcribed by author November 15–30, 2018.

Horwood, Stanley William. Registration Birth. 26008/1904. Births Deaths and Marriages Victoria.

Horwood, Stanley William. Registration Death. 2499/1957. Births Deaths and Marriages Victoria.

Horwood, Stanley William and Emily Irene Hansen (nee Wood). Registration Marriage 19552/1956. Births Deaths and Marriages Victoria.

Lust, Benedict, ed. *Universal Naturopathic Encyclopaedia and Buyers Guide 1918–1919.* Butler, NJ: Benedict Lust MD, ND, 1918, 84 and 1149. Accessed November 17, 2024. http://archive.org/details/universalnaturop00lust.

McAlister, Alistair Graham. Registration Birth, 23714/1915, Births Deaths and Marriages Victoria.

Mortelliti, Ann. Interview by Strachan June 26, 2018.

NAA MT1486/1. Bowen, William Arthur.

Natures Path to Health, various editions January/February 1937, November–December 1937, Christmas, 1937. September 1, 1938, October 1939, December 1939, January–February 1941 and February/March 1949, November–December 1937, November 1939 Collection held at Alfred Deakin Library, Waterfront Campus, Geelong, location ADPML SPC 613.05 Fgr/Npt.

Notable Citizens of Sydney (Sydney: Notable Publications of Australia, 1940).

Osteopathy, Massage and Manual Therapeutics. Psychic Research Company, Temple Chambers, London 1900. Accessed November 17, 2024. https://archive.org/details/homestudycoursei00lond.

PROV. Masseurs Registration Bill – G. E. Saunders VPRS6345/P/, Unit 64, General Correspondence Files 1094/4, Letter from the Victorian Massage and Physiotherapy Association to the Hon. H. Bolte, Premier April 14, 1957 and letter Massage Registration Board – Victoria to the Hon. E. P Cameron, Minister for Health, April 19, 1957.

PROV. Chiropractic Treatment – Letters and Reports, Pt 1. VPRS 6345/P/, Unit 155. General Correspondence Files, Letter Jacka to Mack Minister for Health, August 25, 1961.

PROV. Chiropractic and Osteopaths Registration Board, VPRS 6345/P/, Unit 556. General Correspondence, Alan Wilkie President of VSSO to Minister Houghton, April 5, 1978.
PROV. Osteopathy, Chiropractic and Naturopathy Committee, VPRS 16439/P1 Committee Records, Goldby transcript: 447–54.
PROV. Osteopathy, Chiropractic and Naturopathy Committee, VPRS 16439/P1, Unit 13, Committee Records, Cogan transcript: 428–35.
PROV. Osteopathy, Chiropractic and Naturopath Joint Select Committee pp. 783–938, VPRS 241/P/, Unit 14, Transcripts of Committee, South Pacific Federation of Natural Therapeutics represented by Janssen, Lucy and Goulson, transcript: 890–914.
PROV. Report and evidence Osteopathy Committee (Pt.1–4), 27/11/975 (Pt. 2) 2261, VPRS 3253/P1/, Unit 47. Original papers tabled in the Legislative Assembly, transcripts of proceedings, Bowen transcript: 672–78.
PROV. Report and evidence Osteopathy Committee (Pt.1–4), 27/11/975 (Pt. 2) 2261, VPRS 3253/P1/, Unit 47. Original papers tabled in the Legislative Assembly, transcripts of proceedings, Doyle transcript: 463–68.
PROV. Report and evidence Osteopathy Committee (Pt.1–4), 27/11/975 (Pt. 2) 2261, VPRS 3253/P1 Unit 47. Report and evidence Osteopathy Committee, Original papers tabled in the Legislative Assembly, transcripts of proceedings, Jacka transcript: 15–29.
PROV. Report and evidence Osteopathy Committee (Pt.1–4), 27/11/975 (Pt. 2) 2261, VPRS 3253/P1/, Unit 50, Original papers tabled in the Legislative Assembly, transcripts of proceedings, McAlister transcript: 3424–60.
PROV Chiropractic Treatments – Letters and Reports, Pt.1, VPRS 6345/P/, Unit 155, Andrew Fraser letter to Sir (Minister for Health), November 22, 1972.
"Routine Orders." AWM 52 8/3/61. Accessed November 17, 2024. https://www.awm.gov.au/collection/C1360730.
Scott, Peter. Interview by author, November 13, 2015. Transcript in Strachan, Shirley. *Healing Hands, Unsung Voices, Thomas Ambrose Bowen Osteopath, 1916–1982.* United Kingdom: Cloister House Press, 2016.
Shaw, Agnes. Interview by Ron Phelan, n.d., 2003. Transcript by Phelan in Strachan, Shirley. *Healing Hands, Unsung Voices, Thomas Ambrose Bowen Osteopath. 1916–1982, Osteopath.* United Kingdom: Cloister House Press, 2016.
Tattersall, Barry. Interview by author, January 9, 2015. Transcript in Strachan, Shirley. *Healing Hands, Unsung Voices, Thomas Ambrose Bowen Osteopath (1916–1982).* United Kingdom: Cloister House Press, 2016.
Vahland, Therese. Interview by author July 1, 2015, transcribed in Strachan, Shirley, *Healing Hands, Unsung Voices, Thomas Ambrose Bowen Osteopath (1916–1982).* Great Britain: Cloister House Press, 2016.
VIC Parliamentary Debates. Legislative Council. Vol. 362. December 9, 1981. Accessed September 27, 2018.
"Wages in Victoria, Average Yearly Wages Factory Workers." State Library of Victoria. Accessed November 17, 2024. https://guides.slv.vic.gov.au/whatitcost/earnings.
Ward Inquiry Report – full title – Victoria Parliament, Osteopathy, Chiropractic and Naturopathy Committee, et al. *Report from the Osteopathy, Chiropractic and Naturopathy Committee: Together with Appendices.* Melbourne: C. H. Rixon, Government Printer, 1975. Accessed November 17, 2024. http://www6.austlii.edu.au/au/other/vic/VicLASelCPubInq/1975/1.pdf.

Secondary Sources

Baer, Hans A. "The Drive for Professionalisation in British Osteopathy." *Social Science and Medicine* 19, no. 7 (1984): 717–25. Accessed November 18, 2024. http://doi.org/10.1016/0277-9536(84)90244-2.

Booth, Emmons Rutledge. *History of Osteopathy and Twentieth Century Medical Practice*. Cincinnati, USA: Jennings and Graham, 1905. Accessed November 17, 2024. https://archive.org/details/historyofosteopa00bootuoft.

Bradbury, Parnell. *Healing by Hand*. London: The Harvill Press, 1957.

Chaitow, Leon, ed. *Naturopathic Physical Medicine*. Edinburgh: Churchill Livingstone, 2008.

Chaitow, Leon with Judith Delaney. *Modern Neuromuscular Techniques*. New York: Churchill Livingstone, 1996.

Collins, Martin. *The British School of Osteopathy, the First Hundred Years*. United Kingdom: Xlibris Publishing 2016.

Devereaux, Edwin, Brian O'Reilly, and John Cice. *History of the Sydney College of Chiropractic*. Sydney: Macquarie Lighthouse Press, 2012.

Dummer, Tom. "History and Development of Osteopathy in the UK." In *Textbook of Osteopathy*. Berrington Press, UK, JoTom Publications, 1999.

Fraser, Andrew. *Osteopathic Natural Treatments*. Geelong: Deakin University Press, 1994.

Gordon, Libby, and Brian Smart. *Tom Bowen Personal Reflections*. Australia: BTAV and BTSA, 1999.

Janse, Joseph, R. H. Houser, and B. F. Wells. "Reflex and Pressure Technics." In *Chiropractic Technic*, chapter IV, 494–511. 1978. Reprint. Chicago, IL: National College of Chiropractic.

Murray, Col. *In Search of Tom Bowen and the Therapy he Inspired and Lots of Other Stuff*. Armadale: Palmer Higgs, Booksonline, 2010.

Murtagh, John. "Musculoskeletal Medicine in Australia, a 50 Year Journey and Perspective." *Australasian Musculoskeletal Medicine* 18, no. 1 (2013): 8–9. Accessed November 17, 2024. https://search.informit.org/doi/10.3316/informit.354643897972196.

O'Brien, John. *Bonesetters: A History of British Osteopathy*. Tunbridge Wells, Kent: Anshan Ltd, 2013.

Phelan, Ron. "Tom Bowen – the Technique Where Did It Come from?" *Bowen News Australia*, December 2009: 29.

Pizzorno, Joseph E., Michael T. Murray, and George W. Cody. "History of Natural Medicine." In *A Textbook of Natural Medicine* compiled by Joseph E. Pizzorno and Michael T. Murray, I: HistNM-17. Seattle, WA: John Bastyr College Publications, 1989.

Pruss, W. "Natural Therapies from the 1890s to the 1950s." *Journal of the Australian Natural Therapists Association* 21, no. 1 (2006): 31–33.

Salvation Army National Headquarters Melbourne. "In the Ranks of the Reservists." *The Musician*, July 1948, 165.

Shurtleff, William, and Akiko Aoyagi. *Soyinfo Center, History of Soybeans and Soyfoods in Australia, New Zealand and Oceania 1770–2010, Extensively Annotated Bibliography and Sourcebook*. Lafayette, CA: SoyInfo Center, 2010. Accessed November 17, 2024. www.soyinfocenter.com/pdf/138/Ocea2.pdf.

Websites

"Commonwealth Reconstruction Scheme." *Australian War Memorial*. Accessed November 17, 2024. https://www.awm.gov.au/collection/LIB23061.

"History of the British College of Osteopathic Medicine." *The British College of Osteopathic Medicine*. Accessed November 17, 2024. https://www.bcom.ac.uk/about-bcom/history-of-bcom/.

National Museum of Australia. "Defining Moments, Great Depression." Accessed November 19, 2024. http://www.nma.gov.au/defining-moments/resources/great-depression.

3 Neuropathy Practice and Pressure Movements Within Early Australian Osteopathy

> It is not necessary to have bony pressure such as is the principle of chiropractic and osteopathy. Contracted muscle can cause the pressure or prolapsed viscera pressing on nerves and nerve plexuses.
>
> FW Collins, *The Dullmage System*[1]

Introduction: FG Roberts – a Cosmopolitan Naturopath

Chapter 2 identified chronological consistencies between Bowen's attempts at study at an English institution (Stanley Lief's British College of Naturopathy concluded from related evidence) along with relevant opportunities available with practitioners connected to the networks of early naturopathic pioneers, namely FG Roberts and Maurice Blackmore, with Roberts more accessible in Victoria. After his pre–First World War training at the London School of Natural Therapeutics (LSNT), Roberts undertook correspondence studies via USA's establishments. Roberts forged strong connections with nature cure leaders, including USA's father of naturopathy, Benedict Lust MD, ND, DO and with prominent leaders in the UK, including Milton Powell of the LSNT and Stanley Lief. As a naturopath, Roberts adhered to this view of naturopathy as a catch-all concept. The vision of Dr Still MD, DO for osteopathy had also vied for recognition as the complete system of medicine but that faded two years before his death in 1917. After the Flexner Report of 1910, a medicalised drug-based and surgically oriented pathway was evident for osteopathy in the USA.[2] Still expressed his concern to Dr Benedict Lust, that osteopathy 'was doomed as the school that could have incorporated all the natural and biological healing arts'.[3]

Naturopathy, the Umbrella for all Healing Arts

Historically until late in the twentieth century, a Doctor of Naturopathy was an umbrella credential that encompassed all other modalities; this was reflected in a document published by ACONPAL, an organisation Bowen joined in the early 1970s, which highlights that in 1931, the US Congress accepted a legal definition of naturopathy as encompassing a range of manual

DOI: 10.4324/9781003602125-4

therapeutics, dietetics, minerals and herbs.[4] An advertisement of 1909 for training at Dr Lust's Naturopathic College in Florida and Yungborn, with home study available, gives an excellent idea of common study subjects of the period that shows a Doctor of Naturopathy qualification embraced all other modalities.[5] The training resulted in several embedded credentials, in addition to neuropath, it included osteopath, chiropractor, hydropath, dietician, electropath, mechanotherapist, zone therapist, mental scientist, and skills in massage, Swedish movements, phytotherapy, phototherapy, heliotherapy and the systems of Kniepp, Lehmann, Khune and Bilz and Schroth.[6] Roberts, reflecting his ongoing training, including with Dr Lust MD, continued to embrace all the manual healing arts and was a catalyst in promoting osteopathy before his college succumbed to the political tide and chiropractic rose to dominate from 1959. Roberts had an accident in 1960 and became less involved in the running of his college and posthumously was adopted by COCA as the figurehead of chiropractic in Australia and remembered in the FG Roberts Memorial address.[7] Osteopathy became an afterthought.[8] This chapter will look at the terminology Bowen used, and others trained in osteopathy with Roberts and how this informs an understanding of origins of his approach.

Neuropathy

During Dr Still MD, DO's lifetime, a dedicated group of his followers advocated neuropathy as a preferable title for his novel system of manual medicine, because 'osteo' implied bone yet the essence of the work was on nerves, hence neuropathy. Nerves controlled blood and lymph flow and their optimal functioning was essential for healthy spinal nerve reflexes to the organs they controlled as well as unimpeded nerve transmission away from the spine towards the peripheral structures. The schools that developed this concept were the nature cure or naturopathic colleges and they are named later. A characteristic of neuropathy was the use of pressure using fingers and thumbs on nerve reflexes and pathways – to induce inhibition of nerve activity (and reduce pain) or a dilatory effect to encourage blood flow and nerve activity. Some schools included ideas about tissue acidity and other elements that are evident in Bowen's work. Neuropathy actions included cross-fibre pressure movements on muscle bellies and influencing tensions on ligaments.

Bowen's Terminology and Approach

Beginning first with Bowen's own terminology, the most useful clues are conveyed by the Ward Inquiry in 1973. Bowen said he worked with 'muscles and nerves', his method was 'through my fingers and nerve pressure' and he knew he was on nerves because 'I get the vibration from the nerve'. Pressure also encompassed the idea of pressure externally applied and from restrictions within the body itself on nerves. Bowen specifically mentions 'nerve pressure on the sacroiliac', 'one finds that the sciatic nerve jumps and you go for it'.

The Panel was intrigued to find out how Bowen actually found nerves since the sciatic nerve is a large nerve, and 'few nerves being big enough'. Bowen responded, 'you get the contraction from the muscle' which he agrees 'is an inference rather than something actually observed'.[9] In his clinic, Bowen simply explained issues to patients 'you have a pinched nerve'.[10] There were also internal structures that could be 'strangulated' such as the stomach, throat and testes. Bowen paid attention to tissue states of warmth, coldness, state of circulation and acidity. Some patients were advised to wear a vest to keep their backs and presumably their kidneys warm.[11] If a patient was acidic, he would recommend an alkalising strategy which suggests he had some introduction to naturopathic ideas.[12] These ideas are found in neuropathy too. Structurally and neurologically Bowen would explain his treatments as 'I have locked it in' or would request patients to return in a week to ensure 'a fix' had 'held'.[13] He paid attention to the pelvis as the primary platform that supports the body against gravity and would generally clear the pelvis first in treatment of someone without a spinal injury before he treated the upper body.[14]

In 1979, Neil Skilbeck DC, ND took up Bowens' invitation through ANTA to observe him at work. Skilbeck remembered Bowen spoke of waiting for tissues 'to fluid' or 'fluid to flow' when he rested his patients after a set of moves.[15] This was a reference to blood and lymph fluid in tissues as osteopaths and neuropaths alike were concerned with freeing venous and lymphatic circulation in tissues – constricted circulation caused contracted muscle which in turn was a form of pressure on nerves. For this reason, Andrew Still had said the 'rule of the artery' was supreme. The key objective was to restore nerve functioning to optimal. Nerves controlled blood and lymph flow. Adequate circulation was required to deliver nutrients to the body's cells and to remove wastes as build-up of wastes was the key factor in disease.[16] Lymphatic drainage is an observed effect of Bowen's work and this was achieved without massaging lymph towards the heart as in Swedish massage. Bowen would also have used 'fluiding' in relation to cerebrospinal fluid (CSF) and this is indicated later in the case of Greg Hutchins, the father of a spina bifida patient in 1978.[17] Bowen practised craniosacral osteopathy which meant he paid attention to the circulation of CSF in the brain and spinal cord. Bowen would also make a diagnosis from swelling: Skilbeck claimed that Bowen would look at swelling on the jaw and figured out a reflex relationship to the body part affected.[18] This evidence confirms Bowen was working with a knowledge of reflex patterns that led him to understand which nerves were irritated or experiencing pressure that enabled him to quickly size up a patient's complaint without being told.

Bowen applied pressure to points along the spine, on the edge or parts of muscle bellies, and ligaments using only his fingers and thumbs and executing a (mostly) rolling cross-fibre move applied with different pressures depending on the desired effect. Observers such as Smeeton confirmed that Bowen's pressures could range from quite light to deep and firm. Although light pressures were mainly used, depth of pressure was important as Bowen was quite specific about which structures he wanted to influence. Sometimes his interventions involved deeper work and directional precision was key overall. Since Bowen said he worked on both muscles and nerves, this makes sense. Bowen's treatments were minimalist and he was sequential in his approach to the body, but not regimented, as his treatments were highly individualised to the patient on the table. Treatments were always conducted in a warmed room under a sheet and Bowen had a dislike of air conditioning presumably because cold air causes the contraction of tissues. Once treatment was completed, some patients were advised to avoid hot showers and all were told to walk around every half hour or so. Those with asthma or migraine were given specific dietary advice, but Bowen was not generally prescribing ingestive remedies like a naturopath. From an experiential perspective, patients remembered him doing 'pressings' on their backs or 'digging fingers in' and many remembered osteopathic lever work as he would 'swing their leg out' when doing work on the pelvis or back.

Bowen's tactile giftedness lay in the ability to feel 'nerve vibration'. Pat Allen, a protégé of Bowen contemporary, Albert (Bert) Donald used the expression in a way that likely have matched Bowen's understanding; to mean how functional nerve activity feels, determined by the presence or absence of vibration, the latter indicating a blockage responsible for pain, 'We activate that nervous system that is not working. We link it up again and get it working'.[19] Doug Sells, a football masseur who worked with Bowen in the early period at Latrobe Terrace, demonstrated similar sensitivity and language.[20] Coupled with this, Bowen had an acute sensitivity to bioelectricity described in Chapter 8. One of the most astounding aspects of Bowen's sensitivity is that it was maintained through his own circulatory problems with chronic atherosclerosis and diabetes, both of which should have negatively impacted his sense of touch. Bowen's sensitivity to nerve vibration led him to assess clients with nervous system issues that affected nerve transmission from the brain into the spinal cord. With patients such as those with polio, spina bifida, cerebral palsy and any forms of paralysis, Bowen would enhance his perception of healthy or absent nerve conduction or 'vibration' by using copper pennies to scan the back and detect where the nerve flow was stopped 'there is where the break is in the spine'.[21] Bowen believed in the power of the body to heal itself.[22] This chapter will demonstrate that his ideas and practice are notably those of neuropathy and incorporate other ideas, mainly osteopathic.

FG Roberts: 'Australia's Leading Neuropath'

One of the interesting new discoveries from the research for this book about FG Roberts is that he promoted himself when first qualified and teaching as a neuropath. In 1931, Roberts first appeared on the electoral rolls after he opened his college in 1929 with this title.[23] A year later, Roberts advertised with the formal initials of ND and DO denoting naturopathic doctor and osteopathic doctor but did not mention neuropath.[24] However, the entry in the electoral rolls was not a typographical error. Roberts advertised again in 1939 in WA with the credentials of ND, DO but describes himself again as 'Australia's Leading Neuropath' and importantly he is lecturing on the subject making it accessible to the general community.[25] Again in Sydney in 1945, he presents as FG Roberts, ND, DO, 'Australia's leading Neuropath and Dietician'.[26] Roberts' advertising indicates he is lecturing on spinal diagnosis and how this links to lumbago (back pain) and health issues related to internal organs such as digestive system, heart and nervous disorders. Roberts trained his family too, and so it comes as no surprise that Fred Roberts (junior) lectured for BAIN in 1935 and describes adjusting vertebrae to remove pain and 'manipulative surgery' as '*by the pressing on the different nerve centres and by relieving congestion*, it was possible . . . to relieve the worst headache, give relief from indigestion' (emphasis added).[27] In the article, manipulative surgery refers to osteopathy and it emphasises the importance of the spine to health.[28] One piece of evidence about the possible work of Fred Roberts junior has survived. Another talented lay practitioner by the name of Ned Thompson was an inspiration to Arthur Wright DO/DC who taught the 'Thompson Technique of Connective Tissue Manipulation'. Wright surmised Thomson had learnt from Fred Roberts in Newcastle. Wright's remarks with respect to Thompson's style are similar to what Smeeton and Neave said about Bowen.[29] Thompson's technique was based on the ability to diagnose and treat aberrations of the fascia with relatively gentle thrusts.[30] Both Thompson and Bowen instilled the awareness not to use too much pressure and to be mindful of the level of intervention in the body's tissues. Wright said, 'It took me a whole year working with Ned before I realised I was going in too deep'. Like Bowen, Thompson was also adept at resetting twisted joints and as Wright said, 'knees were a snack to Ned'.[31] Like Bowen, Thompson did not name anatomical parts. According to Wright, everything was 'sinews' to Thompson.[32]

The influence of FG Roberts dates from 1929 in Victoria and elsewhere through to at least the late 1940s, after which time he wound down his Roberts Health Service on the eastern seaboard and focused on his Melbourne factory on soy products, his business in Melbourne. As described in Chapter 1, Roberts' college was evolving in a chiropractic direction around 1959 and BAIN became COCA before finally becoming the CCA in the late 1970s, synonymous with the International Institute of Chiropractic. As time went on, Roberts appears on the electoral rolls as a dietician and naturopath and this continued into the early 1970s when he first appears as a chiropractor. The shift to chiropractor reflects the background politics that forced Australian colleges to align with chiropractic to secure better chances of registration as moves towards regulation became a reality. Reflecting his naturopathic education that encompassed neuropathy, in 1951, Maurice Blackmore, a contemporary of FG Roberts, was also described as a neuropath in the press when he was fined for using the title of 'doctor'.[33] Later, when over a decade retired from his teaching, Blackmore presented to the Ward Inquiry in 1973 and said:

> Naturopaths use a certain amount of manipulation and there is a specific naturopathic type of manipulation aside from chiropractic manipulation. It tends to lean towards the naturopathic point of view. *It is actually on pressure points rather than on heavy manipulation* [emphasis added].[34]

Blackmore makes no mention of shiatsu to suggest he meant any reference to Eastern manual medicine. In fact, neither shiatsu nor acupressure seems to have come up in any discussions between the Ward Inquiry and participants. The list of references at appendix R to the Inquiry report reveals no effort went to sourcing any literature on these topics.[35] Acupuncture was discussed with some participants and the panel did source a copy of Worsley's *Everyman's Guide to Acupuncture*. Additionally, the ACONPAL publication makes no mention of shiatsu and acupressure, only acupuncture citing one article that presents acupuncture as acupuncture-neuropathy.[36]

Early Roberts Trained Practitioners and Neuropathic Language

Agnes Cogan of Ballarat was the earliest Roberts School graduate found so far in a reading of Ward Inquiry transcripts. Her first contact with Roberts was in 1933 as a patient and she eventually qualified after five years full-time as an ND and added DC in 1973. Cogan was working as a dietician by 1942, the identity she maintained on the electoral rolls.[37] Cogan too spoke of 'pinched nerves' and 'nerve pressure' and 'leveraging pressure off the problem', the problem being pressure on nerves 'because bones had slipped out'.[38] Nigel Love was a Bowen observer trained later at the Roberts College also qualifying as a naturopath and chiropractor in 1958.[39] In 1973, he said to the Ward Inquiry 'I am here to treat spinal misalignments and nerve pressures'.[40] Although Love described himself a DC, in the electoral rolls he is an osteopath suggesting he (and Cogan too) adopted a chiropractic identity for registration. Both Cogan and Love use the nerve-pressure terminology as a result of their training though chiropractors generally assumed that nerve issues were caused by bony misalignments or 'subluxations' specifically of spinal vertebrae and that osseous adjustments were required to realign bones. Osteopath-Neuropaths would consider nerve pressure on any areas and joints of the body and the notion it was soft tissue restrictions and tight muscles impinging on nerves and pulling bones out of place. As described next, this recognition led to some schools of thought challenging the term *osteopathy* as 'osteo' implied bones, and many wished to embrace neuropathy instead which better reflected nerves.

Bowen Patients Remember Nerves as the Focus of His Treatments

Aligning with notions of 'pinched nerves' Bowen's patients thought his work was 'putting nerves back in place' or in one instance 'putting [nerve] communications together'.[41] Former patient Cec Capon said:

> Most of it was manipulation and moving nerves type of thing than clunking bones. Tommy never seemed to get you and go 'crunch'. He'd run his hand down you and whatever. Things would get a jar and things would feel better . . . but he wasn't a 'cruncher', He was a manipulator. That was quite interesting.[42]

Brian Munns echoed Capon:

> He did a lot of manipulation, just manipulating, probably a mixture of pressures. To me it was obviously all about nerves. It was to do with nerves, that's what it was all about, what they were doing and if they were in the right spot or whatever. That's my feeling he just knew where each nerve went and what it did. He'd manipulate down the back or your leg and neck. I think he just knew what he needed to do.[43]

Likewise, Thérèse Vahland recalled 'Mr Bowen explained to me that he was treating the nerves that were out of place. They had to learn to stay in better position but kept slipping back'.[44] Bowen's approach is entirely consistent with neuropathy and in removing pressure on nerves. Doug Sells said that Bowen considered that eye dullness was a sign the ovary or testes on that side was to do with restricted nerves.[45] Bob Lucy who also observed Bowen for a period makes these observations in his training video on Myorthotics, presumably taken from Bowen as the observation sits outside of iridology, one of Lucy's areas of expertise.[46] In babies, any blueness of hue in the sclera was a sign of compression of nerves in the neck (in allopathic medicine, this hue is considered normal by doctors and simply due to the sclera being thinner in an infant).

Development of Neuropathy vs Osteopathy

In 1901, it was considered that osteopathy was a derivative of 'mechanoneuropathy' and the term neuropathy preferable to osteopathy. The Columbian Home Study Course on Osteopathy sheds light:

> This name [osteopathy] has been adhered to by his followers, notwithstanding the fact that the advancement in the science have shown that the real osteopathic treatment consists principally in the treatment of nerves, and, strictly speaking the term 'neuropathy' would be far more appropriate, although the original name will probably be adhered to, as the public have become accustomed to it, and a change in names at this time would create confusion.[47]

By 1917, Lust's *Encyclopaedia* recognised five American schools of neuropathy: the American College of Neuropathy in Philadelphia was led by Dr WW Fritz; the Chicago College by William Havard and Brightside Sanatorium by Marc Blochwitz.[48] Another advertisement identified seven 'Professors' of neuropathy without naming schools: 'Drs Lahn, Struch, [Henry] Lindlahr, Carl Schultz, [Dr FW] Collins, Deninger, [Andrew P] Davis and [William] Havard'.[49] Writings from these professors are sparse. Davis wrote two books, the first, *Neuropathy* in 1909.[50] *Neuropathy Illustrated* followed in 1915.[51] Before then, in 1899, Davis had written *Osteopathy Illustrated*.[52] Throughout the works of Davis, 'nerve pressure' appears as a predominant concept. Havard wrote an article for Lust's *Encyclopaedia*.[53]

Dr FW Collins wrote many articles on systems of painless adjusting that were based on soft tissue methods to relieve pressure.[54] In 1946, Thomas T Lake ND/ DC (originally trained with Fritz and later Dean of his College) published a collation of material on neuropathy providing a history of key writers. In the philosophy and principles chapter, he confirms the emphasis on nerve health:

> If a nerve is not functioning properly the organ controlled by that nerve is not performing its function, therefore if a nerve is abnormal the organ controlled by that nerve is abnormal. As the nerve is, so is the organ it controls, and every part of the body can be reached and controlled, directly or indirectly, by the Neuropathic Treatments.[55]

Lake's work also captured the thinking of Havard – an adherent of Fritz and highlighted the importance of treating nerve centres to control circulation by normalising vasomotor nerves to improve circulation:

> Neuropathic treatment is directed to the nerve centers controlling circulation for the purpose of restoring the normal activity to the vasomotor nerves, and of relieving either active or passive congestion by establishing better lymphatic drainage.
>
> The treatment itself consists of simple manipulations, which are varied for the purpose of achieving three main effects. The first is merely mechanical and consists of propelling the lymph through the lymphatic vessels and glands, and of emptying congested tissues of their infiltrations. The other effects are accomplished as the result of altering the reflexes by influencing the vaso-motor mechanisms, and even the myo-motor.[56]

Treatments were given in accordance with the presenting conditions and a general physical examination that paid attention to reflexes. An additional insight into Lake's approach as principal of the Philadelphia School is recorded by Yergin.[57] Yergin published facial points used by Lake. Pressure could be put on facial points related to cranial nerves or points related to spinal nerves. Some had a dilatory effect, others were constrictors, thereby influencing nerve reflexes and circulation. For instance, pressure on cranial point 10 acted as a dilator.[58] Yergin also published Collins' diagram of spinal centres.[59] This includes two images side by side. Table 3.1 represents the labelling – the first is labelled normally with the cervical, thoracic and lumbar spine and sacral spine given the numbering of normal anatomy today. The other had different codes shown in column three:

According to the Lake system described under Yergin's entry on Neuropathy, pressure on D4 to D8 (number of segments shown under 'Thoracic' on the left in column two) acted as a constrictor for the lungs and bronchial tubes. Some points had both effects, for instance, pressure on D5 to D7 in

Table 3.1 Dr FW Collin's Spinal Segments Labelled for Neuropathy in Yergin with Extra Column Added to Interpret Codes

	Normal label	*Neuropathy points*	*Likely reflex /plexus decoding*
Cervical	1	AtP	Atlas
	2	AxP	Axis
	3	MCP	Middle Cervical
	4	MCP	Middle Cervical
	5	LCP	Lower Cervical
	6	LCP	Lower Cervical
	7VP	VP	Vagus?
Thoracic	1	AP	
	2	HP	
	3	LuP	Lung
	4	LiP	Liver
	5	CP	Cardiac
	6	SP	
	7	SP	
	8	SP	
	9	SplP	Spleen?
	10	KP	Kidney
	11	KP	Kidney
	12	KP	Kidney
Lumbar	1	UPP	Urinary?
	2	UPP	Urinary?
	3	MPP	
	4	LPP	Lumbar Plexus?
	5	LPP	Lumbar Plexus?
Sacrum		SACP	Sacral Plexus
	Coccyx	Cx,P.or Cc.P	Coccyx

the Thoracic area were both constrictors and dilators for the kidneys.[60] Davis also illustrated the relationship between spinal segments and organs but with traditional correlations of spinal nerve reflexes to the organs innervated.[61]

Bowen's Osteopathy Aligns with Neuropathy

Bowen's appreciation and focus on the nervous system sit very comfortably within neuropathy and associated 'nerve pressure theory' as explained by the neuropathy schools. According to Smeeton, Bowen was fully cognisant of spinal nerve segments and the reflex relationships to both internal organs and muscles. According to Smeeton, Bowen would clear the spinal area first before moving to the periphery. Bowen would do direct visceral manipulations too, presumably to take the pressure off nerves; he would address nerves related to the gall and urinary bladder. Kidney work was also very important with attention paid to whether they had been opened or closed – presumably a reflection of dilation and constriction ideas described about reflex effects of neuropathy and pressure on segments. However, according to Smeeton, Bowen's work with kidneys as opened or closed (closed being important at the end of treatment) was also important for his ideas about linkages to the brain, especially when working with those with neurological disabilities.

Neave DC recalled that Bowen would say you could control a nosebleed with pressure on the neck vertebra at the level of cervical 3 (C3).[62] Bowen's questioning to Brian Anderson who became paralysed in 1963 is confirmatory. Bowen sought to eliminate which part of Anderson's back was injured by eliminating the segments that were not affected by the injury causing paralysis when he said, 'Can you see straight or have you got . . . a side vision? . . . Can you wee alright?'[63] Bowen's treatments restored Anderson to full movement and he did so without any aggressive adjustments, simply 'he'd get the fingers in'.[64] Smeeton said Bowen had the ability to trace nerves to the periphery.[65] As Munns said, 'He just knew where all the nerves went'.[66] The importance of nerves to osteopathy is reflected in a dissection done by Still's students in 1902, available on the internet.[67] Bowen educated himself by visiting abattoirs to study animal carcasses, especially pigs as they were closest to human.[68]

The notion of 'pressure on points', therefore, is a feature of neuropathy which was in existence long before Eastern manual medicine was popular in the west. Soft tissue techniques used by neuropaths were varied and used by osteopaths. Neuropathy offers a comfortable fit as an original influence on Bowen's style of work and it is hypothesised, given the available evidence and parallels in symbolism, that Roberts (and to an extent, Maurice Blackmore) were the most likely earliest disseminators of this knowledge in Australia. Alongside the concepts of neuropathy, pressure on reflex points is also a feature of Neuromuscular Technique developed by Stanley Lief who was originally inspired by Varma's work on Pranotherapy. Pranotherapy recognised nerve flows, bio-electrical currents and vibration in the body and the need to balance the current so the vibration is regular and of average amplitude.[69]

The evidence of course readings for Roberts' trained osteopaths of the 1950s is slim. In his 1970s transcript, McAlister reflecting on his studies with Roberts in the 1950s said he read Stoddard, Downer and Cyriax which indicates an alignment with texts used in the elite mainstream schools overseas. Michael Chadwick (a BSO graduate) outlined his reading material to the Ward Inquiry and these sources repeated Stoddard.[70] ACONPAL literature likewise.[71] Alan Stoddard was a lecturer at the BSO and his *Manual of Osteopathic Practice* has endured as an authoritative source. Neuropathy, osteopathy and chiropractic all recognise reflexive neurological relationships which underpin the philosophy of reciprocal relationship between structure and function.

Kevin Ryan DO who obtained his qualifications through the Southern School of Natural Therapies thought Bowen's awareness was innate and that he had a natural grasp of the relationship between structure and function as understood by osteopaths and chiropractors.[72]

Romney Smeeton, a chiropractor graduated from Roberts' College in 1976 and longest Bowen observer from 1977, was most surprised at Bowen's 'lack of osseous adjustments' and he elaborated:

> The more I got into watching Tom work the more I realised that the principles he worked under were the same principles I'd learned as a chiropractor and what osteopaths learned in their course . . . . The results were remarkable, a lot quicker that what chiropractic results were. Tom would see people usually for a minimum of twice, one week apart. A third treatment could be made if he wasn't happy with the progress but that was at the discretion of the patient.[73]

Neuropathy was lost and discarded by the 1970s and by then, none of Bowen's Roberts' college-trained observers remarked on the similarities of Bowen's work to neuropathy, it was only those who studied with Roberts' college in the pre-chiropractic period who shared similar language of 'nerve pressure'. When the Roberts' college 1970s-trained chiropractors Davis and Neave presented Bowen's work to the Sydney College of Chiropractic seminar in 1979, the workshop was entitled 'The Muscle Techniques of Ted [*sic*] Bowen'.[74] It is telling, however, that Smeeton recently said to understand Bowen's work, 'Learn your neurology'.[75]

The practical delivery of neuropathy could incorporate osteopathic ideas of gentle two-handed thrusts on the spine to push bones back into place.[76] Early on Bowen apparently did not advocate any robust thrusts on vertebrae. Ron Garner the masseur who worked with Bowen from the late 1950s would use this technique to elicit a 'click' but Bowen showed him how to use the leg lever instead.[77] Bowen said that the thrusts like this should be avoided as they could damage nerves.[78] Techniques used in neuropathy did not necessarily employ fixed pressure on points. This is illustrated in the descriptions by Andrew P Davis. Davis, a medical doctor, was one of the first graduates in 1894 of A T Still's ASO and an early teacher and board member too.[79] According to Keating who describes Davis an 'itinerant schoolman', Davis also graduated in 1898 from the Palmer Chiropractic School.[80] Davis does not appear to have written on chiropractic. Rather Davis viewed neuropathy as the umbrella system and all else subservient: 'Osteopathy, Chiropractic, Ophthalmology, Suggestion or Magnetism, designate how it [Neuropathy] is applied'.[81] The motto of the Davis College of neuropathy was 'lift the pressure' as espoused by the 'nerve pressure theory' of disease:

> It will be remembered that all diseases are products of nerve disturbance or impeded circulation of the fluids of the body. The science of neuropathy, properly applied, removes the pressure which causes all pathological conditions in the easiest, the best and most rational way of any system or method ever known or used by any physical manipulator.[82]

Other than this method of spinal adjusting with gentle thrusts, the neuropathy texts described that manipulations were otherwise done solely with thumbs and fingers to influence nerve centres:

> Treatment is directed to nerve centers and lymph drainage . . . . All peripheral irritations produce nerve reflexes, all central irritations produce sensory reflexes or motor disturbances in both.[83]

In the Davis school, the focus was on removing muscle contractions as he considered these put pressure on nerves. The techniques utilised were gradual massage, direct thrusts involving stretching for a moment and frequently repeating sudden stretching and heat.[84] These thrusts included both thrusts on vertebrae and thrusts on tissues. This description of thrusts implies manipulations that are isolated and do not involve continuous contact with the skin as in massage. Davis describes that the origins and insertions of muscles are to be located and 'it should be an easy matter to make the thrust in such a manner that the contraction be overcome and the normal condition reestablished'.[85] Here Davis is describing a cross-fibre mobilisation which is entirely consistent with Bowen's style. Anatomically, the positioning of Bowen's gentle soft tissue thrusts were alongside spinal segments with cervical 3, thoracic 9 and 12 or lumbar 3 common and on peripheral muscles.

William Havard's neuropathy school ascribed instead to the notion of controlling the vasoconstrictor mechanism and spoke only of manual manipulations directed to the nerve centres controlling circulation. Irritations of the central and peripheral nervous system produced nerve reflexes leading to constriction.[86] The fundamental idea was to 'normalise the activity of the constrictor mechanism throughout the body' and to lift the pressure from nerves.[87] The neuropath was expected to notice evidence in tissues of inflammation, congestion, passive infiltration and constrictor fatigue of the blood vessels of the spinal cord and anywhere on the body. Hyperactive nerves were calmed and hypoactive nerves were stimulated to restore balance. All of these elements are also consistent with Bowen's work. Bowen would observe heat and swelling and where the body was cold. To some patients, Bowen recommended they wear a vest to keep their kidneys warm (to improve circulation).[88]

Bowen's personal style of intervention or thrust simply involved him making contact with the muscle belly or edge and without any exaggerated drag or slide, he simply pushed down to the desired depth to influence a particular physical and neurological level. He would then nudge or slowly thrust the fibres precisely in the direction necessary, usually across-fibre though sometimes it would be along-fibre according to Smeeton.[89] Transverse actions across muscle bellies generally relax muscles and this sort of cross-fibre mobilisation work is not unique at all to Bowen but is ubiquitous in manual therapy traditions around the world. The work of Lauren Berry (1917–1983) combining corrective cross-fibre tissue work with structural balancing.[90] Pat Allen, a younger protégé of Bert Donald, a contemporary of Bowen, uses cross-fibre 'flicking' as did the famous Swedish healer Ernst Kjellberg in Queensland.[91] Kevin Ryan pointed out 'flickers' were commonplace'.[92] Sometimes very firm pressure was used; Gary Bovine described the work of the Scottish William Rae, the Blantyre bonesetter, 'He used his thumb and forefinger . . . and would work hard over a painful region of the spine, inch by inch with his thumb and finger until relief was felt'.[93]

Antii Hernesniemi recorded traditional Finland bonesetters whose tactile work was more sensitive.[94] Other features of Bowen's tactile approach involved his thumbs working together in synchrony: one slightly ahead of the other, with the following thumb checking on the soft tissue state achieved by the grading of the first. Directional subtleties existed depending on the response Bowen sought in removing a somatic disturbance of nerve vibration he could feel. Precision was key in other aspects and Bowen (like Ned Thompson mentioned earlier) would regularly pull his apprentices up on being too firm or too deep, as Neave recalled:

> But with Tom's technique [compared to mine], he's using the weight, he'd make his contact . . . to be moved . . . he just thumbed the area, and just move it gradually to do the thing. When initially I started doing Tom's work with hard like that, I put my hands in like that and I was going to start treating and he put his hand on mine. He said, 'Don't hurt the fellow!' I said, 'Why, what do you mean Tom?', he said, 'That's much too heavy'.[95]

Neave elaborated further on the quality of Bowen's touch:

> Really soft, really soft to the point you feel something radiating from the touch you know. He'd like, he'd put your hand on, on there and you'd wait, and just gradually put a little bit more pressure on . . . and he'd say, 'You've got it'. Any time he said, anytime I'd, 'Got it', with Tommy I knew I didn't have to go beyond that point.[96]

Others commented on the relaxing quality of Bowen's touch – Phil Dower recalled a childhood sense of a miracle happening and John Garner who described the pulsating effect when Bowen and his father worked together on him.[97]

Neuropathy practice of the Davis school specifically allowed for variations in pressure depending on the hardness or soreness of muscle tissue: some treatments were to be effected using light pressure where deeper would be 'injurious' and other times more strength with terminology such as 'stand strong' and 'vigorous'. Treatments varied depending on whether presentations were acute or chronic and whether internal organs were involved in the complaint.[98] Consistent with neuropathy, Bowen was noted to apply tissue thrusts at particular points along the spine. Evidently, the thinking was that releasing tight muscles immediately parallel to the spine also released pressure on the nerves at that segment. Bowen's style was perceived as gentle because he did not do robust adjustments that would elicit a 'crack' from joints whether spinal or in the limbs. However, depending on the presenting complaint his treatments could be painful.

Bowen's Practice Aligned to Osteopathy

Bowen's treatment approach not only resonates strongly with 'neuropathy' as an enclave within osteopathy, but with the traditional practice of Dr Still MD, DO along with elements in the origins of NMT. Still's original work was largely soft tissue manipulations and this is revealed in *The Original Moves taught by Andrew Taylor Still to Dr Charles F Haverin*.[99] A particular section of *Original Moves* will be described later with reference to Bowen's pelvic work. Dr Lust's osteopathy lessons, published in 1937, describe kneading and stretching muscles as for massage but of most interest regarding Bowen's style of manipulations he echoes the neuropathy of Davis:

> Stretching of the muscle consists in forcibly pulling the insertions away from the origin, *or it may be done by applying pressure across the muscle while the two ends are stationary.* [emphasis added][100]

Using neuropathy as a reference and readings of Still confirm Bowen's approach to be aligned with neuropathy practised in the context of osteopathic philosophy and tenets. Andrew Still spoke of the distinction between massage and osteopathy in terms of osteopathy freeing nerves and working with a plan and the work of a masseur as unstructured:

> Our work is done when we leave open the nerve channels to the perfect eye of Nature's inspection . . . freedom is given to the nerves to act . . . . He [the operator] is dealing with cause and effect.[101]

Bowen exhibited the professionalism and rationale of a three-tiered approach of palpation, working diagnosis and intervention with a view to a 'fix' that should 'hold'.[102] Osteopaths embraced the concept of a reciprocal relationship between structure and function and Bowen demonstrated an informed grasp of this concept to his college-trained observers.[103] Bowen would not treat a patient if he did not have a clear idea of how to proceed. His daughter Heather remembered when her father was perplexed in one case, he said, 'I couldn't fix her I don't know what's wrong with her, I've told her to come back in a week's time and so maybe I'll think of something'.[104] By the following week, Bowen would have it figured out and came home happy that he had 'fixed' his patient. Ryan confirmed 'Every response that occurred under Tom Bowen's hands was the result he expected to occur'.[105] Talking about Bowen's requirement to have patients return the following week, according to Ryan, Bowen would explain what he had done in terms of 'locking in' an intervention, that the treatment involved more than just superficially addressing tension in an area of the body, it was designed to rectify the cause of a problem. Bowen would balance the lower body first and if the client presented with issues in ribcage or neck he would address the lower back first.[106]

Nerve activity can be over-stimulated or under-stimulated and techniques were designed to calm or stimulate activity depending on presentation. Pressure on a nerve has an inhibiting or calming effect. Slow moves are calming, faster moves are stimulating. Janse, whose work was a resource for FG Roberts after 1939, dedicated a chapter to reflexes and describes a variety of practitioner approaches and sets out the principle 'The whole of the periphery is a 'switchboard' of innumerable reflex circuits which extend to and influence all parts of the body.[107] A description by Columbia College is apt regarding neuropathy and Bowen's work that the client spoke of in terms of the notion of putting nerves back in place:

> Our student, like the skilled linesman, first finds out where the wires are crossed or interfered with, and starts in to adjust them he extends the contracted muscle or reduces the slight dislocation which has caused a pressure upon the nerve and has shut off its current, and by so doing he restores the line to working order and gives the suffering organ or part the perfect service it deserves.[108]

Bowen included in his work moves called 'stoppers' at the start of a treatment. These, according to a remark he made to Keith Davis ND, DC, he apparently learned from Ernie Saunders. Stoppers were a thrust, or pressure movement made over the muscles near the spine at the level of lumbar 3 and at the level of thoracic 7 before working on the rib cage. There has been much debate on what the purpose of the 'stoppers' or 'blockers' was but the name implies that the soft tissue thrust applied was to 'stop' or 'block' signalling of some kind. Nerve signalling is the obvious conclusion for therapies intended to address painful conditions. No specific use of 'stoppers' has been found in neuropathy texts though the concept aligns with the neuropathic practice of using pressure to inhibit nerve action. For a master of muscle and cartilage like Saunders, the use would have been related to the motor system and muscles of the lower body. Chapter 4 illustrates that, unlike Bowen's work, there is no evidence at all that Saunders was concerned with reflex relationships related to internal health issues.

Bowen had an awareness of other relationships that for his time were traditionally the preserve of osteopathic training. Bowen was renowned for his extensive neck work and was aware that his manipulations of the neck and cervical spine had a neurological influence on seizures and epilepsy and other related bodily functions. Bowen was also aware of the osteopathic sacro-occipital relationship between the cervical 3 on the neck (C3) and the coccyx (tailbone) as accepted in craniosacral therapy (CST).[109] For instance, Greg Hutchins took his daughter Renée to Bowen as she suffered from spina bifida:

> The other thing to me that was really interesting was that Renée's spina bifida is on the lumbar four/five, right? The thing that always made me think was, 'Why is he working there (the neck)?'[110]

At the very outset, Bowen determined whether or not he could assist Renée but the fact that doing a move on her neck elicited a physical response when her foot flicked about one centimetre. Bowen said to the father 'If you believe in me, give me time, and do whatever I ask you to do I'll get this girl walking'.[111] The Hutchins had been told their daughter would never walk and Bowen's treatments defied this prognosis.[112] Bowen said, 'I've got to get the fluid flowing'.[113] In Bowen's disability clinic, this can also be a reference to CSF as well as the circulatory fluids of lymph and blood. To Bettye LeMarquand's mother, Bowen said, 'I have joined up all of Bettye's communications' and from that Bettye's movement palsies abated and were more controllable; she improved in kidney functioning and in hormonal functioning with the return of menses. Her improvement was noted by her physician, Doctor Gooch.[114] Significantly, when working with patients with spinal injury or movement debility caused by disruption to nerve transmission in the central nervous system, Bowen would not apply the stoppers or nerve blockers that were a standard part of his general practice. With these patients, he wished no impediment to nerve signalling.[115]

In 1979, Ryan DO noted Bowen was practising CST.[116] He also suggested Bowen demonstrated a superior shortened process to CST.[117] William Garner Sutherland, a student of Andrew Still, first introduced his ideas in 1929.[118] *The Cranial Bowl* was published in 1939.[119] Sutherland observed that the sutures of the skull were mobile and not fused as assumed by conventional medical anatomy. From this, CST evolved with the concept of a 'respiratory mechanism'. Tactile contact with the bony skull allows the mechanism to be felt through pulses and rhythms of CSF and this is used to assess the health of CSF flow in the brain and spine.[120] There is no specific mention of CST in the selection of Roberts' magazines inspected for 1928–1952, nor in the 1960s, curricula of COCA and PAX nor in SCC courses of the 1970s.[121] CST is also absent in the bibliography published by ACONPAL in the 1970s.[122] Considering that CST was not widely publicised until after Bowen's death with John Upledger's work in the 1980s, how did Bowen became aware of this new therapy? It appears that Stanley Lief's BCNO graduates were teaching CST in the 1950s.[123] This suggests Bowen acquired the knowledge through connections with BCNO which as determined in Chapter 2 is the most likely institution Bowen had started, but not completed, his correspondence studies in osteopathy.

Bowen's style with pelvic adjusting has some similarities to the *Original Moves* published by Dr FW Collins but a stronger resonance with the

Dullmage System described later that did not involve any bony thrusts. Most of Dr Still MD, DO's work was soft tissue and stretching work, on occasion utilising bony thrusts. With respect to adjusting of the sacroiliac joint which Bowen did with his patient's prone, he achieved his results with soft tissue work alone and use of the leg as a lever to relieve tension. In *Original Moves*, Dr FW Collins describes the technique for addressing sacroiliac lesion by operating from the left side of a prone patient, putting right hand under the patient's knee and lifting it up of the table with a lever movement towards the operator and use the left hand to remove tension on the right ilia by applying a thrust.[124]

Bowen's pelvic adjusting as practised by Smeeton DC does not involve raising the leg or doing a thrust, the left leg is similarly used as a lever moved by the right hand without lifting the leg, while the fingers and thumbs of his left hand put pressure on ligaments and points around the sacrum to adjust sacral and sacro-iliac tensions. Lever work follows on the right side with finger and thumb placements to achieve the desired result. Lust's osteopathy lesson reprinted in Roberts' NPH in 1937 describes similar positioning except for use of thrust but distinguishes the positions for a hip tilted anterior (forwards) or posterior (backwards).[125] For the former, the patient lay on their back and only the knee on the symptomatic side was taken to the chest not both.[126] Raising the knee to the shoulder with a person supine brings the hip into a more posterior alignment. *The Dullmage System of Pelvic Adjusting* was promoted by Dr FW Collins who operated a neuropathy college. The *Dullmage system* did not involve bony thrusts or joint cracking. The importance of the sacroiliac joint (SIJ) to functioning above and below the pelvis is highlighted and the system was focused on removing soft tissue pressures on sciatic and pelvic nerves. Collins described the system as 'entirely different from Osteopathy, has nothing to do with Chiropractic and could well be defined under Naturopathy, and is not known to medical science'.[127] Talking neuropathically, Collins said, 'It is not necessary to have bony pressure such as is the principle of chiropractic and osteopathy. Contracted muscle can cause the pressure or prolapsed viscera pressing on nerves and nerve plexuses'.[128] Although the Dullmage technique involved using sandbags under the hips to induce a passive stretch to the ligaments of the SIJ and pelvis, Bowen was not observed to do this.[129] At the Ward Inquiry, Bowen specifically spoke of taking nerve pressure off the sacroiliac. Bowen's changes to ligament tensions were induced by placing thumb pressure on the ligaments of the sacrum in combination with a leg lever motion. Tissue changes were sensed by the working hand and when the desired tissue release felt, Bowen would say 'you've got it' and the leg was brought down. The move took pressure off nerves affected by any structural strain on the joint.

Key to Bowen's style was minimalism and a sequential approach that incorporated highly individualised and creative soft tissue interventions tailored to his patient. Already in existence in osteopathic and nature cure circles was the Universal Natural Tonic Treatment Tonic (UNTT) developed by Dr FW

Collins and a roundtable of leaders and students of Still including Drs Charles F Haverin, Andrew Victory, EK Stretch and Jacob Lang who endeavoured to restore Still's principles to osteopathy.[130] The roundtable was concerned that the general osteopathic treatments contained too many moves and stimulated hyper reflexes. The roundtable reviewed the work of Still, Barber, Murray, McFadden and German texts on manual therapies to develop the UNTT. The UNTT involved a minimalist sequence of moves that effected comprehensive therapeutic benefit.[131] The UNTT was applied in a sequence which was not prescriptive allowing for variation in how the sequences were applied to specifically cater to patients' unique needs.[132] Applied over six to eight minutes, specific lesions were then to be addressed to take care of individual issues affecting the patient. Dr Collins added, 'With hygiene and proper combination of food, this treatment will remove (cure) about ninety-five percent of the troubles the human family is heir to'.[133] Bowen's sequencing and minimalist approach can be viewed as a derivation of UNTT since he was adamant about not 'over treating' the patient which fits with minimising hyper reflexes. This is congruent with Still's precepts captured in the UNTT and specifically with Andrew Davis who said with respect to neuropathy, as few osteopathic moves as possible were required so as not to exhaust the patient.[134] As a minimalist, Bowen reflects Stills' adage of 'Find it. Fix it and Leave it Alone.'[135] The rest of the statement less quoted was 'and Nature will do the Rest':

> Then the engine goes into the hands of the engineer, who waters, fires, and conducts this artificial being on its journey. As osteopathic machinists we go no further than to adjust the abnormal conditions back to the normal. Nature will do the rest.[136]

Leon Chaitow DO described that as well as correcting specific lesions found, the manner of delivery of treatment in the UNTT provided for simultaneous diagnosis.[137] As observed by Smeeton, this was an element that challenged observers of Bowen; differentiating whether a hand movement was a therapeutic intervention or whether Bowen was just simply assessing and diagnosing tissue states. Bowen's work was so subtle and he worked so swiftly it was difficult to follow without close attention to what he was doing. Interestingly, Chaitow also stated the UNTT or General Naturopathic Tonic Treatment (GNTT) was represented in a few manual therapy movements, including Bowen Technique, Reflexology and Neuromuscular Technique (NMT), all of which he also considered to be 'constitutional therapies'.[138]

To minimise hyper reflexes, Bowen would also allow the tissues to rest and integrate before doing further work and observers confirm rests took place, but not in a predetermined way and only after a sequence of moves.[139] Bowen was resting patients at the start of his work in the early 1960s in football rooms and patients just assumed Bowen had 'gone off for a smoke'.[140] Bowen was so attuned to what was going on with his patients he could tell if any interference had occurred while he was out of the room. Rob McPherson remembered a situation in the 1970s:

> There was one time when Tom had an apprentice with him and Alice [Rob's wife] was sitting up and Tom did something at the neck on one side of her spine and you could see the ripples running down her back from her neck. He said he'd need to, 'Block that as it could hurt her'. When Tom treated her and left the room, he left an apprentice in the room and when he came back he said, 'Did you touch her back? I told you not to touch her back'. Tom could tell when he came back in that her back had been touched while he was out of the room.[141]

Still would advocate not to treat the spine more than once a week because it was irritating to the spinal nerves; Bowen too with general patients would only treat a week apart. The second treatment was also to ensure that the first 'fix' had 'held'.

Like Bowen's methods, NMT addresses biomechanics and releases held patterns of restriction.[142] Ryan noted that when Bowen had completed a treatment with patients he would ask them to sit up on table, put both feet on the floor at the same time and stand up. The purpose relates to understanding the relationship between doing balancing in postural work as the influence of gravity is key.[143]

Still said, 'nature has no apology to offer. It does the work if you know how to line up the parts; then food and rest is required'.[144] There are numerous examples where Bowen concerned himself with alignment. On the table, he would check the levels of the gluteal crease as an indicator of pelvic imbalance. His daughter Heather remembered:

> He used to be able to tell what was wrong with a person by looking at them. I remember walking down Malop Street, and he'd diagnose people walking towards him, he'd say, 'That man's got his hip out of joint', 'That lady needs her back looked at' and he'd tell you as we were walking down the street. Gee he was annoying! he just told you what was wrong with everybody! I guess that's probably why he went through the number of patients he did, he just knew.[145]

Laymen like William (Bill) Mitchell observed posture and gait too. However, seen in the context of his overall practice, Bowen's biomechanical work was done consciously within the grasp of knowledge drawn from the osteopathy/neuropathy concept.

The body's various internal ducts and tubes are surrounded by smooth muscle and governed by nerves of the autonomic nervous system. Bowen used the term 'strangulation' for the stomach (and 'twisted gullet'), gall bladder and testes.[146] The use of 'strangulated' in medical literature is common with respect to hernias. In neuropathy, Andrew Davis makes it clear that synonyms are 'occlusion', 'obstruction' and 'invagination' and discusses the 'occlusion of the bowel'.[147] Dr Still MD, DO used the term 'strangulation' more widely including the effect of gravity as a 'hangman's rope' creating congestion and tumours in relation to 'bladder, womb, bowels, kidneys, appendix, pancreas, stomach, gall sac, liver, spleen, heart, lung and brains'.[148] To his daughter Heather who was nursing a screaming newborn suffering colic, Bowen quizzed her on what happened at birth and remarked on the habit of turning the infant upside down 'it was the worst thing you could do as it kinks the gullet'.[149] Bowen would inspect infants for 'strangulated' testes. Terminology supported in old medical literature referred to undescended tests and 'twists' of the epididymis or cord.[150] Much of Bowen's successful fertility work was aimed to free restrictions in fallopian tubes that could be twisted and blocking the successful passage of ova (eggs) to the uterus.[151] This is confirmed by the fact that the intervention involved a soft tissue intervention on the front of the body at the position of the ovary in the pelvis. Bowen also addressed any restriction on nerves at the spinal level that reflexed to the ovary if he thought this was an issue.[152]

Bowen had an individualised approach to his patients. Bruno Chikly quoted JL Dickey DO and emphasised that Still was not prescriptive about specific techniques that should be used to address patients' issues, only that they were applied in the service of the philosophy and principles. Still had *The Philosophy and Mechanical Principles of Osteopathy* recalled because the book contained descriptions of techniques and Still did not want to advocate specific manipulations. Instead, the physician was expected to draw on their understanding of the body and its physiology to arrive at the optimal approach for the patient before them.[153]

Bowen's work looked simple to the uninformed observer. Early osteopaths recognised that some osteopathic movements could 'look' the same but in fact at the micro level, quite different somatic dysfunctions were being addressed according to the patient's presentation. It was important for the student to use their mental faculties and rather than copying any other physician, think about where the interventions are to be applied in each individual case, '*instead of yielding to the pernicious habit of passing each of his cases through the routine of an unvarying set of manipulations*' [emphasis added].[154]

Smeeton considered that any one of Bowen's treatments of a patient was but a snapshot of his vast repertoire.

> It might have looked like it was the same, he would be looking in similar areas, yet there were variations in everything that he did. Where I often explain it every patient Tom treated was a snapshot of his work, so see the whole of his work, you put all those snapshots together you'll get what Tom was doing in his clinical work.[155]

Keith Davis said that other than the use of the stoppers Bowen was very 'changeable' and that he [Davis] 'would never stop being amazed' at Bowen's creativity depending on a patient's issues.[156] For Bowen who identified as an osteopath, it would have been anathema to him to simply copy another or expect anyone to directly copy him. As Dain Tasker said in 1916:

> Do not copy anybody's movements. Learn the principles, then apply them in the manner most satisfactory to yourself and helpful to the patient. To understand the principles and apply them intelligently, one cannot know too much concerning all the subjects which are the basis of a broad medical education.[157]

Other Pressure Movement Systems

Other 'pressure movement' systems existed around the turn of the century and taught in nature cure establishments such as those of Andrea Rabagliati (1843–1930). Stanley Lief was a known star pupil of McFadden before he set up BCN in the 1920s.[158] These were self-administered systems that recognised the reflex relationship between painful points on the skin and internal organs. Rabagliati wrote two books.[159] The first, *Initis*, was published in 1905 and was Rabagliati's term for 'congestion of the body's tissues'. *Initis* similarly involved a kind of connective tissue technique using isolated thumb and finger pressures on tender spots designed to remove congestion caused by a build-up of too much lymph fluid. Echoing neuropathy on removing nerve pressure, *Initis* entailed 'lifting pressure' off nerves by applying pressure work and using 'pressure movements' to muscles and their surrounding connective tissues to reduce congestion responsible for blockages that affected nerve activity and circulation of lymph, 'and that the pressure movements will be gradually extended to parts of the limbs, so as to dissipate the congestion and tenderness which weight them down'.[160]

Sutherland, writing for a medical, rather than nature cure audience on Rabagliati's death, said, Rabagliati's books did not reach a wide circle of readers.[161] However, Rabagliati advertised *Initis* in Lust's Encyclopaedia of 1917 and *Initis* would have been known and accessible to an international community of nature cure leaders and advocates. Allen Pattreiouex offered *Initis* on the curriculum alongside massage, osteopathy and other nature cure subjects at his well-known Therapeutic Institute in Manchester mentioned in Chapter 2.[162] Lief and Boris Chaitow combined the ideas of Rabagliati with the Indian ayurvedic techniques of Dr Varma to develop NMT before the Second World War.[163] Varma stated 'Our method of treatment by the removal of all obstacles to the flow of nervous current (Pranotherapy) allows creation to proceed unimpeded'.[164] This flow was downward (through deep-seated nerves for muscle contraction) and spiral (superficial for surface warmth and sensitivity).[165]

Summary

Neuropathy and Dr Still MD, DO's original moves and tenets echo strongly in Bowens' work. The popularised view of Bowen is he developed his techniques and approach all by himself. This chapter has illustrated that Bowen's work sits very comfortably with approaches already documented for the first quarter of the twentieth century following the development of neuropathy and osteopathy as systems of manual medicine. Adjunct techniques such as *Initis* and Pranotherapy influenced the development of Lief and Chaitow's NMT. Attention to Bowen's language in the Ward Inquiry and how he is remembered in the symbolic interaction of oral histories viewed together with characteristics of his treatment style have proved invaluable in contextualising Bowen's style of work in historical terms.

In particular, Bowen's work is strongly congruent with the philosophy and principles of neuropathy as promoted and taught by various schools, including Lust, Davis, Havard, Collins and Lake whereby nerve pressure was reduced by various recognised means. These include applying pressure to points to change vasomotor reflexes and dilate or constrict activity as required, the application of thrusts on muscles near nerve roots and the use of soft tissue stretches to release contracted muscle and free nerves. Bowen's neuropathy was practised aligned with osteopathic principles of minimising reflexes and doing minimal work as reflected in the short treatments of the UNTT. Bowen combined his neuropathic approach with the use of osteopathic long levers, but he did not utilise bony thrusts as was the norm to adjust the pelvis and spine. Bowen was highly adept at using soft tissue approaches alone and his work implied an expectation of more lasting change at a neurological level beyond the superficial relief normally achieved by massage.

It has been hypothesised that Bowen somehow gained access to Roberts or knowledge of neuropathy through his network, including through individuals trained with Marcus Blackmore though he was chiropractic in his focus from the beginning. The work of an osteopath and neuropath was expected to result in more than a change in tissue tone but to remove interferences on nerves.[166] Bowen has emerged so far undeniably osteopathic or, more precisely, neuropathic and also utilising osteopathic ideas. Bowen worked solely with fingers and thumbs and the palm of the hand was not in contact with the body as for massage. The following chapter will now look at Bowen in relation to the legendary football masseur Ernest (Ernie) Saunders who has been popularly assumed to be Bowen's mentor and to the claim that Saunders introduced Japanese acupressure techniques to his students, Bowen included.

Later, Chapter 8 on medical pluralism and beyond considers the unique positioning of football masseurs in Australian culture and offering consumers a philanthropic health service.

Notes

1 F. W. Collins, *The Dullmage System of Pelvic Adjusting*, n.p., n.d., Reprint (Pomeroy: Health Research Books, 1993), 1.

2 Abraham Flexner, *Medical Education in the United States and Canada* (New York City: Carnegie Foundation for the Advancement of Medical Teaching, 1910), 258.

3 Joseph E. Pizzorno, Michael T. Murray, and George W. Cody, *A Textbook of Natural Medicine* (Seattle, WA: John Bastyr College Publications, 1988), I: HistNM-16 (this relates to an editorial to the June 1937 edition of Lust's *Naturopath* and *Herald of Health*).

4 "Philosophy of Natural Therapeutics," in *Natural Therapeutics* (Melbourne: Australian Chiropractors, Osteopaths and Naturopathic Physicians Association Limited, 196-?)., 1.Note, though this document is of uncertain date, research has shown it was written after ACONPAL established a branch in Melbourne in 1971 and for submissions for government enquiries commenced in 1973.
5 Louis Khune, *Neo-Naturopathy* (Butler, NJ: Benedict Lust MD, ND, 1909), advertising section post page 277, section not paginated. Louis Khune, *Neo-Naturopathy.*
6 Khune, *Neo-Naturopathy.*
7 B. F. Walker, "FG Roberts Memorial Address," Murdoch University Research Portal, 2015.
8 The views of VSSO men in Chapter 7 who completed studies with Roberts in the early 1950s are relevant.
9 PROV, VPRS 3253/P1/, Unit 47. Bowen transcript, 674.
10 Romney Smeeton personal communication to author.
11 Gerald Arnold personal communication to the author.
12 Smeeton personal communication.
13 Kevin Ryan, "Working alongside Tom Bowen," in Shirley Strachan, *Healing Hands, Unsung Voices, Thomas Ambrose Bowen Osteopath (1916–1982)* (United Kingdom: Cloister House Press, 2016), 239–52.
14 Smeeton personal communication; Ryan, "Working alongside Tom Bowen."
15 Neil Skilbeck, "A Typical Day Working with Tom Bowen," *Vic Bowen News* 1, no. 2 (May 1998): 3.
16 Andrew Taylor Still, *Osteopathy Research and Practice* (Kirksville, MO: A T Still, 1910), 270.
17 Greg Hutchins interview by author, transcript in Strachan, *Healing Hands*, 174.
18 Skilbeck, "A Typical Day Working with Tom Bowen," 3–4.
19 Pat Allen, interview by author, transcript in Strachan, *Healing Hands*, 257.
20 Doug Sells, interview by author, July 27, 2018.
21 Rene Horwood, interview by Ron Phelan, September 11, 1998, transcript extract in Strachan, *Healing Hands*, 33; Doris Robbins personal communication to author, May 3 and 10, 2016.
22 Phil Dower, interview by author, transcript in Strachan, *Healing Hands*, 210.
23 *Australia, Electoral Rolls 1903–1980*, available on Ancestry.com.
24 "Advertising," *Morning Bulletin (Rockhampton)*, September 7, 1936: 2.
25 "Advertising," *Mirror, (Perth)*, October 21, 1939: 22, (col.6).
26 "Advertising," *Sydney Morning Herald*, December 1, 1945: 45, (col.1).
27 "Manipulative Surgery," *Maryborough Chronicle, Wide Bay and Burnett Advertiser (Qld)*, August 17, 1935: 10.
28 "Manipulative Surgery."
29 Arthur Wright email message to the author, April 28, 2017; Smeeton personal communication to author.
30 "Graduate News from Arthur Wright Our First Graduate, Class of 64," *Chirobiz* 3, no. 2 (July 2010).
31 Wright email message to author.
32 Wright email message to author.
33 "Neuropath Fined for Using the Title 'Doctor'," *Brisbane Telegraph*, April 5, 1951: 2.
34 PROV, Osteopathy, Chiropractic and Naturopath Joint Select Committee pp. 783–938, VPRS 241/P/, Unit 14, Transcripts of Committee, Blackmore transcript, 857.
35 Ward Inquiry Report, appendix R.
36 The article listed in Natural Therapeutics under "Acupuncture" was "Modern Acupuncture-Neuropathy" from an unreferenced *Journal of the International Congress of Acupuncture and Moxibustion, Tokyo.*

37 PROV, VPRS 16439/P1/, Unit 13, Cogan transcript: 428–35, 429, 430; *Australia Electoral Rolls 1903–1980.*
38 PROV, VPRS 16439/P1/, Unit 13, Cogan transcript: 429, 430.
39 PROV, Osteopathy, Chiropractic and Naturopath (Joint Select Committee), pp. 652–78, VPRS 241/P/, Unit 14, Transcripts of Committees. Love transcript: 655.
40 PROV, VPRS 241/P/, Unit 14, Transcripts of Committees. Love transcript: 655.
41 Romney Smeeton interview by author, 230; Hutchins interview by author, 173; Brian Munns interview by author, January 9, 2015 transcript in Strachan, *Healing Hands*, 117–19: 118; Therese Vahland interview by author, 81; Bettye Le Marquand interview by author, 96, all transcripts in Strachan, *Healing Hands.*
42 Cec Capon interview by author, transcript in Strachan, *Healing Hands,* 85.
43 Munns, interview by author in *Healing Hands*, 117.
44 Vahland, interview by author in *Healing Hands*, 81.
45 Sells, interview by Shirley Strachan, February 24, 2018.
46 Robert Lucy, "Myorthotics," Training Video, 2.30–3.05 (Sydney: College of Somatic Studies, 1991).
47 Columbia College of Osteopathy, *Home Study Course in Osteopathy* (Chicago, IL: Columbia College of Osteopathy, 1902), 7–8.
48 Lust, ed., *Universal Naturopathic Encyclopaedia,* 800; Brightside Sanatorium operated as a home for epilepsy sufferers between 1910 and 1915 under Marc Blochwitz.
49 Louis Khune, *Neo-naturopathy, a New Science of Healing* (Butler, NJ: Benedict Lust MD, ND, 1917), 311.
50 A. P. Davis, *Neuropathy* (Cincinnati, Ohio: F L Rowe, 1909), 8.
51 A. P. Davis, *Neuropathy Illustrated, the Philosophy and Practical Application of Drugless Healing* (Long Beach, CA: Grave and Hersey, 1915), 4.
52 A. P. Davis, *Osteopathy Illustrated* (Cincinnati, Ohio: Fred L. Rowe, 1899), 603, 638 and 757.
53 William Havard, "Neuropathy," in *Universal Naturopathic Encyclopaedia*, ed. Lust, 702–7.
54 F. W. Collins, *The Naturopathic Method of Reducing Dislocations after the Great French Physician LeGrange* (Newark, NJ: United States School of Naturopathy, 1924); Collins, *The Dullmage System of Pelvic Adjusting.*
55 Thomas T. Lake, "Philosophy and Principles of Neuropathy," Book 1, Chapter 2 in Lake, *Treatment by Neuropathy and the Encyclopedia of Physical and Manipulative Therapeutics.*
56 Lake, *Treatment by Neuropathy and The Encyclopedia of Physical and Manipulative Therapeutics*, chapter VI.
57 M. E. Yergin, *This Book Is Mine* (Newyark, NJ: Dr. M. Erskine Yergin, 1925), entry 1059- Neuropathy.
58 Yergin, *This Book Is Mine.*
59 Yergin, *This Book Is Mine.*
60 Yergin, *This Book is Mine.*
61 Davis, *Neuropathy Illustrated*, 27.
62 Kevin Neave interview by Vicki Mechner, March 14, 2003.
63 Brian Anderson interview by author, March 1, 2015, transcript in Strachan, *Healing Hands*, 98–103: 99.
64 Strachan, *Healing Hands*, 101.
65 Smeeton interview by author, transcript in Strachan, *Healing Hands*, 229.
66 Brian Munns interview by author, transcript in Strachan, *Healing Hands*, 117.
67 Image available at the Museum of Osteopathic Medicine, Kirksville, Missouri catalogue number [1999.08.01].

68 Rene Horwood interview by Ron Phelan July 15, 1998 transcript extract by Phelan in Strachan, *Healing Hands*, 34; Horwood interview by Phelan, July 15, 1998, notes by author.
69 Dewandchand Varma, *The Human Machine and Its Forces* (London: Health for All Publishing), 1937.
70 PROV, VPRS 3253/P1/, Unit 50, McAlister transcript, 3426; Ward Inquiry Report, appendix R.
71 *Natural Therapeutics* (Melbourne: Australian Chiropractors' Osteopaths' and Naturopathic Physicians Association Limited, 196-?).
72 Ryan, "Working alongside Tom Bowen," transcript by author in Strachan *Healing Hands*, 242.
73 Romney Smeeton interview by author, transcript in Strachan, *Healing Hands*, 225.
74 Devereaux et al., *History of the Sydney College of Chiropractic*, 187.
75 Smeeton interview by author, transcript in Strachan, *Healing Hands*, 229.
76 John Garner interview by author, in Strachan, *Healing Hands*, 42.
77 Garner interview by author, in Strachan, *Healing Hands*, 42.
78 Garner interview by author, in Strachan, *Healing Hands*, 42.
79 Emmons Rutledge Booth, *History of Osteopathy and Twentieth Century Medical Practice* (Cincinnati, USA: Jennings and Graham, 1905), 81, accessed June 1, 2016, http://archive.org/details/historyofosteopa00bootuoft.
80 Joseph Keating Jr, "A Hundred Years Ago in Chiropractic," accessed March 20, 2018, http://www.chiroweb.com/archives/16/09/11.html; Joseph Keating Jr, "Show Me Chiropractic," *Dynamic Chiropractic* 23, no. 5 (February 26, 2005), accessed March 20, 2018, http://www.dynamicchiropractic.com/mpacms/dc/article.php?id=50095.
81 Davis, *Neuropathy, New Science of Drugless Healing*, 8.
82 Davis, *Neuropathy Illustrated*, 4.
83 Havard, "Neuropathy," 705.
84 Davis, *Neuropathy Illustrated*, 183.
85 Davis, *Neuropathy Illustrated*, 184–85.
86 Havard, "Neuropathy," 705.
87 Havard, "Neuropathy," 705.
88 Gerald and Coleen Arnold personal communication to author.
89 Smeeton personal communication to author.
90 "History" Berry metho.
91 See biographical entries at appendix one.
92 Ryan, "Working alongside Tom Bowen," 241.
93 Gary Bovine, "Blantyre Bonesetter, William Rae's Rise to Fame in the Popular Press," *Scottish Medical Journal* 57 (2012): 103–6.
94 Ante Hernesniemi, "Presentation of Bonesetter-Patient Collaboration through Positiographical Analysis" (Medical Thesis, University of Oulu, 1999), chapter 6, 116, accessed March 27, 2018, http://www.researchgate.net/publication/23153681.
95 Kevin Neave interview by author, transcript in Strachan, *Healing Hands*, 219.
96 Kevin Neave interview by author, transcript in Strachan, *Healing Hands*, 219.
97 Phil Dower, interview by author in *Healing Hands*, 121 and John Garner interview by author, in Strachan, *Healing Hands*, 39.
98 Davis, *Neuropathy Illustrated*, 472.
99 F.W. Collins, *The Original Moves Taught by Andrew Taylor Still to Dr Charles F. Haverin*, 9th ed. (Mokelumne Hill, CA: Health Research Books, n.d.).
100 *Natures Path to Health*, November–December 1937, 39.
101 Andrew Taylor Still, *Philosophy and Mechanical Principles* (Kansas City, MO: Hudson Kimberley Pub Co, 1902), 40.

102 Still, *Philosophy and Mechanical Principles.*
103 Smeeton interview by author, 229; Ryan, "Working alongside Tom Bowen," 242.
104 Edmonds interview by author, 71.
105 Ryan, "Working alongside Tom Bowen," 243.
106 Ryan, "Working alongside Tom Bowen," 250.
107 Janse, Houser and Wells, "Reflex and Pressure Technics," chapter IV, 494–511.
108 Columbia College of Osteopathy, *Home Study Course in Osteopathy* (Chicago, IL: Columbia College of Osteopathy, 1902), 6.
109 Ryan, "Working alongside Tom Bowen," 249; John Upledger, *Craniosacral Therapy* (Berkley, CA: North Atlantic Books, 2001), 12.
110 Hutchins, interview by the author, in Strachan, *Healing Hands*, 175.
111 Hutchins, interview by the author, in Strachan, *Healing Hands*, 175.
112 Hutchins, interview by the author, in Strachan, *Healing Hands*, 173.
113 Hutchins, interview by the author, in Strachan, *Healing Hands*, 173.
114 Bettye LeMarquand interview by author, April 16, 2015, transcript in Strachan, *Healing Hands*, 95.
115 Smeeton personal communication to author.
116 Ryan, "Working alongside Tom Bowen," 249.
117 Ryan, "Working alongside Tom Bowen," 249.
118 "Cranial Osteopathy," accessed December 2, 2018, http://osteodoc.com/cranial-osteopathy/.
119 William Sutherland, *The Cranial Bowl* (Los Angeles, CA: Free Press Company, University of California, 1939).
120 John Upledger, *Craniosacral Therapy* (Berkley, CA: North Atlantic Books, 2001), 60–66 and 67–69.
121 Devereaux et al., *History of the Sydney College of Chiropractic*, 368–72, 379–82.
122 *Natural Therapeutics*; Note research has indicated the publication date would post-date 1971 when the Victorian branch was formed and this document was created for the government enquiries of the early 1970s.
123 Pamela Snider and Roger Newman Turner, "Nature Cure in Europe: The Transatlantic Journey from Pragmatism to Principles," *Naturopathic Doctors News and Reviews*, October 2, 2010; Carolann Bailey-Lloyd, "Neuromuscular Therapy," *Massage Magazine*, November 16, 2008.
124 Collins, *Original Osteopathic Moves Taught by Dr Andrew Taylor Still to Doctor Charles Haverin, 5.*
125 "Home Study Course of Naturopathy – Osteopathy Lesson XXII, Pt II," *Natures Path to Health*, November–December, 1937, 39.
126 "Home Study Course of Naturopathy – Osteopathy Lesson XXII, Pt II."
127 Collins, *The Dullmage System of Pelvic Adjusting*, 1.
128 Collins, *The Dullmage System of Pelvic Adjusting*, 1.
129 Collins, *The Dullmage System of Pelvic Adjusting*, 6.
130 Chaitow, *Naturopathic Physical Medicine,* 70.
131 Chaitow, *Naturopathic Physical Medicine,* 70.
132 Chaitow, *Naturopathic Physical Medicine*, 300–1.
133 Chaitow, *Naturopathic Physical Medicine*, 70–71.
134 Davis, *Neuropathy Illustrated*, 141.
135 Image in the Collection of the Museum of Osteopathic Medicine, Kirksville, MO [1975.67.02.02].
136 Andrew Taylor Still, *Philosophy of Osteopathy*, 1946 Reprint (Kirksville, MO: A.T. Still, 1899), 21.
137 Chaitow, *Naturopathic Physical Medicine*, 71.
138 Chaitow, *Naturopathic Physical Medicine*, 70.
139 Neave notes of meeting by Mechner; Smeeton interview by author, 227–28.
140 Capon interview by author, in Strachan, *Healing Hands*, 88; Tattersall interview by author, January 9, 2015, transcript in Strachan, *Healing Hands*, 6.

141 McPherson interview by author, in Strachan, *Healing Hands*, 109.
142 McPherson interview by author, in Strachan, *Healing Hands*, 301.
143 Ryan, "Working alongside Tom Bowen," 250.
144 Still, *Osteopathy Research and Practice*, 25.
145 Edmonds interview by author, in Strachan, *Healing Hands*, 69.
146 Smeeton personal communication to author.
147 Davis, *Neuropathy*, 627.
148 Andrew Taylor Still, *Philosophy and Mechanical Principles of Osteopathy* (Kansas City, MO: Hudson Kimberley, 1902), 179, 241.
149 Edmonds interview by author, in Strachan, *Healing Hands,* 67.
150 Vahland interview by author, in Strachan, *Healing Hands*, 84; Smeeton personal communication to the author; Charles E. Farr, "Strangulation of the Undescended Testes," in *Annals of Surgery*, Vol. XLVI, Lewis Stephen Pilcher (London etc: Cassell and Company, 1907), 849, 838–52.
151 Smeeton personal communication to the author.
152 Smeeton personal communication to the author.
153 Bruno J. Chikly, "Manual Techniques Addressing the Lymphatic System: Origins and Development," *Journal American Osteopath Association* 105, no. 10(2005): 457–64.
154 G. D. Hulett, *Textbook of the Principles of Osteopathy*, 5th ed. (A.T. Still Research Institute, 1922), 149.
155 Smeeton interview by author, 228.
156 Murray, *In Search*, 166.
157 Dain Tasker, *Principles of Osteopathy* (Los Angeles, CA: Bireley and Elson Printing Co, 1916), 442.
158 Chaitow with Delany, *Modern Neuromuscular Techniques*, 19–21.
159 Andrea Rabagliati, *On Some Symptoms Which Simulate Disease of Pelvic Organs in Women and Their Treatment by Auto Piesto Kinetics* (New York: William Hood and Co, 1895); Andrea Rabagliati *Initis, Congestion of the Connective Tissues Pioneers of Manual Therapy Volume II* (Great Britain: Masterworks International, 2012).
160 Rabagliati, *Initis*, 105.
161 "Obituary Andrea Rabagliati," *British Medical Journal*, December 10, 1930: 1067.
162 Lust ed., *Encyclopaedia*, 1075.
163 Thomas Dummer, *The Lief Neuromuscular Technique* (Maidstone, Kent, 1991), 1 (unpublished).
164 Dewandchand Varma, *The Human Machine and Its Forces* (London: Health for All Publishing, 1937), 18 reproduced in Phil Young, ed., *Pranotherapy and the Origins of Polarity Therapy and European Neuromuscular Techniques,* by Dewandchand Varma and Dr Randolph Stone, Pioneers of Manual Medicine, Vol. 1 (Great Britain: MWI Publishing, 2011), 45–47 (note reproduction is inserted between this pagination).
165 Varma, *The Human Machine and Its Forces*, 19–24.
166 J. H. Kellogg, *Art of Massage* (Battle Creek, MI: Modern Medicine Publishing Co, 1895), 164.

Bibliography

Newspapers

"Advertising." *Morning Bulletin Rockhampton*, September 7, 1936: 2 (col.2). Accessed November 17, 2024. http://nla.gov.au/nla.news-article54973782.
"Advertising." *Mirror, Perth*, October 21, 1939, 22 (col.6). Accessed November 17, 2024. http://nla.gov.au/nla.news-article75865425.

"Advertising." "F G Roberts, ND DO." *Sydney Morning Herald (Sydney),* December 1, 1945: 45 (col.1). Accessed November 17, 2024. http://nla.gov.au/nla.news-article27921891.

"Advertising." "Shops, Factories &c, To Let." *Argus* February 11, 1937: 2 (col.7). Accessed November 17, 2024. http://nla.gov.au/nla.news-article11967941.

"Manipulative Surgery." *Maryborough Chronicle, Wide Bay and Burnett Advertiser (Qld),* August 17, 1935: 10. Accessed November 17, 2024. http://nla.gov.au/nla.news-article149964460.

"Neuropath Fined for Using the Title 'Doctor'." *Brisbane Telegraph,* April 5, 1951: 2. Accessed November 17, 2024. http://nla.gov.au/nla.news-article212087365.

Primary Sources

Allen, Pat. Interview by author. Transcript in Strachan, Shirley. *Healing Hands, Unsung Voices, Thomas Ambrose Bowen Osteopath (1916–1982).* United Kingdom: Cloister House Press, 2016.

Ancestry.com [database on-line]. Provo, UT, USA: Ancestry.com Operations, Inc. *Australia Electoral Rolls 1903–1980.*

Capon, Cec. Interview by author. Transcript in Strachan, Shirley. *Healing Hands, Unsung Voices, Thomas Ambrose Bowen Osteopath (1916–1982).* United Kingdom: Cloister House Press, 2016.

Collins, F. W. *The Dullmage System of Pelvic Adjusting.* n.p., n.d. Reprint. Pomeroy: Health Research Books, 1993.

Collins, F. W. *The Naturopathic Method of Reducing Dislocations after the Great French Physician LeGrange.* Newark, NJ: United States School of Naturopathy, 1924. Accessed November 17, 2024. http://www.mcmillinmedia.com/eamt/files/collins/naturo.htm.

Collins, F. W. *The Original Moves Taught by Andrew Taylor Still to Dr Charles F. Haverin.* 9th ed. Mokelumne Hill, CA: Health Research, n.d.

Columbia College of Osteopathy. *Home Study Course in Osteopathy.* Chicago, IL: Columbia College of Osteopathy, 1902. Accessed November 17, 2024. https://archive.org/details/homestudycourse00ostegoog/mode/2up.

Davis, A. P. *Osteopathy Illustrated.* Cincinnati, Ohio: Fred L. Rowe, 1899. Accessed November 17, 2024. https://archive.org/details/osteopathyillust00daviuoft.

Davis, A. P. *Neuropathy, New Science of Drugless Healing Amply Illustrated and Explained.* Cincinnati, Ohio: F. L. Rowe, 1909. Accessed November 17, 2024. https://archive.org/details/neuropathy00davigoog.

Davis, A. P. *Neuropathy Illustrated, the Philosophy and Practical Application of Drugless Healing.* Long Beach, CA: Grave and Hersey, 1915. Accessed November 17, 2024. https://archive.org/details/neuropathyillust0000andr.

Dower, Phil. Interview by author. Transcript in Strachan, Shirley. *Healing Hands, Unsung Voices, Thomas Ambrose Bowen 1916–1982, Osteopath.* United Kingdom: Cloister House Press, 2016.

Edmonds, Heather. Interview by author. Transcript in Strachan, Shirley. *Healing Hands, Unsung Voices, Thomas Ambrose Bowen 1916–1982, Osteopath.* United Kingdom: Cloister House Press, 2016.

Farr, Charles E. "Strangulation of the Undescended Testes." In *Annals of Surgery,* Vol. XLVI, Lewis Stephen Pilcher (London etc: Cassell and Company, 1907). Accessed November 17, 2024. http://archive.org/details/p2annalsofsurgery58philuoft.

Garner, John. Interview by author. Transcript in Strachan, Shirley. *Healing Hands, Unsung Voices, Thomas Ambrose Bowen 1916–1982 Osteopath.* United Kingdom: Cloister House Press, 2016.

Havard, William. "Neuropathy." In *Universal Naturopathic Encyclopaedia and Buyers Guide 1918–1919*, edited by Benedict Lust, 702–7. Butler, NJ: Benedict Lust MD, ND, 1918. Accessed November 17, 2024.

Hernesniemi, Antii. "Presentation of Bonesetter-Patient Collaboration through Positiographical Analysis." Medical thesis, University of Oulu, 1999. Accessed November 17, 2024. hhttp://www.researchgate.net/publication/231536811.

Horwood, Rene. Interview by Ron Phelan, September 11, 1998 transcribed by author November 15–30, 2018.

Hulett, G. D. *Textbook of the Principles of Osteopathy*. Kirksville, MO: Journal Printing Company, 1906. Accessed November 17, 2024. https://archive.org/details/textbookofprinci00hule.

Hutchins, Greg. Interview by author. Transcript in Strachan, Shirley. *Healing Hands, Unsung Voices, Thomas Ambrose Bowen 1916–1982, Osteopath*. United Kingdom: Cloister House Press, 2016.

Kellogg, J. H. *Art of Massage*. Battle Creek, MI: Modern Medicine Publishing Co, 1895. Accessed November 17, 2024. https://archive.org/details/in.ernet.dli.2015.510534.

Khune, Louis. *Neo-naturopathy, A New Science of Healing*. Butler, NJ: Benedict Lust MD, ND, 1917. Accessed November 17, 2024. https://archive.org/stream/neonaturopathyne00kuhn.

Lake, Thomas T. "Philosophy and Principles of Neuropathy." In *Treatment by Neuropathy and the Encyclopedia of Physical and Manipulative Therapeutics*, compiled by Thomas T. Lake, Book 1, chapter 2. 1946 republished online. Accessed November 17, 2024. http://www.mcmillinmedia.com/eamt/files/lake/lakecont.html.

Lake, Thomas T. *Treatment by Neuropathy and The Encyclopedia of Physical and Manipulative Therapeutics*. Chapter VI, 1946 republished online. Accessed November 17, 2024. https://www.mcmillinmedia.com/eamt/files/lake/lakecont.html.

Le Marquand, Bettye. Interview by author. Transcript in Strachan, Shirley. *Healing Hands, Unsung Voices, Thomas Ambrose Bowen 1916–1982, Osteopath*. United Kingdom: Cloister House Press, 2016.

Lucy, Robert. *Myorthotics*. Sydney: College of Somatic Studies, 1991.

Lucy, Robert. *Myorthotics*. Training Video. Sydney: College of Somatic Studies, 1991.

Lust, Benedict, *Universal Naturopathic Encyclopaedia and Buyers Guide 1918–1919*. Butler, NJ: Benedict Lust MD, ND, 1918. Accessed November 17, 2024. https://archive.org/details/universalnaturop00lust.

McPherson, Rob. Interview by author. Transcript in Strachan, Shirley. *Healing Hands, Unsung Voices, Thomas Ambrose Bowen 1916–1982, Osteopath*. United Kingdom: Cloister House Press, 2016.

Munns, Brian. Interview by author. Transcript in Strachan, Shirley. *Healing Hands, Unsung Voices, Thomas Ambrose Bowen 1916–1982, Osteopath*. United Kingdom: Cloister House Press, 2016.

Natural Therapeutics (Melbourne: Australian Chiropractors, Osteopaths and Naturopathic Physicians Association Limited, 196-?).

Neave, Kevin. Interview by Vicki Mechner. March 14, 2003. Transcript in possession of author.

Neave, Kevin. Interview by author. Transcript in Strachan, Shirley. *Healing Hands, Unsung Voices, Thomas Ambrose Bowen 1916–1982, Osteopath*. United Kingdom: Cloister House Press, 2016.

"Obituary Andrea Rabagliati." *British Medical Journal*, December 10, 1930, 1067 Accessed November 17, 2024. http://www.bmj.com/content/2/3650/1067.2

PROV. Osteopathy, Chiropractic and Naturopathy Committee, VPRS 16439/P1, Unit 13, Committee Records, Cogan transcript: 428–35.

PROV. Osteopathy, Chiropractic and Naturopath Joint Select Committee pp. 783–938, VPRS 241/P/, Unit 14. Osteopathy, Chiropractic and Naturopath Joint Select Committee, transcripts of Committee, Blackmore transcript: 857–61.

PROV. Report and evidence Osteopathy Committee (Pt.1–4), 27/11/975 (Pt. 2) 2261, VPRS 3253/P1/, Unit 47. Original papers tabled in the Legislative Assembly, transcripts of proceedings, Bowen transcript: 672–78.

PROV. Report and evidence Osteopathy Committee (Pt.1–4), 27/11/975 (Pt. 2) 2261, VPRS 3253/P1/, Unit 50, Original papers tabled in the Legislative Assembly, transcripts of proceedings, McAlister transcript: 3424–60.

Rabagliati, Andrea. *On Some Symptoms Which Simulate Disease of Pelvic Organs in Women and Their Treatment by Auto Piesto Kinetics.* New York: William Hood and Co, 1895. Accessed November 17, 2024. http://archive.org/stream/onsomesymptomswh00raba.

Rabagliati, Andrea. *Initis, Congestion of the Connective Tissues Pioneers of Manual Therapy Volume II.* Great Britain: Masterworks International, 2012.

Ryan, Kevin. "Working alongside Tom Bowen." Presentation to National Conference of Bowen Interest Groups, August 21, 1999. Transcript in Strachan, Shirley. *Healing Hands, Unsung Voices, Thomas Ambrose Bowen 1916–1982, Osteopath.* United Kingdom: Cloister House Press, 2016.

Smeeton, Romney. Interview by author. Transcript in Strachan, Shirley. *Healing Hands, Unsung Voices, Thomas Ambrose Bowen 1916–1982, Osteopath.* United Kingdom: Cloister House Press, 2016.

Still, Andrew Taylor. *Philosophy of Osteopathy.* Kirksville, MO: A. T. Still, 1899. 1946 Reprint. Accessed November 17, 2024. https://archive.org/details/64340710R.nlm.nih.gov.

Still, Andrew Taylor. *Philosophy and Mechanical Principles of Osteopathy.* Kansas City, MO: Hudson Kimberley, 1902. Accessed November 17, 2024. https://archive.org/details/philosophymecha00stil.

Still, Andrew Taylor. *Osteopathy Research and Practice.* Kirksville, MO: Andrew Taylor Still, 1910, 25. Accessed November 17, 2024. http://archive.org/stream/osteopathyresea00stilgoog.

Sutherland, William. *The Cranial Bowl.* Los Angeles, CA: Free Press Company, University of California, 1939.

Tasker, Dain. *Principles of Osteopathy.* Los Angeles, CA: Bireley and Elson Printing Co, 1916. Accessed November 17, 2024. https://archive.org/stream/principlesosteop00taskiala/principlesosteop00taskiala_djvu.txt.

Tattersall, Barry. Interview by author. Transcript in Strachan, Shirley. *Healing Hands, Unsung Voices, Thomas Ambrose Bowen 1916–1982, Osteopath.* United Kingdom: Cloister House Press, 2016.

Vahland, Therese. Interview by author. Transcript in Strachan, Shirley, *Healing Hands, Unsung Voices, Thomas Ambrose Bowen Osteopath (1916–1982).* Great Britain: Cloister House Press, 2016.

Ward Inquiry Report – full title – Victoria Parliament, Osteopathy, Chiropractic and Naturopathy Committee, et al. *Report from the Osteopathy, Chiropractic and Naturopathy Committee: Together with Appendices.* Melbourne: C. H. Rixon, Government Printer, 1975. Accessed November 17, 2024. http://www6.austlii.edu.au/au/other/vic/VicLASelCPubInq/1975/1.pdf.

Secondary Sources

Bailey-Lloyd, Carolann. "Neuromuscular Therapy." *Massage Magazine*, November 16, 2008. Accessed November 17, 2024. http://www.massagemag.com/neuromuscular-therapy-3050/.

Booth, Emmons Rutledge. *History of Osteopathy and Twentieth Century Medical Practice*. Cincinnati, USA: Jennings and Graham, 1905. Accessed November 17, 2024. https://archive.org/details/historyofosteopa00bootuoft.

Bovine, Gary. "Blantyre Bonesetter, William Rae's Rise to Fame in the Popular Press." *Scottish Medical Journal* 57 (2012): 103–6. Accessed November 17, 2024. https://doi.org/10.1258/smj.2012.012008.

Chaitow, Leon, ed. *Naturopathic Physical Medicine*. Edinburgh: Churchill Livingstone, 2008.

Chaitow, Leon with Judith Delaney. *Modern Neuromuscular Techniques*. New York: Churchill Livingstone, 1996.

Chikly, B. J. "Manual Techniques Addressing the Lymphatic System: Origins and Development." *The Journal of the American Osteopathic Association* 105, no. 10 (October 2005): 457–64. PMID: 16314678.

Columbia College of Osteopathy. *Home Study Course in Osteopathy*. Chicago, IL: Columbia College of Osteopathy, 1902. Accessed November 17, 2024. http://archive.org/details/homestudycourse00ostegoog.

Devereaux, Edwin, Brian O'Reilly, and John Cice. *History of the Sydney College of Chiropractic*. Sydney: Macquarie Lighthouse Press, 2012.

Dummer, Tom. *Lief Neuromuscular Technique*. Maidstone, Kent, 1991 (unpublished).

Flexner, Abraham. *Medical Education in the United States and Canada*. New York City: Carnegie Foundation for the Advancement of Medical Teaching, 1910, 258. Accessed November 17, 2024. https://archive.org/details/medicaleducatio00flexgoog.

"Graduate News from Arthur Wright our First Graduate, Class of 64." *Chirobiz* 3, no. 2 (July 2010). Accessed March 12, 2017, http://archive.chiro.mq.edu.au/Alumni/ChirobisJuly10.pdf (note website carries a not secure warning now)

Janse, Joseph, R. H. Houser, and B. F. Wells. "Reflex and Pressure Technics." In *Chiropractic Technic,* chapter IV, 494–511. 1978. Reprint. Chicago, IL: National College of Chiropractic.

Keating, Joseph Jr. "Show Me Chiropractic." *Dynamic Chiropractic* 23, no. 5 (February 26, 2005). Accessed November 17, 2024. http://www.dynamicchiropractic.com/mpacms/dc/article.php?id=50095.

"Modern Acupuncture-Neuropathy." *Journal of the International Congress of Acupuncture and Moxibustion* (Tokyo: Japanese Acupuncture and Moxibustion Society). Listed in *Natural Therapeutics* under "Acupuncture" with no other details but believed to be published as part of several articles in the journal in 1965.

"Philosophy of Natural Therapeutics." In *Natural Therapeutics*. Melbourne: Australian Chiropractors, Osteopaths and Naturopathic Physicians Association, 196-?

Skilbeck, Neil. "Typical Day Working with Tom Bowen." *Vic Bowen News* 1, no. 2 (May 1998): 3.

Snider, Pamela, and Roger Newman Turner. "Nature Cure in Europe: The Transatlantic Journey from Pragmatism to Principles." *Naturopathic Doctors News and Reviews*, October 2, 2010. Accessed November 17, 2024. http://ndnr.com/education-web-articles/nature-cure-in-europe-the-transatlantic-journey-from-pragmatism-to-principles/.

Still, Andrew Taylor. *Philosophy of Osteopathy*. Kirksville, MO: A.T. Still, 1899, 21. 1946 Reprint.

Still, Andrew Taylor. *Osteopathy Research and Practice*. Kirksville, MO: A T Still, 1910. Accessed November 17, 2024. http://archive.org/stream/osteopathyresea00stilgoog.

Upledger, John. *Craniosacral Therapy*. Berkley, CA: North Atlantic Books, 2001.

Varma, Dewandchand. *The Human Machine and Its Forces*. London: Health for All Publishing, n.d. Reproduced in *Pranotherapy and the Origins of Polarity Therapy and European Neuromuscular Techniques, by Dewandchand Varma and Dr Randolph Stone, Pioneers of Manual Medicine, Volume 1,* edited by Phil Young. Great Britain: MWI Publishing, 2011.

Walker, B. F. "F G Roberts Memorial Address." Murdoch University Research Portal, 2015. Accessed November 17, 2024. https://researchportal.murdoch.edu.au/esploro/outputs/conferencePresentation/FG-Roberts-Memorial-Address/991005544101207891.

Websites

Berry Method. "History." Accessed November 17, 2024. https://www.theberrymethod.org/history.

Brightside Sanatorium. Accessed November 17, 2024. http://www.asylumprojects.org/index.php/Bright_Side_Sanitarium.

4 Bowen and the Influence of Saunders

Australia's Herbert Barker

> I recognise that there is room for a difference of opinion as to whether a person who has not passed a theoretical examination can be considered competent to practice massage or osteopathy. There are men who are particularly gifted, whether with animal magnetism or something else, so that they are able to effect many cures where others although apparently equally qualified would fail.
>
> The Hon W J Beckett in Legislative Council, October 15, 1935[1]

Neuropathy in Practice Could Look Like Pressure Movements of Eastern Manual Medicine or German Stress Points

Bowen identified with and expressed his style of practice and symbolism using the knowledge base of osteopathy and this formed the case made in Chapter 3 that Bowen came in contact directly or through intermediaries with the early osteopathic practice of neuropathy. Neuropathy was brought to Australia by the naturopathic pioneers who had trained overseas; namely, the Tasmanian FG Roberts who trained at the London School of Natural Therapeutics (LSNT) and with Benedict Lust's college in the USA and Maurice Blackmore who studied at the British Naturopathic College – concluded to be Stanley Leif's BCN before emigrating to Australia in 1923. The descriptions of neuropathy available from the various American neuropathy schools would indicate that in practical application, it could look like pressure movement/pressure point work of Eastern manual medicine or German pressure work on stress points now called trigger points. In some neuropathy sources such as AP Davis, his work is combined with well-illustrated depictions of osteopathic stretches and lever work. However, these movements to lift pressure off nerves were ostensibly of western and not eastern origin and conceived of within an osteopathic framework and taught by Australia's early naturopathic pioneers. Not all of Bowen's skills and techniques can be sourced to neuropathy and osteopathy and he integrated other influences throughout his formative informal years among football masseurs and from later osteopathic developments in his formal clinic years.

DOI: 10.4324/9781003602125-5

Bowen the Football Masseur and Ability to Rectify Ligament Problems

For instance, from the outset before he set up in business, Bowen had the ability to deal swiftly with injured and strained ligaments on the football and sports field and kept the players in play. His patients understood this to be putting things back in place, ligaments and nerves. Bowen was connected with Victorian Football League (VFL, now AFL) under-eighteens football and before going into formal business in 1959 had made the acquaintance of Ernest Saunders a senior VFL trainer and before Saunders' death in 1951. Later in his career in the 1970s, Bowen was training Melbourne VFL trainers with masseur friend and football trainer Ron Garner.[2] This chapter will focus on Bowen's early period that involved contact with the legendary older-generation football masseur Ernest (Ernie) Malcolm Clement Saunders (1880–1951). Posthumously, because of this contact and Saunders' stature, Saunders not only has been erroneously popularised as Bowen's mentor but also is claimed to have introduced Bowen to Japanese acupressure techniques, leading to assumptions that Eastern Medicine was foundational to Bowen's work. This chapter focuses on evidence that highlights the skills that led Saunders to be regarded in parliament akin to the famous English bonesetter Herbert Barker. The research presented in this chapter also leads to debunking claims of Saunders and Eastern medicine influences and focuses on Saunders' imparting his legendary ligament and joint aligning skills. Chapter 8 will look at other famous football masseurs of Bowen's own generation, some of whom also went on to self-identify as osteopaths and others who were community legends and did not establish businesses, but received donations and were renowned as gifted healers, masseurs or chiropractors. Some of these men entertained ideas and demonstrated expert practise addressing nerves issues that resonate with Bowen, though none delivered their techniques within an osteopathic frame and recognisable osteopathic professionalism like Bowen did.

Training Standards of Officially Registered Masseurs: Swedish Massage

To provide context for what is known of the techniques of these legendary masseurs and their approach, it is worth considering the training standards of the formally qualified and government-registered masseurs of the time. Many of these individuals operated in football clubs too. Fay's book *Scientific massage for Athletes* written first around 1905 describes him as 'the Australian Authority on massage for athletes'.[3] Massage was to remove wastes and bring nutrients to muscles.[4] Although he did not credit sources, Fay, a former athlete, essentially described the principles and techniques of Swedish or Classic massage which involve effleurage (stroking), frictions (rubbing), petrissage (kneading) and tapotment (striking). Striking can encompass the stimulating moves of cupping, hacking and pounding. Vibrations can be added. These movements were core to massage writings of the nineteenth and twentieth centuries, many of them by early medics and nature cure doctors who wrote knowledgeably on the subject. There is some debate regarding the originator of these techniques as discussed by Calvert.[5] The techniques now known as Swedish massage are usually attributed to Ling who pioneered scientific approaches to physical culture, leading to Swedish gymnastics and movement cures. Calvert drew on research of Emil Kleen and Richard Hael to conclude it was Ling's follower, the Dutch practitioner Johan Georg Metzger (1838–1909), who deserves the credit for developing massage therapy as a standalone healing art.[6] Lauren Berry was influenced by 'Swedish movements' from a Finnish source and Ernest Kjellberg the Swede was trained at the Wahroonga Sanatorium in Sydney and also utilised Swedish massage methods at his healing centre in Millaa Millaa.[7] The use of targeted pressure and thrusts on points or reflex segments as evident in neuropathy is absent in Swedish or classic massage.

When Saunders was twenty-seven years old, the members of the new Australian Massage Association (AMA) sought legislation and 'Swedish movements' were the hallmark of professionalism.[8] A major influence on the AMA was Victoria-based Alfred (Alf) Peters (1871–1944) who served as president of the Old Players and Playgoers Association.[9] Peters' 1890 book also references the Swedish movements.[10] His Institute featured contemporary appliances for physiotherapy.[11] This reveals the adoption of Swedish massage and Western methods in the network of football masseurs formally trained and accredited for association membership. A 1906 image of The Council of Interstate Delegates of the AMA features five Germans, and includes Herr Best (Treasurer), Herr Schuch (Sydney), Miss McAuley, Dr Hugh Murray, Mr Teepoo Hall (secretary), Herr Grund, Mr Alfred Peters, Miss Develaqua (Adelaide), Herr Nystrom, Dr Springthorpe (President), Miss Armstrong (Sydney) and Hugo Leschen (Adelaide).[12] Leschen had trained at the Dresden Royal Institution of Gymnastics and learned massage in 1890 from Professor Von Reyher in Germany.[13] Leschen is claimed in the press to be the founder of the AMA.[14] Football masseurs benefitted from Leschen's instruction in South Australia around 1908 but the styles of massage described are Swedish with the principle of massage towards the heart.[15] Hodges of North Adelaide described Leschen as 'the best masseur in Australia'.[16] Hot towels and showers were considered improvements.[17] Leschen's colleague Teepoo Hall (1856–1909) is also recognised as the founder of the Australian Massage Association and pioneer of physiotherapy in Australia.[18] Hall is pictured teaching in 1905.[19] Hall had practised massage in military hospitals in colonial India and Swedish exercises are mentioned.[20] Like Leschen, Hall worked as an honorary football masseur, in his case to Port Melbourne Football Club.[21] Ernie Saunders was backdoored into registered status in December 1935 without formal training and the parliamentary discussion in the lead-up focused on his ligament manipulation skills. When the later titled Massage and Physiotherapy Association objected to the proposals for Ernie's son George to also be registered without qualifications, the training material submitted to the government continued to uphold Swedish massage.[22] Together this research reveals a strong picture of the adoption of Swedish massage and Western methods in the network of professionally accredited masseurs, many of whom worked with football clubs.

Oral Histories of Saunders' Influence on Bowen

Proof of contact between Saunders and Bowen originates from two oral history sources – Keith Davis DC, one of Bowen's clinic observers in the 1970s (who credited Bowen's success to Saunders) and Bowen's daughters. With the latter, there are issues with the remembered timeline of contact and the places of contact as these also introduce another man, the osteopath Alister McAlister discussed in Chapter 7. Among Bowen's college-trained observers, Keith Davis DC is interesting because he had a genuine interest in prominent lay healers in the community and reportedly is the only one who struck up exchanges with Bowen about Saunders. The close connection of Roberts' graduates to the Blackmores concern is illustrated by the previous membership of Davis DC of Blackmores NANOC and he originally used Blackmores remedies in his naturopathic prescribing before switching to the Sydney-based Martin and Clarke company.[23] By the time of the 1973, Ward Inquiry, Davis bridged the old and emerging regulated professional world and was a member of both ACONPAL and the UCA (later to become the UCAA from 1975).

Davis learned of Bowen's contact with Ernie Saunders directly from Bowen – specifically in relation to a technique that Saunders was strict about which involved lumbar moves he called 'putting the stoppers on' before a treatment began. These were medial moves on both sides of lumbar 3. Davis also met a contemporary of Saunders, Leslie (Les) Edward Dettman (1888–1972) eight years junior to Saunders. Dettman is the sole source of the account of going to America with Saunders to learn Japanese acupoints between the wars.[24] This has resulted in popularised claims of Saunders passing knowledge of Eastern medicine to his protégés. The assumption of Saunders as Bowen's mentor does not stand up to historical scrutiny when his style of work described next is compared to Bowen's described in Chapter 3.

Saunders' Reputation as a Football Masseur and Registration Without Credentials

Ernie Saunders was a legend and enjoyed a significant profile in the press and in political circles. He had an association from the early 1900s with Collingwood, South Melbourne, University and Brunswick Football Clubs, before joining Richmond as a trainer in 1923/24, a position held until late 1935, before he resumed it after the Tokyo Olympics were cancelled in 1940. Saunders had attended the 1936 Berlin Olympiad and was approached to attend Tokyo. Massage was regulated last century nationally from the early 1900s and in Victoria from 1922 to 1978. Eligibility provisions in the original act set out requirements for registration of masseurs. A technical issue (and some evidence of discrimination on the part of the secretary of the association who held a masseur role at the same club as Saunders) had resulted in Saunders' application being rejected by the Masseurs Board in 1928. Saunders' autodidact career underwent significant change after he appealed the Board's decision to reject his registration. His standing in treating powerful figures in high places in parliament and the police force, as well as popular sports' heroes, is reflected in the political backing he received that resulted in Saunders' appeal culminating in a Bill being introduced in parliament on July 11, 1935, by the Honourable Henry Bailey MLA. The Bill was to amend Section 10 of the *Masseurs Act* 1928 'to provide for the registration of certain persons as masseurs'. The issue received animated debate in parliament and attentive press coverage.[25] The Honourable R Kilpatrick said, 'they call this "the Saunders Bill"'.[26] After months of deliberations, the Bill became law. The opportunity in 1935 was not a free-for-all. Colonel Harold Cohen was keen to prevent 'mutts' getting through the back door.[27] Parliament had anticipated that the door would be opened to about seven masseurs who were expected to gain entry to the register without being qualified and four of them expected to be football trainers.[28] Along with Saunders who was gazetted first on December 10, 1935, the other football trainers who benefitted from Saunders' case were Henry Ross Sampson (East Brunswick, registered January 9, 1936); Frederick John Wren (1885–1960) (Seddon; masseur to Footscray Football Club, registered March 9, 1936) and Houston Owen Elliston Trappes (1899–post 1977) (Essendon; masseur to Essendon Football Club, registered on May 14, 1936).[29] These men were connected as among the leading trainers of twelve leagues that had formed the Victorian Football League Head Trainers Association formed in 1933. The first formal head trainers' dinner was chaired by Henry (Harry) Sampson.[30] The trainers met in the city so were socially acquainted, but more importantly, Wren, Trappes and Sampson would have been indebted to Saunders as they benefited from his fight in parliament to gain registered professional status. The association of Wren with Footscray is returned to later in the text. Saunders left his role as trainer/masseur to Richmond Football Club and was appointed soon after as honorary masseur to the Australian team for the Berlin Olympiad in 1936.[31] Ernie had been in the running for the Tokyo Olympics in 1940 too, but the Second World War resulted in cancellation.[32] Before Ernie's death in February 1951, and no doubt due to his failing health, his son George had taken over from his father and attended the 1950 Empire Games held in New Zealand. George's own reputation with the Olympic committee was such that another piece of legislation was specially proclaimed in 1957 to also allow him, like his father, to be formally registered as a masseur without the requisite formal qualifications.[33] These special legislative arrangements attest to the talent of father and son at this time.

Evidence of Bowen's Contact With Saunders

Ernie Saunders' case in parliament is useful as alongside newspaper references his style of work can be gauged. Except for evidence of Bowen's skill in swiftly dealing with twisted or injured ligaments on the football field and the implementation of cross-fibre lumbar movements that Ernie called 'stoppers', Saunders' style does not emerge as a match for Bowen's soft tissue style of working at all. Heather Edmonds, Bowen's youngest daughter, asserted that her father's contact was with Saunders senior and not the son George (1914–1981) who was of Bowen's generation.[34] Linked in her mind to her father's visits to Footscray, to meet up with other men, Edmonds indicates that her father's connection with Saunders was short-lived:

> Now, Ernie Saunders, another man and dad, there was definitely three guys who met together in Footscray and I think that would have been in the '50s and they would 'chew the fat' or so I'm told. This happened for a couple of years I think, then dad left the group and developed things on his own. I'm told that happened as his thinking was ahead of the others. So, he broke away from those two guys and did his own thing.[35]

Bowens' contact with Saunders senior logically would have occurred before Ernie's death in early 1951. Saunders' 1950 press profile only featured two stories about treating athletes and his son George attended the Empire Games in New Zealand, which suggests Ernie was slowing down and handing the reins over to his son. This means the 1940s are more plausible than the 1950s as the timescale for the Bowen-Saunders' contact. Edmonds also concurred the contact phase could have been earlier.[36] Bowen's personal circumstances also point to the later 1940s as plausible for connecting with Saunders as he had more freedom when his disapproving father moved out of the McDougall Street Bowen family home to Clarence Street and his eldest children were no longer toddlers and by the late 1940s around five to six years old. Bowen always said he 'found his gift in the war'.[37] The popular narrative is that Bowen found his ability from having to help his wife Jessie who suffered from asthma. In addition, there are two war period scenarios worth highlighting, provided a stimulus and likely opportunities to see masseurs in action and apply his own techniques. Oral history indicates Bowen became active in the 1940s as Bowen was 'good mates' with Jonathon Robert (Bob) McHenry a champion foot runner who ran at the Stawell Gift and other Gift races including Port Fairy in 1947 and winning the 1948 Geelong Gift.[38] McHenry was also a football player for Fitzroy in 1943 and Geelong in 1944 and acted as board director for the Geelong Umpires Football League in 1950. Geelong Football Club went into recess during the war which forced McHenry to play for Fitzroy. McHenry's son, Greg, said Bowen treated his father and this definitely occurred during the war.[39] The other wartime linkage is the presence of both Bowen and later football masseur and Footscray Football Club osteopath Alister (Lal) Graham McAlister (1915–2011) at Mount Martha where both were stationed during the war. McAlister was winning soldier races and had already established a reputation as a talented masseur.[40] McAlister will be returned to in Chapters 7 and 8 as he was living with his parents until 1943 in West Melbourne, just over a kilometre in a straight line from the Footscray Football Club and moved to Moonee Ponds in after his spell as osteopath at Footscray

Football Club between 1960 and 1964. Bowen's daughters also remembered Moonee Ponds as a place visited by their father to meet with others.

Footscray and the Footscray Football Club

The 1940s also make sense as a timeframe for Bowen's contact with Saunders as Fred Wren who benefitted from Saunders' registration was masseur at Footscray where he received most press coverage in the 1940s, though the last entry was as a veteran aged seventy in 1956.[41] Wren died in 1960 and McAlister took over as an osteopath in 1962. Additionally, the Footscray Football Club would have been a select venue for football trainers and progressive masseurs to gather and learn from each other. The club established itself as early as 1931 with a prominent profile. The press stated:

> No club in Australia can boast of better premises than Footscray . . . . What is most impressive, however, is the club's medical room, fitted up by Mr Wren, the club masseur. There is an operating table with perfect lighting facilities. A special apparatus gives special ray treatment. A player badly hurt on the field can be whipped straight into this room and examined or operated upon if necessary by Dr [Kevin] McCarthy, the club's president or any other medical officer present.[42]

These amenities would undoubtedly have been a drawcard to the men backdoored into registration in 1935/36 and they may have collaborated to share ideas to keep abreast of professional developments and present a strong professional image and reputation – especially given the massage association's vehement antipathy to their success. With his registered status since December 1935, there was no impediment to Saunders passing on skills to others in the 1940s. The club medic then was McCarthy a skilled doctor and his role with the team received honourable mention along with other doctors including Dr Piper of Geelong who supported Ernest (Ern) Davie, the Geelong Football Club head trainer. In 1938, Wren was photographed with ray lamps.[43] FG Roberts is credited with bringing ray lamps to Australia after studying in Britain between 1918 and 1920.[44] Wren may be an early adopter in 1938 for football injuries since the next specific press article on their use for bruises, strains and sprains for footballers is dated 1952.[45]

Except for Bowen's passing mention to Keith Davis DC that his practice of using lumbar 'stoppers' was imposed on his thinking from Saunders, it seems odd, given Saunders' standing and celebrity status, that if Saunders was a key influence on Bowen, Bowen solely volunteered mention of him to Davis. Neither the others college-trained nor the attending football masseurs such as Douglas (Doug) Windsor Sells (1936–2019) a younger football masseur who assisted Bowen in the evenings at 283 Latrobe Terrace between 1967 and 1973 knew of Bowen's contact with Saunders. Sells said Saunders was a household name, but had no knowledge at all that Bowen had spent time with him, yet Bowen and Sells often enjoyed a beer together.[46]

Evidence of Saunders' Style

What is known of Saunders' treatment style? The cricketer Donald Bradman is stated in some sources to have suffered from fibrositis (fibromyalgia) and was treated by Saunders in the 1940s. The robustness of Saunders' treatments is evident in Bradman's account of, 'steel like fingers' running down his back and 'agonies' of treatment because Saunders said, 'I believe in nature' and did not use anaesthetic.[47] Despite the pain, Bradman said, 'after my first visit the relief from searing muscle pain was like a draught of ice cold water in a heat wave'.[48] Bradman went on to return to cricket.[49] It is known that Ernie used oils and jealously guarded his secret recipes.[50] A journalist to his clinic after his death revealed his son George also used oils and foments and said, 'the smell of liniment smote me'.[51] In stark contrast to Bowen's oil-free exquisite minimalism and seven-day intervals for treatments, Saunders' work could be intensive running continuously over days.[52] During the parliamentary debate on his registration, Ernie Saunders was reportedly self-taught and in 1935 he said that he learned his craft from 'desultory reading of books'.[53] Later on in 1946, he indicated physiotherapy and massage books.[54] Saunders never mentioned any interest in osteopathy nor neuropathy and there is no evidence whatsoever of him working with spinal segments and reflex or pressure points to influence visceral or other systemic complaints; the reported benefits of his work were entirely musculoskeletal with what was regarded a bone-setting gift to correct twisted ligaments and reset joints.

There is no contest that both Ernie and his son George had standout bone-setting skills in swiftly rectifying ligament injuries and restoring joint mobility. Credence may be given to Muscle Energy Techniques (MET) as Professor John Murtagh said of Ernie's son George Saunders when associated with the Melbourne Football Club in the 1970s and used MET.[55] Saunders could run on the field during a game and rectify a ligament problem on the spot. He 'liked to catch them hot' and Bowen too expressed the necessity of having this kind of injury addressed instantly with similar language.[56] Saunders' treatments for these were fast, one attendee at a game had a limp fixed in ten minutes and another had cartilage treated in 'record time'.[57] Bowen too could successfully address acute injuries swiftly but could also address a chronic problem on the spot. There is an account of when he was in hospital and a male in the next bed to him had a problem knee awaiting medical attention and Bowen reportedly got out of bed, attended to it and successfully addressed the problem quickly without any fuss.[58] The parliamentary debate in 1935 and press articles on Saunders as a masseur in the lead-up to registration confirms Saunders' abilities. Dr Shields said of Saunders, 'He is especially skilful in those cases . . . more particularly of derangement of the cartilage of the knee'.[59] Saunders was attributed with 'sensitive fingers' for putting cartilage back in place.[60] Other cases were cited by Mr Jewell of Brunswick of three-minute treatments for those unable to walk that Saunders restored to movement and Mr Barry of Carlton who was personally saved by Saunders of an operation from a slipped knee cartilage which Saunders fixed in five minutes.[61] In 1947, he rectified 'a twisted sinew' in the foot of runner Pianta.[62] In 1950, he 'snapped' a knee cartilage back into position for rugby player Johnny Hawke who decided an operation was no longer necessary.[63] Again that year in Western Australia, an article talks of how 'Saunders clicked something and there was immediate relief' and Saunders said a ligament in the ankle was out of place and to remedy it he had to 'break the adhesions'.[64] The Honourable Dr Harris spoke of a case where a doctor put a patient under chloroform to 'break adhesions' and stated Saunders [without anaesthesia] 'knows how to deal with this matter of adhesions'.[65] Pulled muscles and joint troubles were Saunders' forte.[66] Cain reinforced Saunders' excellence as a bonesetter dealing with limb injuries 'he does the job, more particularly in connexion [*sic*] with the treatment of joints and hundreds of people go to him on the recommendation of the medical profession'.[67] Foot runners in the Stawell gift would seek Ernie Saunders' services: Sprague required foot strapping for a fallen arch and Tommy Deane injured a hamstring. Recorded in Perry's book on the Stawell Gift, Deane remembered Saunders being an old man in an old house telling him he had a badly torn hamstring and be cautious, 'Don't get out of your holes too quick'.[68]

Ernie recommended washing soda packs for swellings and Bowen did likewise and this was a common remedy at the time.[69] Though the Honourable HI Cohen was strongly opposed to Saunders being registered and unkindly said he 'would not call him to a pet dog' in the Legislative Assembly, Mr Cain said of Saunders:

> He is one of the most qualified men of his type in the State. His association with sporting bodies has revealed him as a master of his art. He exercises his manipulative skill as does the great Barker in London.[70]

Sir Herbert Barker was trained by his cousin John Atkinson the famous English bonesetter.[71] Barker was knighted in 1922 after years of persecution by the medical mainstream. In 1932, Barker's attempts to demonstrate his techniques to doctors were rejected.[72] In 1939, however, FG Roberts mentioned Barker had made a film of his techniques of manipulative surgery for orthopaedic doctors.[73] The footage from these demonstrations has survived and is now on YouTube.[74] Any viewing of Barker's work reveals him to be directly adjusting joints and treating the body using quite robust movements though Atkinson taught him 'skill in place of force'.[75] The robustness of Saunders' methods is reflected in impressions of the work of his son George who learned his techniques and is provided in testimony to the Ward Inquiry. During interview, Evans, an American-trained osteopath, responded to the mention of Saunders and referring to George (as Ernest was deceased), also likened George, akin to his father, to Herbert Barker the bonesetter, as developing 'a wonderful gift' having an ability 'to juggle joints and a sisard [*sic*] [wizard] on certain things'. Evans acknowledged Saunders' lack of anatomical training but that 'he had a feel for this art and could intelligently interpret a lot of cases'. Evans admitted to admiration and would follow his work, remarking 'he [George] was not frightened to tear into tissues'.[76] George's skills saw him in demand with the Australian Olympic Team, a position he held solo until Montreal in 1976 when a physiotherapist, David Zuker, attended the Games for the first time.[77] Saunders looked after many athletes and treated the champion runner Marjorie Jackson at several events. At the 1951 Empire Games in New Zealand, Saunders stated he 'examined Marjorie Jackson's left ankle and her defeat in the 100 yards and put a ligament back in place'; after the 220 yards, he found it to be 'definitely torn, strapped it up and advised Ms Jackson to see a doctor'.[78] Saunders' attendance at Jackson's wedding to Olympic cyclist Peter Nelson signals the athletes' regard for him and the press described him as a 'world famous'.[79]

In addition to apparently very firm and deep massages, all of the patients seen by the Saunders' duo were treated mostly for restrictions on functional joint or muscle movement. Saunders also fixed a groin injury for Australian cricketer Arthur Morris.[80] Did Bowen learn his ability to align joints and ligaments from Saunders? This is highly likely given Saunders stature and reputation in this area. Bill Mitchell described in Chapter 8 had this ability too. At the 1973 Ward Inquiry, Bowen indicated his more limited scope of his knee work and said he mainly treated ligaments but 'cartilage was a doctor's job' he would not touch a joint that was 'locked' and he said he referred dislocations of knees, elbows and cartilage to doctors.[81] 'Saunders was a "master of muscle and cartilage" who gave magical massage and muscle manipulation'.[82] The press description of Saunders curing Quist of tennis elbow focuses on muscle connections too.[83] Bowen also knew how to address tennis elbow, restricted shoulders, injured wrists, twisted ankles, club foot and knees. Regardless of the source of these skills, they go beyond the remit of pressure movements of neuropathy and lifting pressure off nerves discussed in Chapter 3.

Garner's Contact With Saunders and Garner's Style

Ron Garner worked with Bowen in the late 1950s and his youngest son John recounted his father also made trips to visit Saunders. According to Ron's wife Nancy, Ron would travel from Sorrento to Newport to meet 'Ernie' and this was in the 1940s.[84] John Garner recounted that his father Ron had a book with Ernie Saunders' name in it which suggests a reasonably close connection between the men.[85] The book was described as having anatomical transparency images when layered created a 3D effect.[86] Garner had also lived on the west side of Melbourne at Newport and started early with the West Newport Football club in the 1930s. Since both Ron and Tom had contact with Saunders, it is revealing that there was no evidence of pressure points in Garner's style, oriental or otherwise. Neither Garner's son, nor John Hine, the Olympic cycling athlete in Ron Garner's care, gave any validation to pressure points being part of Ron's work.[87] Ron Garner's style was different to Bowen's.

For spinal adjustments, John Garner said his father used to cross hands and put on pressure on the back to get a 'click'. Also according to John, Bowen did not like spinal adjustments as 'they could damage nerves', it was important to 'get the nerve out of the way first'.[88] Tom showed Ron 'how to adjust with the leg levers and move the sciatic nerve out of the way'.[89] Logically, it stands to reason that Bowen must have learnt this from a source other that Saunders as if this was in the Saunders' repertoire, Ron would already have been aware of this technique from his earlier 1940s sessions with him too. Bowen's technique reflects osteopathic practice in the use of the legs as levers for pelvic/lumbar adjusting and points to another influence than Saunders. In 1960, the Olympian cyclist John Hine first received treatments from Garner (who became his personal masseur), Garner was already working with Bowen's approach. Hine had a scoliosis and remembered Ron would work on the lower back using the legs as levers causing the pelvis on one hip then the other to rise off the table while manipulating the leg forward and back would work with the fingers of the other hand [in Hine's mind] 'to open up the vertebrae and put things back in place'.[90] Ron could also manipulate a tendon back into alignment.[91] Ron worked with neatsfoot oil and occasionally penetrine and Finalgon on sore spots.[92] Ron didn't rest Hine between movements as Bowen did.[93] He also did spinal adjustments combined with breathing techniques. In line with scientific massage, according to Hine, Garner adapted firmness of massage depending on whether it was a pre or post-event treatment but his treatments were not as painful as Bowen's.[94] Other than incorporating Bowen's method for pelvic and spinal adjusting, Garner did not change his style. According to his son, Ron learned his gift from his grandmother Amy Jane Sayer who was a colonial masseur and had operated a funeral parlour in Bendigo.[95]

Unlike Ron's approach, Hine recalled Bowen's work as targeted and, bearing in mind Hine had a scoliosis, he described painful spots as 'pressure points'. He said, 'Tom just got to point, went straight in and "bang!" . . . "Seven Days." You'd sort of stagger out and ache somewhere he'd puts his vicious thumbs or fingers or whatever and just on a pressure point'.[96] Hine also referred to Tom's practice of 'stripping' described to him from Ron. It was intended 'to take all the stresses and strains off the body and allow it to recuperate of its own accord. It was pressure points or trigger points or something like that and he would work and just with those fingers – a push here, a push there, and you would feel completely and utterly useless for a while after a week or so'.[97]

Referring to his experience in football rooms of the same 1960 period, Cec Capon said of Bowen's style, 'Most of it was manipulation and moving nerves type of thing than clunking bones Tommy never seemed to get you and go "crunch". He'd run his hand down you and whatever. Things would get a jar and things would feel better . . . but he wasn't a cruncher'.[98] These descriptions of push-thrust techniques with leg lever work also point to an osteopathic source. Combined with evidence of Bowen's formal attempts and ongoing self-study in Chapter 2 and his known contact with the masseur turned osteopath Alister McAlister (later DO), these emerge more likely to be the conduit of these techniques than Saunders. As a later Olympian cyclist, knowledgeable sports performance and the effect of massage on his body, Hine clearly saw pressure points as painful spots, there was no suggestion of specifically Eastern concepts.[99] John Garner dismissed outright that anything oriental lay at the heart of Bowen's work and Tattersall, a family friend and early Bowen patient from 1956 also discounted such influences as 'rubbish'.[100] Other than the working styles of his son George, Garner and Bowen, little survives of others trained by Saunders. The press features only one other Saunders' apprentice, Raymond ('Bluey') Mervyn Hunter, head trainer for Acton in 1952 as 'a disciple of Saunders the famous Richmond Trainer and brings a skill to the game rare in Canberra'.[101] The article only highlights that Hunter 'has installed a 'hot box' [sauna] and other modern equipment as well as teaching masseurs to aid him'.[102] The use of saunas had been popularised in Berlin when arrangements were made to have one constructed for the Finnish team.[103]

Bowen's soft tissue 'stopper' moves were made across the lower lumbars and lower thorax areas. According to Smeeton DC, the effectiveness of these 'stoppers' was of short duration and Bowen would reapply them if more than five minutes had elapsed if he had not completed the necessary procedures on the relevant section of the body.[104] Smeeton also recalled Bowen did not use these when working with children and adults with neurological issues from spinal or brain conditions. A more elusive element attributed to both Bowen and Saunders was their sensitivity of touch. Saunders was attributed with magnetic healing and spoke of vitamins as imparting electricity to the body and Bowen was possessed of a sensitivity to bioelectricity. Other than aspects of joint setting, and the use of stoppers, and fleeting reference to Bowen doing push-thrust work described as stripping, what is recorded of Saunders and Bowen show the men to have quite different styles and there is no substantiation whatsoever of Japanese acupoint influences on Saunders or Saunders teaching these to others. The symbolism around Saunders is therefore more that of a bonesetter-masseur concerned with expert treatment of musculature, ligaments, cartilage and joints overpaid with the attribution of unusual powers of sensitivity.

German Massage in Saunders' Circle of Football and Sports Masseurs: Pleass and Gill

Swedish massage would have been the style Saunders would have encountered in his 'desultory reading of books' and he would have known this to be the standard of training for registered masseurs at the clubs where he was engaged as a trainer. Ernest Saunders worked in a culture where non-registered and well-known masseurs were described or known to have used German methods. German systems of massage utilised pressure points with the objective of inhibiting nerve activity in the interest of resetting pain. German influences do stand out in the world of football and sports massage and especially in the older group of football and sports masseurs at this time. A key figure was Frederick

Norman Pleass (1880–1960) head trainer for Richmond before Ernie Saunders and who held the head trainer position with the Melbourne 'Demons' for some twenty-three years from 1924 till his retirement in 1947.[105] Pleass was masseur to both the Melbourne Football Club and the Melbourne Cricket Club and enjoyed a high profile; 'Mr Pleass who has had such champions as Bradman, Kippax, Roy Cazaly, Laurie Nash, V Richardson and a host of others through his hands.[106] In addition to masseur abilities, he was an organiser who 'puts the boys in order'.[107]

According to his family, Pleass learned German massage methods when he served in the Boer War.[108] A record of service cannot be found, but there is a suggestion he falsified some details so he could enlist. Pleass is recorded on the First World War Rolls and he fell ill in France and sent home.[109] Beforehand, he spent time at a hospital in the UK and it is known that towards the end of the First World War, German internees and Prisoners of War (POW) were used in various employments.[110] It is understandable that masseurs would have been indispensable assisting with those wounded and requiring rehabilitation. Pleass enjoyed his masseur role without any conflict with the Authorities recorded in the press, presumably he worked without financial recompense as he escaped any court action. Supporting practices included baths and mechanical hot air.[111] Pleass taught physical culture to a methodist school as well.[112]

There were other senior men active as masseurs in the football community both unregistered and registered who are connected with the Saunders story. In the lead-up to his honorary appointment, Ernest Saunders had enjoyed professional contact with the younger Ted Gill (1903–nd, post-1989).[113] Edwin (Ted/Eddie) Gill was head trainer of Prahran at the same time Saunders was trainer for Richmond.[114] Gill was also former coach-masseur to the 1932 Los Angeles Olympics.[115] Gill was a member of the Victorian Physical Culture Teachers Association.[116] Gill was also an advocate of German methods and was regarded as very well studied in training methods and massage, with 'the German method' held in the highest esteem.[117] The press reported, 'He has made a special study of the latest methods of massage, particularly those of the Germans, which are considered to be the last word in this science'.[118] Gill had been a favourite for the 1936 Berlin Olympics but turned it down for business reasons.[119] Gill also missed out on the formation of the formal head trainers' association activities as he relocated to Sydney in late 1932 but the professional Saunders-Gill contact continued.[120] Then men referred high-profile clients to each other, notably cricketers Donald Bradman and Stan McCabe.[121] Alongside were the older Melbourne community of masseurs including Wren, Trappes, and Peter McColl, and the Scottish-born Neil Smith Snodgrass Morrison and Leslie Edward Dettman mentioned earlier, all of who enjoyed high profiles. Whatever style of work Saunders practised before his trip to Berlin, it would have been unavoidable for him not to witness German masseurs at work on the Australian athletes. Assuming Saunders was not already aware of German massage methods from his acquaintance with Gill and other masseurs among football trainers such as Pleass, he would surely have taken an interest at Berlin. The masseur Fred McKay was ill on the outward voyage and for the duration of the Berlin games, the team manager was required to engage German masseurs to help Neil Morrison with the workload.[122] The German masseurs were members of Reich Association of Professional Masseurs.[123] No specific record of the styles, the German masseurs is described only the complaint from the Olympics Team who found their styles too heavy.[124] Before the games, the Victorian Swimming Association expressly wanted Ernie and no strangers 'tinkering' with the athletes.[125]

'Reflex massage' was developed in Germany as a system of pressure point massage. Alfons Cornelius wrote about 'Druckpunktes' (stress/pressure points) in 1902 and images in Cornelius show individual point patterns and the quality of radiating pain in migraine, epilepsy and neurasthenia cases.[126] Other than Dettman who put pressure on points on the back of the neck for migraine, and the report of Bowen putting pressure on the cervical three to control nose bleeds, pressure point work is overtly non-existent in available evidence among Bowen's contemporaries.[127] It was established Albert (Bert) Donald, the western district autodidact healer-masseur did not use pressure points, a fact confirmed his daughter, Barbara Hewitt.[128] Further evidence of German influence on masseurs of Bowen's generation is imparted by Bert Donald who was learning about neurology from a German, Pastor Schroeder, while held a prisoner of the Japanese at Papua New Guinea during the Second World War.[129] However, though Donald did not use pressure points, like Bowen, he showed an interest in acupoints when they became topical in the 1970s.[130] Donald's work in the hands of protégé Pat Allen revealed rapid cross-fibre movements to release nerves and utilising an awareness of the concept of nerve vibration described earlier.[131] Allen does not use pressure points either.[132] According to Donald's son Lance, his father trained a number of other individuals. In addition to Allen, these include his Pat's brother Leo Allen, Harold Wilson of Stawell, Karen and Raelene Pohlner, Oswald Rentsch of Hamilton and Lil Scott.[133]

During the Second World War, Jack Meagher, an American, met a German POW masseur who practised German 'stresspoints' or 'pressure point' massage.[134] Meagher, already trained in Swedish massage, used this and developed a system of 'sportsmassage'.[135] Meagher identified reoccurring stresspoints individual to specific sports based on the regular muscles used and he also applied a similar system to horses. Individual stress points were massaged using direct pressure, cross-fibre frictions (described as an offshoot of 'direct pressure') and Cyriax is referenced on the role of deep cross-fibre frictions in addressing adhesions and reducing spasm.[136] Meagher's stress points are mapped in muscle bellies, at junctions of muscles and tendons, or at muscular junctions and at the origin or insertions of tendons, some occurring along the spine too. Some Indian Ayurvedic marma points follow a similar logic. However, these do not feature meridians.[137] However, Meagher did not publish his books until after Saunders' death and it is not known if his ideas were circulating in the massage community after the war. Pressure point massage was not a term encountered in discussions on massage in Australia in Saunders' time. Those better informed on technique adopted 'scientific massage' used by the professionally trained masseurs. When Saunders was establishing his mark as a masseur, the Swedish system of movements prevailed as 'scientific massage'. In this period, the scientific knowledge of massage, especially sports massage was not yet developed. The examinations set by Langridge in 1936 for those contending for the role of Olympic Masseur are informative on requirements to address staleness and stiffness, pulled muscles, ligament issues, sprains and diet.[138]

Summary

Ideas that Bowen's work was founded in Eastern acupoints and inspired by his connection with Saunders are not supportable, given the historical research and evidence found so far, especially since the Dettman story has been researched. Any undocumented use by Saunders of pressure point work is more likely to have been drawn from Western practices whether German or from sources such as McFadden who was popular in the American Young Men's Christian Association (YMCA) movement, an organisation Saunders was involved with and would have been among the athletic clubs on his overseas itinerary and study tour in 1936. Bernarr McFadden, a student of Lust, developed a style of pressure movements focused on the viscera and used the whole hand or a clenched fist on parts of the body.[139] McFadden aimed to ensure internal organs were kept in the right position but did not involve direct influence of spinal nerves.[140] A distinguishing feature of these movements is that there is no rub or slide involved, but they involve a sinking into tissues, with full hand, fist or fingers and thumbs.

A historical review by Travell and Simons in their manuals on trigger points developed in the 1940s referenced sources dating from 1843, including German that described tender spots that referred pain.[141] They discuss Melsack et al. on the high correspondence (71 per cent) between trigger points and acupoints.[142]

In the historical long view, eastern ideas would have flowed to the west and could have influenced the development of Western pressure point systems of manual therapy. However, these did not adopt the concept of energy meridians that attends Chinese Eastern anatomy involving acupoints. German pressure point is also related to the reflex zone therapy that has a history of origins to Egypt.[143] Other systems were developed by Fitzgerald, a medical specialist and ear nose and throat surgeon, who simply found 'the making pressures over certain parts of the body would enable him to do minor operations on the nose and throat without using cocaine or any other local analgesic'.[144] The next chapter will address the Eastern Medicine theme and recontextualise the change in symbolism that occurred around Bowen's practice in the 1970s.

Notes

1 VIC, Parliamentary Debates, Legislative Council, Vol. 197, October 15, 1935, 3494.
2 John Garner, interview by author, transcript in Shirley Strachan, *Healing Hands, Unsung Voices, Thomas Ambrose Bowen Osteopath (1916–1982)* (United Kingdom: Cloister House Press, 2016), 44.
3 H. Joseph Fay, *Scientific Massage for Athletes* (London: Athletic Publications, n.d.).
4 Fay, *Scientific Massage*, 18–24.
5 Robert Calvert, *The History of Massage* (Rochester, VT: Healing Arts Press, 2002), 93: Robert Calvert, "Pages from History, Swedish Massage," *Massage Magazine*, April 24, 2014.
6 Calvert, *History of Massage*, 93; Calvert, "Pages from History."
7 "The Medical and Surgical Sanatorium Training School for Nurses."
8 "Australian Massage Association," *Evening Journal (Adelaide*), April 23, 1907: 3.
9 "Obituary," *Age (Melbourne),* July 24, 1944: 2.
10 Alfred Peters *Massage, Its History, Its Curative Uses, and Its Practical Results* (Melbourne: Peter and Knapton, 1890), 3.
11 "A Noted Institute," *Prahran Telegraph (Vic*), January 27, 1906: 3.
12 "The Northern Territory," *Leader (Melbourne),* February 24, 1906: 3. (Council of interstate delegates).
13 "Mr. Hugo Leschen, "*Chronicle (Adelaide*), October 30, 1926: 22.
14 "Physical Culture," *Mail (Adelaide),* August 23, 1913: 5.
15 "Behind the Scenes," *News (Adelaide*), May 20, 1926: 10.
16 "Work of League trainers," *News (Adelaide),* June 21, 1928, 14.
17 "Work of League Trainers."
18 Joan McMeekin, "How an Anglo Indian Man Made Australian Therapy Great," *History.Physio*, May 13, 2020; Bentley and David Dunstan, *The Path to Professionalism, Physiotherapy in Australia to the 1980s* (Melbourne, Victoria: Australian Physiotherapy Association, 2006), xxi.
19 "No Title," *Weekly Times (Melbourne),* September 30, 1905: 12.
20 "Massage," *Wodonga and Towong Sentinel (Vic),* November 20, 1903: 2.
21 "Port Melb. Football Club," *Standard (Port Melbourne*), March 2, 1907: 4.
22 PROV, Masseurs Registration Bill VPRS6345/P/Unit 64, Pamphlet, Training in Massage, Masseurs' Registration Board.
23 PROV, Osteopathy, Chiropractic and Naturopath, Joint Select Committee pp. 1003–56, VPRS 2341/P, Unit 14, Transcripts of Committee, Davis transcript: 1038–39.
24 Murray, *In Search*, 123.
25 "Masseurs Board," *Age (Melbourne),* September 30, 1934: 10; "Letters to the Editor," *Age (Melbourne),* July 25, 1935: 15; "Masseurs Bill," *Age (Melbourne*), August 21, 1935: 10.
26 VIC, Parliamentary Debates, Legislative Council, Vol. 197, October 15, 1935: 3490.
27 VIC, Parliamentary Debates, Legislative Assembly, Vol. 197, August 29, 1935: 2319.
28 VIC, Parliamentary Debates, Legislative Assembly, Vol. 197, August 20, 1935: 2033.
29 'Register of Masseurs for 1937," *Victorian Government Gazette*, no. 75, May 5, 1937, 1239.
30 "Head Trainers' Dinner," *Sporting Globe (Melbourne),* November 4, 1933: 6; "Head Trainers' Dinner," *Sporting Globe (Melbourne*), November 11, 1933: 5.

31 'Register of Masseurs for 1936," *Victorian Government Gazette*, no. 102, May 20, 1936, 1200–2.
32 "Percentage Lead by St Kilda," *Argus (Melbourne)*, May 1, 1939: 18.
33 *An Act to provide for the Registration of a Certain Person as a Masseur under the Masseurs Acts.*
34 Gordon, "A Glimpse of Tom Bowen," in *Tom Bowen Personal Reflections* (Australia: BTAV and BTASA, 1999), 7.
35 Heather Edmonds interview by author, transcript in Strachan, *Healing Hands*, 65.
36 Edmonds interview by author, transcript in Strachan, *Healing Hands*, 66.
37 Garner personal communication to author.
38 McHenry interview in Strachan, *Healing Hands*, 1–4.
39 McHenry interview in Strachan, *Healing Hands*, 2.
40 "Soldiers' Sports, McAlister Wins at Mount Martha," *Argus*, November 21, 1940, 14; Heather Hay personal communication to author, February 19, 2019.
41 "What Goes On," *Argus*, April 16, 1956: 1.
42 "An Eye-Opener," *Sporting Globe (Melbourne)*, July 8, 1931: 8.
43 "Science as Aid to Footballers," *Courier-Mail*, May 31, 1938, 14.
44 William Shurtleff and Akiko Ayoyagi, *Soyinfo Center, History of Soybeans and Soyfoods in Australia, New Zealand and Oceania 1770–2010, extensively annotated bibliography and Sourcebook*, (Lafayette, CA: SoyInfo Center, 2010), 372.
45 "Ray Lamp for Footballers," *Circular Head Chronicle*, May 14, 1952: 3.
46 Doug Sells, interview by author October 31, 2016.
47 "Sir Donald Bradman's Farewell to Cricket – II," *Courier-Mail (Brisbane)*, November 17, 1949: 2.
48 "Sir Donald Bradman's Farewell to Cricket – II."
49 "Sir Donald Bradman's Farewell to Cricket – II."
50 "Men Who Have Never Played the Game!" *Table Talk (Melbourne)*, September 7, 1933: 35.
51 "Silent Fan," *Argus (Melbourne)*, June 30, 1956: 1.
52 "'Miracle Man' May Cure Stan McCabe," *Sunday Times (Perth)*, February 24, 1946: 3.
53 VIC, Parliamentary Debates, Legislative Assembly, Vol. 197, August 20, 1935: 2035.
54 "Saunders' "Miracles" Cost Five Shillings Each," *Daily Telegraph (Sydney)*, January 6, 1946: 22.
55 John Murtagh email message to author, October 13, 2015.
56 There are numerous accounts of Bowen standing by at football matches ready to tend to a player who was injured. Sometime he would get the player off the field first if he observed an imbalance in their performance, Barry Tattersall remembered Bowen would say, 'Barry, get him off' – Tattersall interview by author, in Strachan, *Healing Hands*, 7. In one case that had become chronic from the previous season, Bowen said to Russell Butcher, he should have come and had his ankle seen to straight away, 'If you'd come and seen me I would have fixed it then' – Butcher interview by author, in Strachan, *Healing Hands*, 130.
57 "Talking Sport," *Herald (Melbourne)*, May 6, 1941: 16.
58 VIC, Parliamentary Debates, Legislative Assembly, Vol. 197, August 20, 1935: 2315.
59 VIC, Parliamentary Debates, 2034.
60 "'Saunders' 'Miracles' Cost Five Shillings Each."
61 VIC, Parliamentary Debates, 2313, 2315.
62 "Stawell Fancy 'Shot' Out," *Sporting Globe (Melbourne)*, March 26, 1947: 11.
63 "Hawke to Test Knee at Training," *Sun (Sydney)*, August 8, 1950: 29.
64 "Victorian Cures McIntosh," *Daily News (Perth)*, July 20, 1950: 18.

65 VIC, Parliamentary Debates, Legislative Assembly, Vol. 197, October 15, 1935: 3494.
66 "Saunders May Get Games Masseur Job," *Daily Telegraph (Sydney)*, January 20, 1948: 15.
67 VIC, Parliamentary Debates, Legislative Assembly, Vol. 197, August 20, 1935: 2037–38.
68 John Perry, *The Quick and the Dead, Stawell and It's Race through Time* (Sydney: UNINSW Press, 2002), 147.
69 Perry, *The Quick and the Dead.*
70 VIC, Parliamentary Debates, 2037.
71 Herbert Atkinson Barker, *Leaves from My Life* (London: Hutchinson & Co, 1927), 29–32.
72 " 'Bonesetter' Knight," *Barrier Miner (Broken Hill)*, September 24, 1932: 1, accessed October 27, 2018, http://nla.gov.au/nla.news-article46666597.
73 *Natures Path to Health*, October 1939, 40–41.
74 Wellcome Library, "Sir Herbert Barkers' Manipulative Technique part 1 (1936)," *YouTube* video, posted January 19, 2011; Wellcome Library, "Sir Herbert Barkers' Manipulative Technique part 2 (1936)," *YouTube* video.
75 Barker, *Leaves from My Life*, 31.
76 PROV, Osteopathy, Chiropractic and Naturopath Joint Select Committee pp. 652–78, VPRS 241/P/, Unit 14, Transcripts of Committee, Evans transcript: 994.
77 Shirley Strachan and Keir Reeves, "Through the Lens of the Trainer-Masseurs: Australia's Incongruous Engagement with the Olympic Amateur Ethos," *The International Journal of the History of Sport* 39, no. 6 (2022): 631–52; Saunders' attendances are documented in Harry Gordon, *Australia and the Olympic Games* (St Lucia, Queensland: University of Queensland Press, 1994), 504, 507, 510, 514.
78 "Surprise Sprint Results," *Sydney Morning Herald*, January 1, 1951: 1.
79 "Marjorie Jackson's Mother Lucky to See Wedding," *Brisbane* Telegraph, November 7, 1953: 2.
80 "Behind the Cricket Scenes", *Daily Telegraph (Sydney)* November 17, 1946: 40.
81 PROV. Report and evidence Osteopathy Committee (Pt.1–4), 27/11/975 (Pt. 2) 2261, VPRS 3253/P1/, Unit 47. Original papers tabled in the Legislative Assembly, transcripts of proceedings, Bowen transcript: 675.
82 "What Goes on? Ernie's Hands Put Athletes Back on Map," *Argus (Melbourne)*, February 21, 1951: 6.
83 "Quist's 'Tennis Elbow' Cured by Masseur," *Daily Telegraph (Sydney)*, December 16, 1945: 24.
84 John Garner personal communication to author.
85 John Garner interview by author, in Strachan, *Healing Hands*, 44.
86 Garner interview by author, in Strachan, *Healing Hands*, 44.
87 Garner interview by author, in Strachan, *Healing Hands*, 44; John Hine, interview by author, in Strachan, *Healing Hands*, 48, 49 and 54.
88 Garner interview by author, in Strachan, *Healing Hands*, 44.
89 Garner interview by author, in Strachan, *Healing Hands*, 42.
90 John Hine interview by author, in Strachan, *Healing Hands*, 51.
91 Hine interview by author, in Strachan, *Healing Hands*, 51.
92 Hine interview by author, in Strachan, *Healing Hands*, 51, 53.
93 Hine interview by author, in Strachan, *Healing Hands*, 51.
94 Hine interview by author, in Strachan, *Healing Hands*, 53.
95 John Garner personal communication to the author, June 28, 2015.
96 John Hine, interview by author, in Strachan, *Healing Hands*, 48.
97 Hine interview by author, in Strachan, *Healing Hands*, 49.
98 Cec Capon, interview by author, in Strachan, *Healing Hands*, 85.

99 Hine interview by author, in Strachan, *Healing Hands*, 48.
100 Garner personal communication to author September 30, 2017; Barry Tattersall, interview by author, in Strachan, *Healing Hands*, 8.
101 "National Football," *Canberra Times (ACT)*, April 1, 1952: 6.
102 "National Football."
103 Michael Mackenzie, "From Athens to Berlin: The 1936 Olympics and Leni Riefenstahl's Olympia," *Critical Inquiry* 29, no. 2 (Winter 2003): 323, https://doi.org/10.1086/374029.
104 Smeeton personal communication to the author.
105 "Fred Pleass Retires," *Age (Melbourne)*, April 12, 1947: 16; "Is Today's Footballer Pampered?" *Sporting Globe*, February 8, 1947: 6.
106 "Football Personality Visits Morwell," *Morwell Advertiser (Morwell)*, September 28, 1944: 7.
107 "Men Behind the Scenes in Melbourne Sport," *News (Adelaide)*, January 5, 1927, 3.
108 Susanne Baessler to author personal communications 2015 and 2017.
109 NAA: B2455 Frederick Norman Pleass.
110 "1914–1918 online," International Encyclopaedia of the First World War.
111 "Round the Training Rooms," *Table Talk (Melbourne)*, June 15, 1933: 10.
112 "Round the Training Rooms."
113 "Sporting Special," *Worlds News*, May 29, 1935: 23.
114 "Wants to Go to Games," *Sporting Globe (Melbourne)*, March 5, 1932: 3.
115 Gill appears in a team photograph: Image National Library of Australia, PIC/15611/9494 LOC Cold store PIC/15611 Fairfax archive of glass plate negatives.
116 "Olympic Trainer," *Sporting Globe (Melbourne)*, April 16, 1932: 2.
117 "Sporting Special."
118 "Australian Olympians Will Be in Good Hands," *Referee (Sydney)*, April 20, 1932: 22.
119 "For Berlin," *Sporting Globe (Melbourne)* February 26, 1936: 10.
120 "Duncan Gray's Trouble," *Referee (Sydney)*, February 8, 1933: 12.
121 "Don And Stan to Play again?" *Sunday Times (Perth)*, April 7, 1946: 8.; " 'Miracle Man' May Cure Stan McCabe," *Sunday Times (Perth)*, February 24, 1946: 3.
122 "Olympic Games," *Sydney Morning Herald* July 6, 1936: 13.
123 *The XIth Olympic Games Berlin, 1936, Official Report Volume 1* (Wilhelm Limpert, Berlin, S. W.68: Organisationskomittee Fur die XI. Olympiade Berlin 1936 E.V, 1936), 190–91, accessed February 10, 2019, https://digital.la84.org/digital/collection/p17103coll8/id/16471/rec/15.
124 Larry Writer, *Dangerous Games, Australia at the 1936 Nazi Olympics* (Sydney: Allen and Unwin, 2015), 176.
125 "German Trainers Advocated," *Herald (Melbourne)*, April 30, 1936: 50.
126 Dr Alfons Cornelius, *Druckpunkte* (Berlin: Verlag von Otto Enslin, 1902), 32–43; J. P. Shah, N. Thaker, J. Heimur, J. V. Aredo, S. Sikdar, and L. Gerber, "Myofascial Trigger Points Then and Now: A Historical and Scientific Perspective," *PM* and *R: The Journal of Injury, Function, and Rehabilitation* 7, no. 7 (2015): 746–61.
127 Kevin Neave interview by Vicki Mechner, March 14, 2003, email to author.
128 Barbara Hewitt interview by author, transcript in Strachan *Healing Hands.*
129 Keith Lockwood, "The Hands That Have Helped Thousands," *Mail-Times*, November 13, 1981: 8.
130 Lockwood, "The Hands That Have Helped Thousands."
131 Pat Allen interview by author, transcript in Strachan, *Healing Hands*, 257–58.
132 Allen interview by author, transcript in Strachan, *Healing Hands*, 259.

133 Letter, Lance Donald (son of Albert Donald) personal communication to author, September 27, 2016
134 Jack Meagher and Pat Broughton, *Sports Massage* (USA: Dolphin Books, Doubleday, 1980).
135 Meagher and Broughton, *Sports Massage*, viii.
136 Jo-Ann Wilson, "The Effects of Sports Massage on Athletic Performance and General Function," *Massage Therapy Journal* (Summer 2002): 90–100, 94.
137 S. V. Govindan, *Massage Therapy for Diseases of Vital Areas: Marma Treatment* (New Delhi: Abhinav Publications, 2005), 26–27.
138 "Olympic Trainer! Experienced." *Sporting Globe (Melbourne),* May 6, 1936: 10.
139 Bernarr McFadden, *Vitality Supreme* (New York City: Physical Culture Publishing Co, 1915), chapter XV.
140 McFadden, *Vitality Supreme*, chapter XV.
141 David Simons, Janet Travell, and Lois S. Simons, *Myofascial Pain and Dysfunction: The Trigger Point Manual, Volume 1. Upper Half of Body*, 2nd ed. (Philadelphia: Lippincott Williams and Wilkins, 1999), 14–18.
142 Simons et al., *Myofascial Pain and Dysfunction*, 41–42.
143 Dwight C. Byers, *Better Health with Foot Reflexology, The Original Ingham Method* (St Peterburg, FL: Ingham Publishing, 1983), 2.
144 W. H. Fitzgerald and Edwin F. Bower, *Zone Therapy* and George Starr White, *Zone Therapy* (Columbus, Ohio: J. H. Long, 1917) reprinted by *Health Research Books* (Mokelumne Hill, CA: Health Research Books, 1972), Part Six, 872.

Bibliography

Newspapers

"A Noted Institute." *Prahran Telegraph (Vic),* January 27, 1906: 3. Accessed November 17, 2024. http://nla.gov.au/nla.news-article144606490.

"An Eye-Opener." *Sporting Globe (Melbourne),* July 8, 1931: 8. Accessed November 17, 2024. http://nla.gov.au/nla.news-article182539965.

"Australian Massage Association." *Evening Journal (Adelaide),* April 23, 1907: 3. Accessed November 17, 2024. http://nla.gov.au/nla.news-article208612461.

"Australian Olympians Will Be in Good Hands." *Referee (Sydney),* April 20, 1932: 22 (cols.5–7). Accessed November 17, 2024. http://nla.gov.au/nla.news-article135327578.

"Behind the Cricket Scenes." *Daily Telegraph (Sydney)*, November 17, 1946: 40 (col.5). Accessed November 17, 2024. http://nla.gov.au/nla.news-article248366157.

"Behind the Scenes." *News (Adelaide),* May 20, 1926: 10 (cols.6–7). Accessed November 17, 2024. http://nla.gov.au/nla.news-article129768551.

Bonesetter' knight." *Barrier Miner (Broken Hill*), September 24, 1932: 1, accessed October 27, 2018, http://nla.gov.au/nla.news-article46666597.

"Don and Stan to Play Again?" *Sunday Times (Perth),* Sport Section. April 7, 1946: 8 (col.2). Accessed November 17, 2024. http://nla.gov.au/nla.news-article59352586.

"Duncan Gray's Trouble." *Referee (Sydney)*, February 8, 1933, 12 (col.4). Accessed November 17, 2024. http://nla.gov.au/nla.news-article135315537.

"Football Personality Visits Morwell." *Morwell Advertiser (Morwell),* September 28, 1944: 7. Accessed August 26, 2017. http://nla.gov.au/nla.news-article66130614.

"For Berlin." *Sporting Globe Melbourne* February 26, 1936: 10. Accessed November 17, 2024. http://nla.gov.au/nla.news-article190319426.

"Fred Pleass Retires." *Age Melbourne*, April 12, 1947: 16. Accessed November 17, 2024. http://nla.gov.au/nla.news-article206018299.

"German Trainers Advocated." *Herald (Melbourne)*, April 30, 1936: 50. Accessed November 17, 2024. http://nla.gov.au/nla.news-article244881874.

"Hawke to Test Knee at Training." *Sun Sydney*, August 8, 1950, 29. Accessed November 17, 2024. http://nla.gov.au/nla.news-article230927398.

"Head Trainers' Dinner." *Sporting Globe (Melbourne)*, November 11, 1933: 5. Accessed November 17, 2024. http://nla.gov.au/nla.news-article181747427.

"Head Trainers' Dinner." *Sporting Globe (Melbourne)*, November 4, 1933: 6. Accessed November 17, 2024. http://nla.gov.au/nla.news-article181746664.

"Is Today's Footballer Pampered?" *Sporting Globe* February 8, 1947: 6. Accessed November 17, 2024. http://nla.gov.au/nla.news-article178131098.

"Letters to the Editor- Amending Masseurs Act." *Age (Melbourne),* July 25, 1935: 15. Accessed November 17, 2024. http://nla.gov.au/nla.news-article203990143

Lockwood, Keith. "The Hands That Have Helped Thousands." *Mail-Times*, November 13, 1981.

"Marjorie Jackson's Mother Lucky to See Wedding." *Brisbane Telegraph*, November 7, 1953: 2 (City Final). Accessed November 17, 2024. http://nla.gov.au/nla.news-article217165326.

"Massage." *Wodonga and Towong Sentinel (VIC),* November 20, 1903: 2. Accessed November 17, 2024. http://nla.gov.au/nla.news-article69571922.

"Masseurs Bill." *Age (Melbourne),* August 21, 1935: 10. Accessed November 17, 2024. http://nla.gov.au/nla.news-article203989842.

"Masseurs Board." *Age (Melbourne),* September 30, 1934: 10. Accessed November 17, 2024. http://nla.gov.au/nla.news-article205873532.

"Men behind the Scenes in Melbourne Sport." *News (Adelaide),* January 5, 1927. Accessed November 17, 2024. http://nla.gov.au/nla.news-article129203502.

"Men Who Have Never Played the Game!" *Table Talk (Melbourne),* September 7, 1933: 35. Accessed November 17, 2024. http://nla.gov.au/nla.news-article147259591.

"'Miracle Man' May Cure Stan McCabe." *Sunday Times (Perth),* February 24, 1946: 3. Accessed November 17, 2024. http://nla.gov.au/nla.news-article59350446.

"Mr Hugo Leschen." *Chronicle Adelaide*, October 30, 1926: 22. Accessed November 17, 2024. http://nla.gov.au/nla.news-article89649552.

"National Football." *Canberra Times (ACT),* April 1, 1952: 6. Accessed November 17, 2024. http://nla.gov.au/nla.news-article2851973.

"No Title." *Weekly Times (Melbourne),* September 30, 1905: 12. Accessed November 17, 2024. http://nla.gov.au/nla.news-article222768669.

"Obituary." *Age (Melbourne),* July 24, 1944: 2. Accessed November 17, 2024. http://nla.gov.au/nla.news-article206002122.

"Olympic Games." *Sydney Morning Herald (Sydney),* July 6, 1936: 13. Accessed November 17, 2024. http://nla.gov.au/nla.news-article17248920.

"Olympic Trainer." *Sporting Globe (Melbourne),* April 16, 1932: 2. Accessed November 17, 2024. http://nla.gov.au/nla.news-article182147006.

"Olympic Trainer! Experienced." *Sporting Globe (Melbourne)*, May 6, 1936: 10. Accessed November 17, 2024. http://nla.gov.au/nla.news-article190325029.

"Percentage Lead by St Kilda." *Argus (Melbourne)*, May 1, 1939: 18. Accessed November 17, 2024. http://nla.gov.au/nla.news-article12123397.

"Physical Culture." *Mail (Adelaide),* August 23, 1913: 5. Accessed November 17, 2024. http://nla.gov.au/nla.news-article63805808.

"Port Melb. Football Club." *Standard (Port Melbourne),* March 2, 1907: 4. Accessed November 17, 2024. http://nla.gov.au/nla.news-article164440912.

"Quist's 'Tennis Elbow' Cured by Masseur." *The Daily Telegraph (Sydney)*, December 16, 1945: 24. Accessed November 17, 2024. http://nla.gov.au/nla.news-article248030417.

"Ray Lamp for Footballers." *Circular Head Chronicle (Circular Head),* May 14, 1952: 3. Accessed November 17, 2024. http://nla.gov.au/nla.news-article163470358.

"Round the Training Rooms." *Table Talk (Melbourne),* June 15, 1933: 10. Accessed November 17, 2024. http://nla.gov.au/nla.news-article149547639.

"Saunders May Get Games Masseur Job." *Daily Telegraph (Sydney)*, January 20, 1948: 15. Accessed November 17, 2024. http://nla.gov.au/nla.news-article248282180.

"Saunders' 'Miracles' Cost Five Shillings Each." *Daily Telegraph (Sydney)*, January 6, 1946: 22. Accessed November 17, 2024. http://nla.gov.au/nla.news-article248473358.

"Science as Aid to Footballers." *Courier-Mail*, May 31, 1938: 14. Accessed November 17, 2024. http://nla.gov.au/nla.news-article40996692.

"Silent Fan." *Argus (Melbourne)*, June 30, 1956: 1. Accessed November 17, 2024. http://nla.gov.au/nla.news-article71811936.

"Sir Donald Bradman's Farewell to Cricket – II." *Courier-Mail (Brisbane)*, November 17, 1949: 2. Accessed November 17, 2024. http://nla.gov.au/nla.news-article49706924.

"Soldiers' Sports McAlister Wins at Mt. Martha." *Argus (Melbourne)*, November 21, 1940: 14. Accessed November 17, 2024. http://nla.gov.au/nla.news-article11319833.

"Sporting Special." *Worlds News*, May 29, 1935: 23. Accessed November 17, 2024. http://nla.gov.au/nla.news-article136320980.

"Stawell Fancy 'Shot' Out." *Sporting Globe Melbourne*, March 26, 1947: 11. Accessed November 17, 2024.http://nla.gov.au/nla.news-article178133279.

"Surprise Sprint Results." *Sydney Morning Herald*, January 1, 1951, 1. Accessed November 17, 2024. http://nla.gov.au/nla.news-article18193430.

"Talking Sport." *Herald (Melbourne)*, May 6, 1941: 16. Accessed November 17, 2024. http://nla.gov.au/nla.news-article244994882.

"The Northern Territory." *Leader (Melbourne)*, February 24, 1906: 36. Accessed November 17, 2024. http://nla.gov.au/nla.news-article198361771.

"Victorian Cures McIntosh." *Daily News Perth*, July 20, 1950: 18. Accessed November 17, 2024. http://nla.gov.au/nla.news-article84469277.

"Wants to Go to Games." *Sporting Globe (Melbourne)*, March 5, 1932: 3. Accessed October 27, 2018. http://nla.gov.au/nla.news-article182143280.

"What Goes on . . ." *Argus*, April 16, 1956: 1. Accessed November 17, 2024. http://nla.gov.au/nla.news-article71797684.

"What Goes on? Ernie's Hands Put Athletes Back on Map." *Argus* February 21, 1951: 6. Accessed November 17, 2024. http://nla.gov.au/nla.news-article23035440.

"Work of League Trainers." *News Adelaide*, June 21, 1928: 14. Accessed November 17, 2024. http://nla.gov.au/nla.news-article129131210.

Primary Sources

Allen, Pat. Interview by author. Transcript in Strachan, Shirley. *Healing Hands, Unsung Voices, Thomas Ambrose Bowen Osteopath (1916–1982)*. United Kingdom: Cloister House Press, 2016.

An Act to Provide for the Registration of a certain Person as a Masseur under the Masseurs Acts, No 6078, June 4, 1957. Accessed November 17, 2024. www.austlii.edu.au/au/legis/vic/hist_act/ma1957271.pdf.

Barker, Herbert Atkinson. *Leaves from My life*. London: Hutchinson & Co, 1927.

Butcher, Russell. Interview by author. Transcript in Strachan, Shirley. *Healing Hands, Unsung Voices, Thomas Ambrose Bowen Osteopath (1916–1982)*. United Kingdom: Cloister House Press, 2016.

Capon, Cec. Interview by author. Transcript in Strachan, Shirley. *Healing Hands, Unsung Voices, Thomas Ambrose Bowen Osteopath (1916–1982)*. United Kingdom: Cloister House Press, 2016.

Cornelius, Alfons. *Druckpunkte*. Berlin: Verlag von Otto Enslin, 1902, 32–43. Accessed September 2018. http://archive.org/details/druckpunkteihre00corngoog.
Edmonds, Heather. Interview by author. Transcript in Strachan, Shirley. *Healing Hands, Unsung Voices, Thomas Ambrose Bowen 1916–1982, Osteopath*. United Kingdom: Cloister House Press, 2016.
Garner, John. Interview by author. Transcript in Strachan, Shirley. *Healing Hands, Unsung Voices, Thomas Ambrose Bowen 1916–1982 Osteopath*. United Kingdom: Cloister House Press, 2016.
Hewitt, Barbara. Interview by author. Transcript in Strachan, Shirley. *Healing Hands, Unsung Voices, Thomas Ambrose Bowen 1916–1982, Osteopath*. United Kingdom: Cloister House Press, 2016.
Hine, John. Interview by author. Transcript in Strachan, Shirley. *Healing Hands, Unsung Voices, Thomas Ambrose Bowen 1916–1982, Osteopath*. United Kingdom: Cloister House Press, 2016.
Letter, Lance Donald (son of Albert Donald) personal communication to author, September 27, 2016
McFadden, Bernarr. *Vitality Supreme*. New York City: Physical Culture Publishing Co, 1915. Accessed November 17, 2024. http://www.bernarrmacfadden.com/vitalitysupreme.pdf.
McHenry, Greg, Interview by author. Transcript in Strachan, Shirley. *Healing Hands, Unsung Voices, Thomas Ambrose Bowen 1916–1982, Osteopath*. United Kingdom: Cloister House Press, 2016.
NAA: B2455. Barcode 8016615. Frederick Norman Pleass.
Natures Path to Health, various editions Jan/Feb 1937, November–December 1937, Christmas, 1937. September 1, 1938, October 1939, December 1939, January-February 1941 and February/March 1949. Collection held at Alfred Deakin Library, Waterfront Campus, Geelong, location ADPML SPC 613.05 Fgr/Npt.
Neave, Kevin. Letter to Ron Phelan, May 9, 2002.
Peters, Alfred. *Massage: Its History, Its Curative Uses, and Its Practical Results* Melbourne: Peter & Knapton, 1890. Accessed November 17, 2024.https://viewer.slv.vic.gov.au/?entity=IE6496247.
PROV. Masseurs Registration Bill VPRS 6345/P/, Unit 64. Pamphlet, Training in Massage, Masseurs' Registration Board.
PROV. Osteopathy, Chiropractic and Naturopath Joint Select Committee pp. 1003–56, VPRS 241/P/, Unit 14. Transcripts of Committee, Davis transcript: 1037–46.
PROV. Osteopathy, Chiropractic and Naturopath Joint Select Committee VPRS 241/P00000 pp. 652–78 Osteopathy, Chiropractic and Naturopath Joint Select Committee Unit 14, Evans transcript: 985–1002.
PROV. Report and evidence Osteopathy Committee (Pt.1–4), 27/11/975 (Pt. 2) 2261, VPRS 3253/P1/, Unit 47. Original papers tabled in the Legislative Assembly, transcripts of proceedings, Bowen transcript: 672–78.
"Register of Masseurs for 1936." *Victorian Government Gazette*, No. 102, May 20, 1936: 1200–2. Accessed November 17, 2024. http://gazette.slv.vic.gov.au/images/1936/V/general/102.pdf.
"Register of Masseurs for 1937." Victorian Government Gazette, no. 75, May 5, 1937: 12e39. Accessed November 17, 2024. http://gazette.slv.vic.gov.au/images/1937/V/general/75.pdf.
"The Medical and Surgical Sanatorium Training School for Nurses." Union Conference Record, January 15, 1899.
VIC. Parliamentary Debates. Legislative Assembly. Vol. 197, August 20, 1935.
VIC. Parliamentary Debates. Legislative Assembly. Vol. 197 August 29, 1935.
VIC Parliamentary Debates. Legislative Council. Vol. 197. October 15, 1935.

Secondary Sources

Bentley, Philip with Dunstan, David. *The Path to Professionalism, Physiotherapy in Australia to the 1980s.* Melbourne, Victoria: Australian Physiotherapy Association, 2006.

Byers, Dwight C. *Better Health with Foot Reflexology, The Original Ingham Method.* St Peterburg, FL: Ingham Publishing, 1983.

Calvert, Robert. *The History of Massage.* Rochester, VT: Healing Arts Press, 2002.

Calvert, Robert. "Pages from History, Swedish Massage." *Massage Magazine*, April 24, 2014. Accessed November 17, 2024. http://www.massagemag.com/magazine-2002-issue100-history100-24026/.

Cornelius, Alfons. *Druckpunkte.* Berlin: Verlag von Otto Enslin, 1902, 32–43. Accessed November 17, 2024. http://archive.org/details/druckpunkteihre00corngoog.

Fay, Joseph H. *Scientific Massage for Athletes.* London: Athletic Publications, n.d.

Fitzgerald, W. H., and Edwin F. Bower. *Zone Therapy* and George Starr White, *Zone Therapy.* Columbus, Ohio: J. H. Long, 1917. Reprinted by *Health Research Books.* Mokelumne Hill, CA: Health Research Books, 1972.

Gordon, Harry. *Australia and the Olympic Games.* St Lucia, Queensland: University of Queensland Press, 1994.

Gordon, Libby. "A Glimpse of Tom Bowen." In *Tom Bowen Personal Reflections.* Australia: BTAV and BTASA, 1999.

Govindan, S. V. *Massage Therapy for Diseases of Vital Areas: Marma Treatment.* New Delhi: Abhinav Publications, 2005. Accessed November 17, 2024. https://archive.org/details/massagetherapyfo0000govi/.

Mackenzie, Michael. "From Athens to Berlin: The 1936 Olympics and Leni Riefenstahl's Olympia." *Critical Inquiry* 29, no. 2 (Winter 2003). https://doi.org/10.1086/374029.

Meagher, Jack, and Pat Broughton. *Sports Massage.* USA: Dolphin Books, Doubleday, 1980.

Murray, Col. *In Search of Tom Bowen and the Therapy he Inspired and Lots of Other Stuff.* Armadale: Palmer Higgs, Booksonline, 2010.

Perry, John. *The Quick and the Dead, Stawell and It's Race through Time.* Sydney: UNINSW Press, 2002.

Shah, J. P., N. Thaker, J. Heimur, J. V. Aredo, S. Sikdar, and L. Gerber. "Myofascial Trigger Points Then and Now: A Historical and Scientific Perspective." *PM* and *R: The Journal of Injury, Function, and Rehabilitation* 7, no. 7 (2015): 746–61. Accessed November 17, 2024. https://doi.org/10.1016/j.pmrj.2015.01.024. http://www.ncbi.nlm.nih.gov/pmc/articles/PMC4508225/.

Shurtleff, William, and Akiko Aoyagi. *Soyinfo Center, History of Soybeans and Soyfoods in Australia, New Zealand and Oceania 1770–2010, extensively annotated bibliography and Sourcebook.* Lafayette, CA: SoyInfo Center, 2010. Accessed November 17, 2024. www.soyinfocenter.com/pdf/138/Ocea2.pdf.

Simons, David, Janet Travell, and Lois S. Simons. *Myofascial Pain and Dysfunction: The Trigger Point Manual, Volume 1. Upper Half of Body.* 2nd ed. Philadelphia: Lippincott Williams and Wilkins, 1999.

Strachan, Shirley, and Keir Reeves. "Through the Lens of the Trainer-Masseurs: Australia's Incongruous Engagement with the Olympic Amateur Ethos." *The International Journal of the History of Sport* 39, no. 6 (2022): 631–52. https://doi.org/10.1080/09523367.2022.2095369.

The XIth Olympic Games Berlin, 1936, Official Report Volume 1. Wilhelm Limpert, Berlin, S. W.68: Organisationskomittee Fur die XI. Olympiade Berlin 1936 E.V, 1936. Accessed February 10, 2019 https://digital.la84.org/digital/collection/p17103coll8/id/16471/rec/15.

Wilson, Jo-Ann. "The Effects of Sports Massage on Athletic Performance and General Function." *Massage Therapy Journal* (Summer 2002): 90–100. Accessed November 17, 2024. http://www.sportsmassageinc.com/EffectsOfSportsMassage.pdf.
Writer, Larry. *Dangerous Games, Australia at the 1936 Nazi Olympics.* Sydney: Allen and Unwin, 2015.

Websites

"1914–1918 Online." *International Encyclopaedia of the First World War.* Accessed November 17, 2024. http://encyclopedia.1914-1918-online.net/article/prisoners_of_war_and_internees_great_britain.
McMeekin, Joan. "How an Anglo Indian Man Made Australian Therapy Great." *History.Physio*, May 13, 2020. Accessed November 17, 2024. https://history.physio/how-an-anglo-indian-man-made-australian-physiotherapy-great/.

Video

Wellcome Library. "Sir Herbert Barkers' Manipulative Technique: Part 1 (1936)." *YouTube* Video. 12.05 Minutes. Posted January 19, 2011. Accessed November 17, 2024. http://www.youtube.com/watch?v=aVYQmJMqxbs.
Wellcome Library. "Sir Herbert Barker's Manipulative Technique: Part 2 (1936)." *YouTube* Video. 10.38 Minutes. Posted January 19, 2011. Accessed November 17, 2024. https://www.youtube.com/watch?v=4Ok410KqD9Q.

5 Recontextualising Bowen and Eastern Medicine

Introduction: The Narrative of Leslie Edward Dettman, Talented Football Masseur and Lay Chiropractor

There is a presumption in posthumous interpretations of Bowen's work that Ernie Saunders, subject of Chapter 4, was Bowen's mentor and introduced Bowen to Eastern medicine and that Eastern concepts of anatomy, including acupoint and energy meridians, are foundational to Bowen's work. The Dettman narrative that gave rise to this is sourced to Keith Davis DC – a Bowen clinic observer who had a great interest in well-known manual healers. Davis practised in Frankston at the opposite eastern side of Port Phillip Bay to Geelong. There, in local newspapers, he read articles about Les Dettman, a lay chiropractor who had developed a strong profile in the community press. Leslie (Les) Edward Dettman (1888–1972) was eight years younger than Saunders and both had sons who were athletes in the Young Men's Christian Association (YMCA) and sporting circuit: Richard Saunders was a comedic high board diver and also featured in swimming and football.[1] Laurie Dettman was regularly profiled as a runner in the press from the mid-1930s and missed out on the Berlin Olympics after being beaten by Gerald Backhouse. Both Saunders and Dettman had reputations as football masseurs though the publicity afforded to Saunders in major metropolitan newspapers was significantly greater in comparison. Saunders' long history was reported in the press and there are multiple articles describing his achievements with athletes as a masseur:

> Ern roved for Collingwood in their first two years in League football to the ruckman of those past champions Ted Murphy and Billy Proudfoot. In those days Collingwood's star kickers were Archie Smith and 'Splinter' Anderson. Ern then played with South Melbourne for 3 years on the same side as Billy Windley that great exponent of the place kick. Following upon which he took up the job of training the University side all the years they were in the league. After 11 years at Brunswick (9 of which he was head trainer) Ern came to Richmond in 1923 to take up his present duties.[2]

DOI: 10.4324/9781003602125-6

Dettman was a well-known lay chiropractor of German descent whose arrival in Australia is not known but grew up in Kyneton, spent his marriage years from 1914 in Port Melbourne, then moved to Malvern in 1942 before settling in Yarra Junction from 1949. Dettman was a runner of profile in his younger years and reported as having set up a physiotherapy business in Melbourne and well-known in football circles.[3] Dettman was also well known in Kyneton as a cross-country coach of runners, including his three sons.[4] At Yarra Junction, Dettman treated the community and footballers such as Bob Skilton; he was well respected and addressed as 'Mr Dettman, the Chiropractor'.[5] The newspaper coverage of him in local Yarra Junction news is not available online at Trove, but clearly, he had a profile for Davis to be interested in meeting him. Both families had a connection with the YMCA, and during the war, the son Laurie Dettman served as commissioner to the YMCA in Papua New Guinea.[6]

Davis DC happened to spot Dettman's name on a fence at Yarra Junction one evening and knocked on his door, was welcomed inside and had a conversation with him. The date of the encounter is not stated, but since Dettman was living alone this post-dates the death of his wife Violet Maude who died on June 8, 1970, and places Dettman in his early eighties. Dettman said to Davis that he and Ernie Saunders had gone to a workshop in America between the wars and learned Japanese acupressure techniques.[7] This later recounting by Davis of what Dettman said and combined with the knowledge that Bowen had made the acquaintance of Saunders and adopted his practice of 'putting stoppers on', allowed the notion to take off that Saunders was Bowen's mentor and wellspring of Bowen's techniques – specifically techniques that justified Bowen's work being assumed to be founded in Eastern medicine.

These conclusions are subject to critical challenge on several fronts. Chapter 4 documented what was publicly known about Saunders' ability and how he described his work in his own words. There is not a trace of any symbolism or influences related to Eastern Medicine. Chapter 2 presented oral histories and evidence of Bowen's unfinished osteopathy studies at an English college, his ongoing self-study and adoption of the title of osteopath. This was not simply a case of assuming an identity to set up in business and Bowen was recognised by his college-trained observers as versed in osteopathic and related chiropractic principles and demonstrated professional discipline in how he approached his patients. Chapter 3 described a field of osteopathy called neuropathy brought to Australia by naturopathic pioneers FG Roberts and Maurie Blackmore both of who held out as neuropaths and offered training in the early period. The congruence with Bowen's language about nerve pressure and his delivery and approach to the practice of pressure movements more closely tie Bowen to neuropathy along with osteopathy than Eastern Medicine – until the 1970s decade arrives. Additionally, Bowen is also connected to Alister McAlister DO (discussed in Chapters 2, 7 and 8), a 1958 Robert's college graduate and earlier known to have provided clinic placements under Blackmores NANOC association/school and later for the Roberts College students in the 1960s.

These elements together are more credible as influences on Bowen than the Japanese acupoints story mentioned by Dettman.

Saunders' Overseas Travel to the Berlin Olympiad and America

Further research did indeed prove Saunders travelled overseas between the wars, specifically in 1936 as an honorary masseur to the Australian athletes competing at the Berlin Olympiad. He was a newly registered masseur and made plans for a study tour of the USA.[8] Research of digitised passenger records online failed to find any evidence of Dettman with Saunders, either on the *Mongolia* for Berlin in 1936, or after on the *Scythia* for New York. Furthermore, Dettman's name is not indexed for any travel to America at any time in the twentieth century either. Added to this, and more telling, is that the Dettman family was contacted via the husband of Dettman's granddaughter who confirmed no family knowledge of such travel either, but the possibility was outright discounted on account of Dettman's domestic and financial circumstances.[9] From family descriptions of Dettman's treatments, Les Dettman did have knowledge of putting pressure on points to treat migraine and knew how to rectify twisted joint ligaments.[10] The family had no knowledge where their relative learned these massage and manipulative skills and they were not aware of any connection with Saunders.[11] The men would have known of each other as prominent football masseurs and through the media exposure of the sporting achievements of their respective sons in the press. Laurie was a foot-runner of note but was not selected for the Games, having been beaten by Gerald Backhouse which further supports the unlikelihood of Dettman making the trip to the Games. Apart from the significant financial cost and the family's advice, there was no personal motivation to do so as Dettman's son Laurie was not competing. Laurie Dettman was a champion foot runner, but it was Gerald Backhouse who competed for Australia at the Berlin Olympiad.[12] At the outbreak of war, Laurie Dettman settled the score and resoundly beat Backhouse.[13] The reasons and motivations for Dettman's remarks will never be known. Dettman was quite elderly at the time and died soon after being brought to Melbourne to be cared for by family members.[14]

The story about a Japanese acupoints workshop only came from one source and if true should have been readily validated, given the availability of passenger lists for Saunders' trip to America in 1936. Saunders was vocal and communicative to the press about observations that could enhance sporting performance and he made no mention of any Japanese acupoint training and showed no interest in Japanese massage techniques at Berlin. Yet, strong attention on the Japanese swimmers was carried through from the Los Angeles Olympics in 1932 to Berlin in 1936.[15] The sensational swimming feats of the Japanese at Los Angeles were remarked on by Ted Gill as coach-masseur to the Australian team and other keen observers. The use of oxygen and a vegetable diet by the Japanese swimmers were all that Saunders noted along with loosening up exercises; there is no intrigue whatsoever with massage being a contributor to their performance.[16] Given his communication style, this would be something he would be expected to comment on. Saunders spoke only of vitamins taken by athletes as retaining 'electricity' in the body and defraying fatigue.[17] Japanese massage was not at all topical in the Australian press either. The previous chapter highlighted the contact the Australian team had with German masseurs in Berlin and the style of massage in Germany called 'Reflex massage' was touched on and developed by writers such as Alfons Cornelius who wrote about 'Druckpuntes' (stress/pressure points) in 1902.[18] Like shiatsu, this kind of pressure-points system bears some similarities with neuropathy in regard to cutano-visceral reflexes but is not delivered within an osteopathic framework, nor does it use the symbolism of neuropathy and 'lifting pressure off nerves'. Chapter 4 outlined the prevalence of German massage utilised by key figures in Saunder's circle of head trainers. The chapter noted the historical review by Travell and Simons in their manuals on Trigger Points developed in the 1940s referenced sources dating from 1843, including German (excluded Cornelius) describing tender spots and referred pain.[19] They discuss Melsack et al. on the high correspondence (71 per cent) between trigger points and acupoints.[20] However, trigger points, German druckpuntes and Indian marma points, do not follow Eastern concepts of energy meridians.

Namikoshi's Shiatsu

Tellingly, the shiatsu book that Bowen held up to Smeeton in the late 1970s with the words, 'this is the basis of the work lad' (and for those who uncritically accept the Dettman story was proof of the Japanese acupressure training story), lacks any reference to acupoints and meridians. The book was written by Tokijuro Namikoshi.[21] Namikoshi's shiatsu is strictly Western in its concepts. There is no mention whatsoever of energy meridians in the explanations of Namikoshi's shiatsu by the developer or his son, the concepts are all based on Western anatomy and the spinal system and cutano-visceral reflexes.[22] Namikoshi's son Toro states his father surmounted difficulties in his study of Japanese anma massage and western massage as he tried to extricate shiatsu from anma massage.[23] Namikoshi established his first shiatsu school in the East in 1925 and the Japan Shiatsu Institute in 1940, but it was not until much later in 1953 that he took shiatsu or finger pressure to the West after he was invited by a group of chiropractic schools to lecture in the USA.[24] Namikoshi was based at the Palmer College of Chiropractic.[25] Namikoshi's first book on shiatsu was first published in the West later in 1969, over three decades after Saunders' last overseas trip in 1936.[26]

The 1970s, Bowen's Interest, Popularity of Eastern Medicine and Use of Finger Pressure Instead of Needles on Acupoints

Did Bowen make a mistake when he obtained Namikoshi's shiatsu and showed it to Smeeton? Did he really intend a source instead based on traditional anma shiatsu that incorporated acupoints and Chinese energy meridians? In Smeeton's view, Bowen just held up the book as a convenient way to fend off questions as the work involved pressure on areas of the body and recognised reflex relationships and that is how he worked.[27] So why was Bowen introducing Eastern medicine into the symbolism of his work in the 1970s? To answer that question, thought needs to be given to information that was trending in Bowen's milieu and professional networks at the time, especially those he operated with as a member of ACONPAL. At the time until 1975, ACONPAL included college-trained practitioners as well as men like Bowen who had passed the required standards. Peter Derig DC/ND was an ACONPAL member and involved with the South Pacific College in Sydney and had been enrolled at the Palmer College in 1963.[28] Derig offered shiatsu as part of his course curriculum at the NSW College of Osteopathic and Naturopathic Sciences (principal Dr D Hamieri) formed as the result of an amalgamation in 1976 of the South Pacific College of Natural Therapeutics and the Derig's NSW College of Naturopathic Sciences.[29] Derig's exposure to shiatsu at Palmer College should logically be Namikoshi's work. However, later on, post-2002 under Nationally Recognised Training, certificate IV courses in shiatsu leaned to anma shiatsu incorporating Chinese Meridians Chi energy flow concepts.[30] Today, this anma view of shiatsu now seems to predominate over Namikoshi's western-focused work.[31]

Bowen undeniably had an interest in acupuncture in the 1970s. In October 1973 at the Ward Inquiry, he indicated to the government panel, he was 'waiting on a book on acupuncture'.[32] Derig also had a strong interest in acupuncture and arranged the first class in 1972 the year before.[33] Attendees included Arthur Wright, Bob Lucy's associate Fred Weston of the Canberra College of Natural Therapeutics and others.[34] Acupuncture became popular in the west after Whitlam and Nixon's visits to China in 1970 and 1971, respectively, and taken more seriously after the televising the use of acupuncture anaesthesia and Derig describes a segment filmed in Australia in 1973.[35] Bowen emerges as a practitioner of his time and someone quick to pick up on what was topical in professional circles around him and to learn more about these trends among his peers. Keith Davis's late wife, Audrey, had some knowledge of acupuncture and Bowen was known to spend time with her discussing the subject when he could.[36]

The Ward Inquiry looked at the topic of acupuncture and only one reference was sourced.[37] Mention was made of acupuncture training available with FG Roberts College and that Frank Hegyi, a chiropractor, was the president of the newly formed Victorian Acupuncture Association.[38] Formed only in 1974, over half of the association members were Victorian Chiropractic Association (VCA – American trained) or the now titled United Chiropractors Association of Australasia (UCAA) – the national body for Australian-trained chiropractors (including those dual-qualified as osteopaths), the rest were naturopaths and osteopaths.[39] There were only seventeen members of the acupuncture association.[40] Frank Hegyi was born in Hungary in 1923 and a child had been manipulated by a Chinese herbalist for a dangerous heart condition and improved.[41] After emigrating in 1949, he completed training with Roberts' CCA in 1967. Hegyi's professional involvement with acupuncture was very recent having involved trips to the Korean Kyung Lee University, considered the best and teaching about ten to twenty groups from around the world. Hegyi also trained with private practitioners in Tokyo and Hong Kong.[42] Frank Hegyi also alluded to the televised segment mentioned by Derig.[43] Barry Jones was specifically interested in classes at South Korea's Kyung Lee University called 'acupuncture and meridian practice'. Hegyi replied (and without reference to shiatsu):

> Acupuncture does not necessarily mean needles are inserted into the body. *It could be done by manipulating the meridian which is part of those points on the particular point to the organ. By finger pressure on the acupuncture point one can obtain the same results as a needle or even better results in some cases*. [emphasis added][44]

The only transcript of much earlier practice of needle acupuncture in Victoria is the transcript of Joseph John Mik who said he was taught in 1920–1925 by a Russian doctor who had been to China before Mik emigrated in 1949.[45] Mik also described 'Eastern manipulation' where he would ask a client 'to put his leg up his back. I touch it with my fingers, but I do not use much pressure'.

Chapter 3 confirmed that Maurice Blackmore like FG Roberts was described a neuropath in the early twentieth century. Blackmore presented to the Ward Inquiry in 1973 and spoke of 'a naturopathic type of manipulation using pressure on points'.[46] Blackmore made no mention of shiatsu to suggest he meant any reference to Eastern manual medicine and no reference to Chinese meridians. This description also mirrors the description in the newspaper advertisement of FG Roberts described in Chapter 3 and leads to a Western rather than Eastern practice as foundational to these techniques. By the time Blackmore presented to the Inquiry, he had been retired from his teaching network for over a decade and was focused on developing his herbal products so it is reasonable to assume he was referring to his earlier knowledge of practice in naturopathic physical medicine drawn from neuropathy. In addition to the lack of reference to shiatsu or acupressure in the Ward Inquiry, it is noted that the ACONPAL publication makes no mention of shiatsu and acupressure, only acupuncture citing one article that presents acupuncture as acupuncture-neuropathy.[47] This would suggest that shiatsu did not have a sufficient market profile at this stage.

Kevin Ryan DO, the only Bowen college-trained observer who was a trained osteopath, said that Bowen stood apart from his peers and said, 'Bowen developed and applied his techniques largely within the postural structural paradigm of osteopathy and always within the framework of osteopathic principles. He also had a well-developed approach to viscero-somatic therapy'.[48] Chapters 2 and 8 consider Bowen in the context of peers in his own generation who were football masseurs and include those who went on to formally qualify after first self-identifying as osteopaths and before regulation. McAlister, in particular, emerges as a key figure most likely to be a Bowen mentor as he developed in his work – a vocation that became home to his unusual sensory giftedness and other esoteric ideas he brought to his practice. The Ward Inquiry Report stated of McAlister, 'He believed that many major diseases originate in the feet'.[49] This seems to be a misrepresentation of reflexology and a possible indication that McAlister was familiar with zone therapy and reflex relationships between areas of feet and structure/organs of the body. In his transcript, he discusses reflex points on the feet suggesting he was versed in the pressure techniques of reflexology.[50]

Applying finger pressure work on acupoints instead of needles and to meridians is evident in transcripts to the Ward Inquiry. Bowen is revealed as someone with an active intelligence attempting to synthesise new ideas and it is clear he was embarking on his own journey of piecing the Western and Eastern anatomical maps together. Frijov Capra explored the parallels between modern physics and Eastern mysticism and quoted semanticist Alfred Korsybski's slogan, 'the map is not the territory'.[51] Excepting unique adaptations to extreme or unusual environments, human bodies share the same gross anatomy and physiology. Different cultures use different conceptual maps to understand how the body works and traditions in manual medicine are uniquely defined by philosophies about the body that give meaning and shape to their unique maps. Bowen had the ability to sense nerve activity and knew how to trace the paths of nerves. Translating the Eastern system to Western physiology, Longhurst explained:

> Modern physiologists have put forward the 'neural hypothesis' stating that the clinical influence of acupuncture is transmitted primarily through stimulation of sensory nerves that provide signals to the brain, which processes this information and then causes clinical changes associated with treatment.[52]

The posthumous interpretations of Bowen's work were born at a time when appropriation of Eastern ideas and practice in the West had become common place. Practitioners already trained in massage or other CAM subjects and embarking on roles as instructors for the various Bowen schools were already exposed to these concepts. It is not surprising that there was a spontaneous tendency to view what was represented of Bowen's work – orphaned from his osteopathic base – in terms that integrated these novel ideas from Eastern medicine. Bowen himself was influenced by these and as described earlier, his symbolism of nerve pressure and pinched nerves used in the Ward Inquiry and described in Chapter 3, started to give way to non-Western frames of reference in the 1970s. This started with the mention of 'waiting on a book on acupuncture' at the Ward Inquiry in 1973 and Davis DC's recounting of Bowen seeking out his wife Audrey to discuss acupuncture. Like many in the chiropractic and osteopathic field at the time, Audrey Davis had learnt acupuncture in the 1970s and Bowen was keen to talk with her on the topic; Bowen showed

Romney the book on shiatsu (a Western anatomical model of Japanese pressure points) in the late 1970s, declaring 'this is the basis of the work lad' and Ann Mortelliti a patient recalled from a social encounter:

> Anyway, so one day while we were talking, I said to Mr Bowen, (my husband had gone out to serve) and I was sitting at the table and I said to him, 'What do you call what you do? 'Well' he said, 'I work on pressure points'. Right? 'On pressure points'. I said, 'Yes, well where did you learn that?' He told me, 'overseas'.[53]

In Smeeton's opinion, Bowen showed the shiatsu book as an easy way of explaining what he was doing and to fend off questions.[54] Just months before his death, Bowen mentioned nothing of Eastern Medicine concepts in the newspaper article in 1982 after he failed the Registration Board's examinations.[55] He spoke simply, 'I only use my ten fingers in my work'.[56] In the article, Bowen says 'Osteopathic,[*sic*] in contrast to chiropractic which involves manipulation of the spinal column, is a system of diagnosis and treatment of disorders by manipulation of muscle and nerve tissue'.[57] None of the former patients interviewed for the *Healing Hands* anthology ascribed any notions of Eastern Medicine to Bowen's work, instead it was dismissed outright. Ryan DO who started observing Bowen later in 1979 recalled that Bowen had books on acupuncture, yet Ryan once noted that the points that Bowen had marked on a physiology book and used for some of his moves were not on acupoints.[58] Bowen maintained a study and library at the Horwood home where he first started his formal practice. When Rene Horwood was asked in 1998 'What sort of books did he . . . was he ever interested in things like acupuncture and things like that? Did he ever look into Chinese type of things?', Horwood answered, 'No, I think he might have in the early days because he used to say his method went back to the osteopath days, really; Chinese sort of, the same points as that for acupuncture'. When pressed further 'But did he know about the points, like do you think he read up about the points, then started to use them and then sort of looked them up?', Horwood just said, 'I don't know where it started from. He seemed to have this feeling in his fingers' and goes on to explain Bowen's use of pennies to detect breaks in nerve conduction in the spine.[59]

From a historical perspective, the trending interests and developments were a result of new boundaries of knowledge opening up to Eastern medicine and professionals taking the lead and following their curiosity. Tom Dummer, dean of the ESO, was integrating ideas from Tibetan Eastern Medicine and Western medicine and later published his ideas in 1988 and dedicated three chapters to osteopathy in this context.[60] Through ACONPAL and having entertained Robert (Bob) Lucy in his clinics, Bowen enjoys a 'six degrees of separation' connection to Dummer and Chapter 6 traces the organisational connections between ACONPAL and its parent South Pacific Body to Dummer as honorary secretary of the International Federation of Practitioners of Natural Therapeutics. The Ward Inquiry sourced John Worsley's book on acupuncture and Worsley earned his Doctorate and Master status in acupuncture between the 1950s and 1960s.[61] From the material in the Ward Inquiry transcripts and the dates of publications – especially of applying pressure to acupoints instead of needles – it is evident that the professional interest in acupuncture/acupressure in the West was very recent. This is consistent with the western popularisation of acupuncture after Whitlam and Nixon's visits to China.[62] Retrospectively, it can be argued that Bowen, on his own intuitive and practical level, was thinking about and attempting to figure out the relationships between Western and Oriental manual medicine. It is interesting to compare the stimulation and inhibition of spinal reflexes featured in neuropathy and osteopathy as described in Chapter 3 with those of Eastern ideas that utilise pressure on acupuncture points without needles, zone therapy which utilised pressure to inhibit painful reflexes and Namikoshi's shiatsu based on Western anatomy.[63] Bowen's college-trained observers attest to Bowen's knowledge of nerve reflexes and not only the location of nerves but also his ability to trace their path to the periphery. Eastern anatomy was in vogue in Bowen's professional networks and allowed him to explore them in the frame of knowledge that was topical. When Bowen said he was 'waiting on a book on acupuncture' to the Ward Inquiry in 1973, this suggests this timing was his first foray into the subject. He did not say he worked with acupuncture or was familiar with related knowledge at all. However, even before Bowen knew what acupoints were, it stands to reason, given his sensitivity to bio-electricity that he would have detected and felt the sites of acupoints before had a knowledge-base to draw on to describe them. This is discussed further in Chapter 8.

It is not surprising that posthumous representations of Bowen's work included features of Eastern medicine and in attempt to integrate them with the Western base that provided the origins of Bowen's work. These interpretations have influenced how Bowen Therapy/Technique is taught and interpreted as part of Complementary Physical Medicine today, though website descriptions tend to focus on the 'Bowen Move', the gentleness of treatment for all ages including babies and outcomes in terms of relaxation and wellbeing along with a list of conditions that benefit from a Bowen treatment. Several posthumous interpretations include Eastern or Asian concepts. These are dually the result of the teachers' own exposure to globalisation in the 1970s and the observation to those trained in Eastern medicine that the Eastern map of the body makes sense in the application of Bowen's techniques. Chapter 6 covers the interest of other contemporary ACONPAL directors in Bowen's work; Bob Lucy and Bill Pruss visited Bowen to watch him work in his clinic with visits occurring from the early 1970s. Reportedly, both were observed to be demonstrating Bowen-like techniques at the South Pacific College in Sydney in the later 1970s. In 1984, two years after Bowen's death, Lucy opened his own college the College of Somatic Studies in 1984, and according to an instructor working for him, as soon as his college was established, from the outset, Lucy offered Myorthotics as part of a naturopathic qualification.[64] The manuals for the early teaching are not in the author's possession, but his

1991 manual and training video are. Lucy's interests were strongly based in naturopathy and he had trained in chiropractic through the Blackmore and Boughen's schools as described in Chapter 6. The name he coined was derived from 'myo' representing muscle and 'orthotics' for supportive and relaxant.[65] After his death in 1999, his college continued to offer Myorthotics as part of the Advanced Diploma of Naturopathy.[66]

Lucy never claimed to be teaching how Bowen practised and he did not use the term 'Bowen Technique' or 'Therapy' but he did acknowledge Bowen's assumed vocational identity as 'one of Victoria's first osteopaths' as the inspiration for Myorthotics. Likely due to his limited number of visits to Bowen's clinic, he described what he had observed as 'effective but unrelated movements applied to areas of the body where pain was present' and that he systematised these and added movements of his own.[67] Lucy's knowledge base and focus is on chiropractic supported by naturopathic principles and this influenced his description of his system based on Bowen's work. Myorthotics featured a mixture of Western and Eastern perspectives. It was described as a relaxing technique for muscles, ligaments and sinews with the purpose of removing uneven strains on spinal vertebrae. Lucy did not consider it needed the same precision as a chiropractic adjustment and Bowen's system would not replace chiropractic theory. He did acknowledge that it was complementary to chiropractic as it dispensed with otherwise painful chiropractic moves on painfully spasmed areas.[68] The manual covers concepts rooted in western anatomy and releasing contracted tissues that could strain the spine with reference to nerve reflexes and internal organs of the endocrine, reproductive and urinary systems – specifically in relation to the thyroid, ovary, prostate, bladder and kidneys. The supporting video produced in 1991 teaches the technique based on holistic principles of body and mind harmony, the importance of spinal alignment and correcting leg-length discrepancies. On the subject of the 'blockers' or 'stoppers' that Bowen said to Davis DC that Ernie Saunders was emphatic be employed, Lucy explains the importance of waiting two minutes after the lumbar blocks were put in so the muscles relax and avoid headaches and likewise, not breaking through the thoracic blocks as tension necks and headaches can result there too. Lucy also expanded the use of blockers to above where any work was done such as the ankle and the knee. His explanation of the blocks or stoppers was the blocks prevented pain from reflexing to other parts of the body causing extra tension or upsetting work done. Lucy's guidelines to an effective treatment are more revealing about the knowledge base he used to understand the work.

Australians who have integrated Western and Eastern ideas into their teachings of Bowen's methods and published books or developed manuals include Robert (Bob) Lucy DC, Graham Pennington, Brian Smart and Kevin Ryan DO and overseas practitioners include USA's Gene Dobkin. Lucy's manual clearly refers to acupoints (and what Lucy termed 'Myorthotic reflex points'). In addition to chiropractic and naturopathic concepts employed, Lucy incorporated polarity therapy and the idea that different parts of our bodies carry different charges – the head being positive, the feet negative, right side being positive and the left negative. Lucy was not the only one to view his interpretation of Bowen's work through the lens of polarity therapy. This is interesting, given that Stanley Lief's development of Neuromuscular Technique (NMT) was derived from pulling together the work of Dewandchand Varma who lived in Paris in the 1930s and was based on Indian Ayurvedic medicine which expounded the existence of bio-currents in the body and the need to balance their amplitude to skin and organs. Varma is a known foundational influence on Stanley Lief's development of NMT with Boris Chaitow between the wars and learned in nature cure circles teaching osteopathy and chiropractic.[69] Ayurvedic medicine also recognises points on the body called Marma points classified into categories of martial/warfare interest, surgical and medical for the treatment, management and diagnosis of diseases that are treated by applying pressure.[70] Marma composition includes muscles and their sheaths, fluids, ligaments and tendons and joints.[71] These are not specifically referred to by Varma, but Raymond Nimmo who developed the USA variant of NMT, recognised the work of Travell and Simons' trigger points and correlations with acupoints as integral to modern NMT.[72] The work of Randalph Stone and polarity therapy is incorporated into a publication on Pranotherapy referred to in NMT textbooks.[73]

Fascial Therapy was established by Graham Pennington in 1992, originally a teaching collaboration with Alf Jacka's college, the Southern School of Natural Therapies and as an elective for six years for students enrolled in naturopathy or massage. There were 260 therapists trained beforehand and an additional estimated 250 students took the opportunity to be trained at this time. The early Fascial Therapy manual (2nd edition 1993) is entirely western though there is a cover sheet that starts to introduce Eastern concepts.[74] Pennington was trained in acupuncture and was developing these ideas at the time, but it was not until he published *A Textbook of the Bowen Technique* in 2012 that he presented fully fledged correlations between Eastern acupoints based on his integration of Bowen methods with his professional clinical practice in acupuncture in the years between.[75] Today, Graham Pennington is an independent instructor teaching Bowen Seminars following the publication of his textbook. He has taught in Australia and internationally in New Zealand, the USA, the UK and with workshops held in 2014 in Croatia, Holland, South Africa and Singapore and later in the USA and Austria, some attended by Smeeton DC to assist with demonstrations of techniques. Smeeton's own conceptual framework about Bowen's work is founded on Western anatomy, but he has an open mind about the integration with Eastern Medicine – firstly because Bowen was known to be interested in Eastern Medicine in the 1970s and secondly because there were aspects of Bowen's approach that could not be explained by Western ideas alone. For instance, Bowen's kidney work involved specifics around when moves would be open or closed; Bowen was adamant that the kidney moves never be left open (brought about by the cross-fibre move being made laterally away from the spine, rather than medially). Most of the moves in the Bowen repertoire are medial moves and he had reasons for an open move with kidneys. Since these moves were done on the back, in Western terms and in the context of neuropathy and spinal reflexes, this was likely intended to increase blood flow and circulation resulting in kidney detoxification and production of urine. In Eastern terms, the kidney meridian is on the front of the body and the meridians influenced on the back would be the governing meridian and the bladder meridian. Smeeton recalled that Bowen's kidney work also integrated with his work on the brain; on a simplistic level, since 'kidney moves' made on the back influence the governing meridian or vessel of Eastern anatomy and the governing vessel relates to the brain, this makes sense.[76] Pennington is an advocate of Eastern Medicine as foundational to Bowen's work and has uncritically accepted the Dettman account about Ernie Saunders that purports Saunders' attendance at a Japanese acupressure course in the USA between the wars, and that Saunders was Bowen's mentor in this regard. This acceptance was due to the fact that he wrote to Davis DC who confirmed the story Dettman told him.[77] Pennington's textbook affirms Bowen's grasp of the osteopathic relationship between structure and function and looks deeper at spinal reflexes to internal organs and highlights that those who watched Bowen work claimed 'he gave special significance to a few areas of the body' and mentions Bowen's 'particular emphasis on restoring function to the sacroiliac joints, the coccyx, the cervical spine and the temporomandibular joint'.[78] Pennington elaborated on the relationship between Bowen's neck moves and cranial bones that are sites of dural attachment and raises awareness of dural drag or dural tension and the effect on health.[79]

Brian Smart, another Australian, developed Smart Bowen in 1992 – a system of more remedial Bowen Therapy procedures based on trigger points and Chinese Acupuncture theory.[80] Smart, who was trained in remedial massage, describes Bowen Therapy as 'a soft tissue, rolling/stretching technique which is applied in mostly two-directional cross-fibre movements using the thumbs or fingers on the skin'.[81] Wherever possible, Smart 'applies Bowen moves to active, satellite and latent trigger points and on acupuncture points selected specifically based on the client's presenting problems'.[82] Travell and Simons' seminal trigger point manuals are used to decide on points to focus on, based on pain patterns.[83]

Bowen observer Ryan DO, a qualified acupuncturist and osteopath developed his own system combining Bowen moves with acupoints drawn from John Worsley's Five Element Theory and currently teaches this work today.[84] On his current website, he describes that on attending for his first clinic with Bowen in 1979, Bowen reportedly said to him that he would have no trouble with his work because Ryan did acupuncture. The timing of this remark is interesting as it post-dates the new legislation and Bowen had his business cards revised to 'natural therapist' as osteopath/DO had become a protected title he was not allowed to use. To Ryan, the trigger points and the blocks and stoppers terms that Bowen used were acupuncture points and Bowen was treating meridians of Eastern Medicine.[85]

Romney Smeeton DC (in partnership with Ross Emmett and developer of Emmett Technique) for a period offered a seminar called 'What Tom said' as part of a course called Tom Bowen Therapy (TBT) 101 that was taught solely through the Emmett School. Today the course is offered through Emmett UK.[86] In 1999, Ross Emmett formalised the establishment of Emmett therapy with registration in Queensland and on a wider scale around 2000.[87] Emmett technique itself is not Bowen Therapy, but it is well accepted as a complementary adjunct to Bowen within the professional Emmett/Bowen community. Emmett Technique involves 'the application of light finger pressure at specific points, referred to as "Emmett points"'. According to Emmett, the points are 'not the same as traditional trigger points or acupressure points or any other points described in any other therapy'.[88] Romney reportedly said of Emmett's work, 'He has an understanding and feeling for Tom Bowen's work that I believe is far greater than anyone I have met, including those of us who actually watched Tom work'.[89]

Overseas instructors of Bowen's techniques also integrated Western ideas with other systems including acupoints. In 1998/99 on the cusp of starting instruction for the Neurostructural Integration Technique (NST) before setting up his own US Bowen school, Gene Dobkin published *The Bowen Companion, Volume 1 and Volume 2*.[90] On his impressions gained of Bowen the man, Dobkin acknowledged his knowledge of Bowen was sketchy and second-hand. He stated contradictions in reports and speculated that Bowen toyed with people 'much like "rascal gurus" (but not in the cultish sense) who don't wish their students to merely copy but instead grasp the core of the work'.[91] Dobkin's *Bowen Companion* written in 1998/99 additionally presented new ideas that correlated hand placements and moves of Bowen Therapy with various points, including Chapman points, neurolymphatic points and acupoints.[92] Similarly to Lucy, he referred to polarity therapy and specifically Randalph Stone's work on Polarity Therapy. This correlation was done in a historical vacuum absent any osteopathic knowledge system used by Bowen and not informed by contact with Bowen's clinician associates whose existence was only becoming known to the international Bowen community at this time. The acupoints' correlation was picked up and in the 1990s, acupoints and meridians were common in workshops and working with Bowen moves and meridians included in nationally qualified training in Australia at least from 2009.[93]

In the UK, Jock Ruddock (1942–2011) and his partner Ivana established VibroHarmonisation Technique.[94] Ruddock already had experience working with wrestlers and in the 1990s trained in the Bowtech interpretation. From there, the Ruddocks developed ideas of using distorted muscle recoil to set up a vibration in soft tissues and incorporated ideas including Eastern from TCM, Dynamic Ki, Isogai and tai chi flow, as well as kinesiology, craniosacral technique, Kahuna and Hyperton-X. By 1999, Ruddock and his partner developed a way of working with pressure points combined with tai chi flow to initiate relaxation and homeostasis. Their work is applied to horse and dogs too.

In 1997, VHT was officially accepted by the Institute of Complementary Health and the British Complementary Medicine Association amongst others.

When Thomas Myers first published *Anatomy Trains* in 2001, he generated some excitement when he presented an appendix that showed the myofascial lines, or anatomy he had discovered as a result of dissection of cadavers, overlaid with Eastern meridian lines.[95] Myers avoided a more definitive response when he was asked questions as Eastern Medicine is not his area of expertise, but he recently recommended a paper included in later additions of his book that clarified the correspondence between acupoints on meridians and trigger points which are known to generate pain patterns.[96] Dorsher, the paper's author, concluded:

> The strong (up to 91%) consistency of the distributions of trigger point regions' referred pain patterns to acupuncture meridians provides a fourth line of evidence that trigger points most likely represent the same physiological phenomenon as acupuncture points in the treatment of pain disorders.[97]

Bowen's work acknowledged myofascial lines in the sense that where a patient was experiencing pain was not necessarily where he applied his treatment. For instance, when clearing the pelvis of imbalance with the patient prone, the hamstrings, iliotibial band, tensor fascia lata and gluteus maximus are addressed before the sacral ligaments are influenced with leg level work. Similarly, when supine, if indicated, muscles below the pelvis such as adductors, vastus lateralis, sartorius and rectus femoris are balanced before inguinal ligaments are influenced with leg work. The growing field of fascia science explains this in terms of the body being a tensegrity structure.[98]

Does it enhance results to integrate Western and Eastern models of anatomy into the interpretation of Bowen's techniques? In practice, this comes down to the expertise and knowledge system that the practitioner works with. Smeeton DC has refined his application of Bowen's techniques for nearly half a century using the western anatomy of his clinical training and with excellent results in long and successful service to a huge client base. Neave DC (dec) and Davis DC likewise continued with western anatomy. Ryan DO, trained in acupuncture and founded his understanding and knowledge base on Eastern anatomy and has developed his training combining Bowen's physical methods with the five-element theory of acupuncture. Chapter 8 also discusses the Eastern theme in the Bowen story under the topic of Medical Pluralism and Beyond.

Summary

There is nothing about Saunders' style of work, how he spoke about it or was described by others that gives any sense that he was working with or imparting to others knowledge of Eastern medicine. Focusing on a Western context, overall, Bowen's knowledge of pressure on nerve segments and stimulation/

inhibition was much more detailed and sophisticated than what is portrayed of Saunders and extended to the viscera as well as muscles. In contrast to Bowen's demonstrable grasp of the workings of the nervous system to manage pain, there is no indication that Saunders' expertise and knowledge extended to a neurological understanding of treating reflexes to organ conditions. This chapter has reframed the Eastern influences on Bowen and his interest in acupuncture as reflective of the influences brought about by the opening up of China to the West at the start of the 1970s decade. Practitioners such as John Worsley pursued interests in acupuncture and trained ten to twenty years earlier, and his 1974 book *The Ward Inquiry* sourced as a reference, but the evidence in transcripts to the Ward Inquiry show the 1970s in Victoria, Australia to be a period of emergence of interest in professional circles. This is signalled by the establishment of the Acupuncture Association of Victoria in 1974 and that idea about using pressure on acupoints instead of needles was topical at this time. This is reflected in transcripts to the Ward Inquiry and the dates of publications that describe acupuncture without needles.

The wider posthumous trajectory into acupoints, meridians and more traditional Chinese systems along with trigger points is a departure from the framework that Bowen worked within, but it can be regarded as an extension of the integrative process that Bowen started himself in the 1970s. In conclusion, there is no solid evidence to support Eastern ideas being consciously foundational to Bowen's approach nor Saunders as an alleged mentor of these after the Berlin Olympiad in 1936. Instead, this research presents Bowen's interest as a developmental and integrative phase in response to new trends dating to the 1970s. All forms of bodywork influence acupoints, but the distinguishing factor between them is the knowledge system and philosophy that informs the practitioner's awareness of what they are doing. Like other leading masseurs described later in Chapter 8, Bowen worked with nerves, but he is unique among them in delivering his work through an osteopathic lens and knowledge system.

Notes

1 "Y. M. C. A. Leads in Victorian Swimming," *Sporting Globe (Melbourne),* December 15, 1928: 6 Note the image appears in an adjacent story. "Rifle Pennant," *Sporting Globe (Melbourne)*, December 15, 1928: 6.
2 "'We Will Not Slip Down the Ladder' Say Richmond Officials," *Sporting Globe (Melbourne),* March 14, 1931: 6; Saunders is noted again as Head Trainer "Football," *Age (Melbourne),* April 20, 1932: 6; Saunders reportedly re-joined Richmond on his return in 1937 "New Players Found," *Argus (Melbourne)*, December 7, 1937: 18; Saunders had been appointed to the head trainer role again but turned it down as he was expecting to be appointed masseur to the Tokyo Olympics – "Percentage Lead By St Kilda," *Argus (Melbourne),* May 1, 1939: 18.
3 "Lure of the West Felt after 58yrs," *Daily News (Perth, WA),* November 2, 1955: 10.
4 "Talking Sport," *Herald (Melbourne),* March 3, 1940: 19.
5 Jill Sebire email message to author January 21, 2015.
6 "Smooth Cooperation of ACF and YMCA in New Guinea," *Proserpine Guardian (Qld)*, October 22, 1943: 2.

7 Murray, *In Search*, 123.
8 "Presentation to Ernie Saunders," *Sporting Globe (Melbourne)*, May 9, 1936: 6; "M. Sheahan Rejects Offer," *Argus (Melbourne)*, May 20, 1936: 12.
9 Mike Dobson personal communication to author, June 25, 2015.
10 Dobson personal communication to author.
11 Dobson personal communication to author.
12 "Backhouse to Have Last Run Before Leaving for Berlin," *Sun News-Pictorial (Melbourne)*, May 16, 1936: 16.
13 "Spotlight on Sport," *Cairns Post (Qld)*, February 29, 1940: 5.
14 PROV, Master of the Supreme Court VPRS 7591/P4/, Unit 264, Wills, item 738/207, Leslie Edward Dettman; Mike Dobson personal communication to author June 25, 2015; Leslie Edward Dettman 6220/1972, Registration Death, Births Deaths and Marriages Victoria.
15 "Oxygen Used by Jap. Swimmers in Berlin," *Evening News (Rockhampton)*, October 27, 1936: 8.
16 "Oxygen Used by Jap. Swimmers in Berlin."
17 "Vitamin Dope to Keep Olympic Men Fresh at Finish," *News (Adelaide)*, October 30, 1936: 3, accessed October 15, 2018, http://nla.gov.au/nla.news-article132031230.
18 Dr. Alfons Cornelius, *Druckpunkte* (Berlin: Verlag von Otto Enslin, 1902), 32–43; J. P. Shah, N. Thaker, J. Heimur, J. V. Aredo, S. Sikdar, and L. Gerber, "Myofascial Trigger Points Then and Now: A Historical and Scientific Perspective," *PM* and *R: The Journal of Injury, Function, and Rehabilitation* 7, no. 7 (2015): 746–61.
19 David Simons, Janet Travell, and Lois S. Simons, *Myofascial Pain and Dysfunction: The Trigger Point Manual, Volume 1. Upper Half of Body*, 2nd ed. (Philadelphia: Lippincott Williams and Wilkins, 1999), 14–18.
20 Simons et al., *Myofascial Pain and Dysfunction*, 41–42.
21 Tokijuro Namikoshi, *Shiatsu, Japanese Finger Pressure Therapy* (New York and Tokyo: Japan Publications, 1992).
22 Namikoshi, *Shiatsu, Japanese Finger Pressure Therapy*, 32.
23 Namikoshi, *Shiatsu, Japanese Finger Pressure Therapy*, 21.
24 Toru Namikoshi, *The Complete Book of shiatsu Therapy* (Tokyo and New York: Japan Publications Inc, 1981), 21; Tokijuro Namikoshi, *Shiatsu, Health and Vitality at Your Fingertips* (San Francisco, CA: Japan Publications Inc, 1969), 11.
25 "About shiatsu Therapy," Shiatsu College (Website).
26 Namikoshi, *Shiatsu, Health and Vitality at Your Fingertips.*
27 Smeeton personal communication to the author, various.
28 Edwin Devereaux, Brian O'Reilly, and John Cice, *History of the Sydney College of Chiropractic* (Sydney: Macquarie Lighthouse Press, 2012), 86.
29 Ward Inquiry Report, 684.
30 Training.gov.au, Health Schools Australia.
31 "What to Know about Shiatsu Massage," *Medical News Today* (Website).
32 PROV, VPRS 3253/P1/, Unit 47, Bowen transcript, 675.
33 Devereaux et al., *History of the Sydney College of Chiropractic*, 87.
34 Devereaux et al., *History of the Sydney College of Chiropractic*, 87.
35 Devereaux et al., *History of the Sydney College of Chiropractic*, 87.
36 Smeeton personal communication to author.
37 John Worsley's *Everyone's Guide to Acupuncture* (no other details), Ward Inquiry Report, 79.
38 Ward Inquiry Report, 37.
39 PROV, Report and Evidence Osteopathy Committee (pt.1–4) 27/11/975 (Pt. 2) 2261, VPRS 3253/P1/, Unit 50, Original Papers Tabled in Legislative Assembly, Hegyi transcript, 3284–96: 3284, 3291.

40 PROV, VPRS 3253/P1/, Unit 50, Hegyi transcript: 3295.
41 PROV, VPRS 3253/P1/, Unit 50, Hegyi transcript: 3284.
42 PROV, VPRS 3253/P1/, Unit 50, Hegyi transcript: 3288–89, 3293–94.
43 PROV, VPRS 3253/P1/, Unit 50, Hegyi transcript: 3295.
44 PROV, VPRS 3253/P1/, Unit 50, Hegyi transcript: 3290.
45 PROV, Osteopathy, Chiropractic and Naturopathy Committee, VPRS 16439/P1/, Unit 12, Committee Records, Mik transcript: 2941.
46 PROV, Osteopathy, Chiropractic and Naturopath Joint Select Committee pp. 783–938, VPRS 241/P/, Unit 14, Transcripts of Committee, Blackmore transcript: 857.
47 The article listed in Natural Therapeutics under "Acupuncture" was "Modern Acupuncture-Neuropathy" from an unreferenced *Journal of the International Congress of Acupuncture and Moxibustion, Tokyo.*
48 Kevin Ryan, "Bowen Methods," *Acupuncture 365* (Website).
49 Ward Inquiry Report, 60.
50 PROV. Report and evidence Osteopathy Committee (Pt.1–4), 27/11/975 (Pt. 2) 2261, VPRS 3253/P1/, Unit 50, Original papers tabled in the Legislative Assembly, transcripts of proceedings, McAlister transcript: 3433.
51 Frijov Capra, *The Tao of Physics, An exploration of the Parallels between Modern Physics and Eastern Mysticism* (Great Britain: Wildwood House, 1975), 36.
52 John C. Longhurst, "Defining Meridians: A Modern Basis of Understanding," *Journal of Acupuncture and Meridian Studies* 3, no. 2 (2010): 67–74.
53 Ann Mortelliti interview by author June 26, 2018.
54 Romney Smeeton personal communication (various) to the author.
55 Jan Breen, "Red Tape Ties Healing Man's Hands," *Geelong Advertiser*, March 31, 1982: 22.
56 Breen, "Red Tape Ties Healing Man's Hands."
57 Breen, "Red Tape Ties Healing Man's Hands."
58 Kevin Ryan personal communication to author October 10, 2015.
59 See Chapter 8 (Biopyschosocial Mystique: The Non-heterodox and Esoteric).
60 Tom Dummer, *Tibetan Medicine and other Holistic Health Care Systems* (London and New York: Routledge, 1988), chapters 14–16, 171–211.
61 "Worsley Classical Five Element Acupuncture History," *Worsley Institute Website*, https://worsleyinstitute.com/pages/history-of-worsley-classical-five-element-acupuncture
62 The Ward Inquiry sourced John Worsley's *Everyone's Guide to Acupuncture*- not dated, but the first edition is dated 1974; 1970s examples of acupressure on acupoints are J. V. Cerney, *Acupuncture Without Needles* (USA: Parker Publishing Company, 1974); Masura Toguchi and Frank S. Warren, *Complete Guide to Acupuncture and Acupressure, Two Volumes* (New York: Gramercy Publishing Company, 1974), 276.
63 Toru Namikoshi, *The Complete Book of Shiatsu Therapy* (Tokyo and New York: Japan Publications Inc, 1981), chapter 1, General Theory, 21–50; Fitzgerald W H and Edwin F Bower, *Zone Therapy* and George Starr White, *Zone Therapy* (Columbus, Ohio: J. H. Long, 1917). Reprinted by *Health Research Books* (Mokelumne Hill, CA: Health Research Books, 1972).
64 Gregory Munro (former national Myorthotics instructor) personal communication to author, March 15, 2019.
65 R. J. Lucy, *Myorthotics* (College of Somatic Studies, 1991), introduction.
66 "Advanced Diploma of Naturopathy," accessed January 19, 2019, http://www.coss.com.au/govt.htm/ (note this link is only workable via the link in the RTO (non-current) listing for COSS at http://training.gov.au.
67 Lucy, *Myorthotics*, introduction.

68 Lucy, *Myorthotics*.
69 Dewandchand Varma, *The Human Machine and Its Forces* (London: Health for All Publishing), 1937).
70 S. V. Govindan, *Massage Therapy for Diseases of Vital Areas: Marma Treatment* (New Delhi: Abhinav Publications, 2005), 26–27.
71 Govindan, *Massage for Diseases of Vital Areas*, 26–27.
72 Leon Chaitow with Judith Delaney, *Modern Neuromuscular Techniques* (New York: Churchill Livingstone), 1996, vii, xi, 25–41, 42–64.
73 Varma, Dewandchand. *The Human Machine and Its Forces* (London: Health for All Publishing, n.d.). Reproduced in *Pranotherapy and the Origins of Polarity Therapy and European Neuromuscular Techniques, by Dewandchand Varma and Dr Randolph Stone, Pioneers of Manual Medicine, Volume 1,* ed. Phil Young (Great Britain: MWI Publishing, 2011), 18 (note reproduction is inserted in between main pagination pp. 45–47).
74 Graham Pennington, *Fascial Therapy*, 2nd ed. (Teaching Notes, 1993).
75 Graham Pennington, *A Textbook of the Bowen Technique* (Warrnambool: Barker Deane Publishing, 2012).
76 Articles that explain the relationship of the governor vessel to the brain include: *Lin-xia Qian et al., "Mechanism of the Acupoints of the Governor Vessel in Treatment of Post-stroke Depression on the Base of the Specificity of Meridian Points," World Journal of Acupuncture – Moxibustion 29, no. 3* (September 1, 2019): 244–48; Xuan Su et al., " 'Governor Vessel-unblocking and Mind-regulating' Acupuncture Therapy Ameliorates Cognitive Dysfunction in a Rat Model of Middle Cerebral Artery Occlusion," *International Journal of Molecular Medicine* 43, no. 1 (2019): 221–32, https://doi.org/10.3892/ijmm.2018.3981.
77 Personal communication to the author.
78 Pennington, *A Textbook*, 65.
79 Pennington, *A Textbook*, 65–66.
80 Brian Smart, *Smart Bowen Therapy, the Practitioners Guide*, 1st ed. (Victoria, Australia: Caroline Springs), iii.
81 Smart, *Smart Bowen Therapy*, 1
82 Smart, *Smart Bowen Therapy*, 1.
83 David Simons, Janet Travell, and Lois S. Simons, *Myofascial Pain and Dysfunction: the Trigger Point Manual, Volume 1. Upper half of body*, 2nd ed. (Philadelphia: Lippincott Williams and Wilkins, 1999) and *The Lower Extremities* ((Philadelphia: Lippincott Williams and Wilkins, 1993), Vol. 2.
84 "Dr Kevin Ryan and Tom Bowen," *YouTube* Video.
85 "Practitioner Workshops, Bowen Methods," *Acupuncture 365*, accessed October 30, 2024, https://acupuncture365.com.au/practitioner-workshops-bowen-methods/.
86 "Tom Bowen's Therapy," *Emmett UK*, https://www.emmett-uk.co.uk/training-courses/tom-bowens-therapy-tbt/
87 "Emmett Technique," http://www.rossemmett.com.au/.
88 "The Emmett Technique," *Emmett Technique Website*.
89 "Tom Bowen's Therapy," *Emmett UK Website*.
90 Gene Dobkin, *The Bowen Companion*, Vol. 1 and 2, 2 (Perris, CA: US Bowen, 1998/99).
91 Dobkin, *The Bowen Companion*, Vol. 1, i.
92 Dobkin, *The Bowen Companion*, Vol. 1 and 2.
93 Training provided by Border College of Natural Therapies, a former Registered Training Organisation (RTO) under the National Training Standards. The RTO status is now acquired by Bowen Training Australia owned by Bowtech school instructors.

94 "VibroHarmonisation Technique History," *VHT World*, accessed October 31, 2024, https://www.vhtworld.co.uk/vht-history/
95 Thomas Myers, *Anatomy Trains*, 2nd ed. (Churchill Livingstone, Elsevier Australia, 2009), Appendix 3, *Myofascial Meridians and Oriental Medicine*, 273–81.
96 Peter Dorsher, "Trigger Point Regions and Classical Acupoints," *Akapunktur, German Journal of Acupuncture and Related Techniques* (2001), https://doi.org/10.1016/J.DZA.2009.01.001.
97 Dorsher, "Trigger Point Regions and Classical Acupoints."
98 Myers, *Anatomy Trains*, 44–61, 229, 230, 283.

Bibliography

Newspapers

"Backhouse to Have Last Run Before Leaving for Berlin." *Sun News-Pictorial (Melbourne),* May 16, 1936: 16. Accessed November 17, 2024. http://nla.gov.au/nla.news-article277236744.

Breen, Jan. "Red Tape ties Healing Man's Hands." *Geelong Advertiser*, March 31, 1982: 22.

"Football-Richmond Clear R O'Neill." *Age (Melbourne),* April 20, 1932: 6. Accessed November 17, 2024. http://nla.gov.au/nla.news-article205097137.

"Lure of the West Felt after 58 yrs." *Daily News (Perth, WA)*, November 2, 1955: 10 (FINAL). Accessed November 17, 2024. http://nla.gov.au/nla.news-article266348272.

"M Sheahan Rejects Offer." *Argus (Melbourne)*, May 20, 1936: 12. Accessed November 17, 2024. http://nla.gov.au/nla.news-article11035977.

"New Players Found." *Argus (Melbourne),* December 7, 1937: 18. Accessed November 17, 2024. http://nla.gov.au/nla.news-article11130428.

"Oxygen Used by Jap. Swimmers in Berlin." *Evening News Rockhampton*, October 27, 1936: 8. Accessed November 17, 2024. http://nla.gov.au/nla.news-ssssarticle201209799.

"Percentage Lead by St Kilda." *Argus (Melbourne)*, May 1, 1939: 18. Accessed November 17, 2024. http://nla.gov.au/nla.news-article12123397.

"Presentation to Ernie Saunders." *Sporting Globe (Melbourne),* May 9, 1936: 6. Accessed November 17, 2024. http://nla.gov.au/nla.news-article190325415.

"Rifle Pennant." *Sporting Globe (Melbourne)*, December 15, 1928: 6. Accessed November 17, 2024.http://nla.gov.au/nla.news-article183970777.

"Smooth Cooperation of ACF and YMCA in New Guinea." *Proserpine Guardian (Qld)*, October 22, 1943: 2. Accessed November 17, 2024. http://nla.gov.au/nla.news-article227415283.

"Spotlight on Sport – Backhouse Beaten" *Cairns Post (Qld)*, February 29, 1940: 5. Accessed November 17, 2024. http://nla.gov.au/nla.news-article42227353.

"Talking Sport." *Herald (Melbourne),* March 3, 1940: 19. Accessed November 17, 2024. http://nla.gov.au/nla.news-article243236621.

"Vitamin Dope to Keep Olympic Men Fresh at Finish." *News Adelaide*, October 30, 1936: 3. Accessed November 17, 2024. http://nla.gov.au/nla.news-article132031230.

" 'We Will Not Slip down the Ladder' Say Richmond Officials." *Sporting Globe (Melbourne)* March 14, 1931: 6. Accessed November 17, 2024. http://nla.gov.au/nla.news-article183017074.

"Y. M. C. A. Leads in Victorian Swimming." *Sporting Globe (Melbourne)*, December 15, 1928: 6. Accessed November 17, 2024. http://nla.gov.au/nla.news- article183970779.

Primary Sources

Cornelius, Alfons. *Druckpunkte*. Berlin: Verlag von Otto Enslin, 1902 32–43. Accessed November 17, 2024. http://archive.org/details/druckpunkteihre00corngoog.
Dettman, Leslie Edward. Registration death. 6220/1972/. Births Deaths and Marriages Victoria.
Fitzgerald, W. H., and Edwin F. Bower. *Zone Therapy* and George Starr White, *Zone Therapy*. Columbus, Ohio: J. H. Long, 1917. Reprinted by Health Research Books. Mokelumne Hill, CA: Health Research Books, 1972.
Lucy, Robert. *Myorthotics*. Sydney: College of Somatic Studies, 1991.
PROV. Master of the Supreme Court, VPRS 7591/P4/. Nit 264. Wills Item 738/207. Leslie Edward Dettman.
PROV. Osteopathy, Chiropractic and Naturopathy Committee, VPRS 16439/P1, Unit 12. Committee Records, Mik transcript: 2941–56.
PROV. Osteopathy, Chiropractic and Naturopath Joint Select Committee pp. 783–938, VPRS 241/P/, Unit 14. Osteopathy, Chiropractic and Naturopath Joint Select Committee, transcripts of Committee. Blackmore transcript: 857–61.
PROV. Report and Evidence Osteopathy Committee (Pt.1–4), 27/11/975 (Pt. 2) 2261, VPRS 3253/P1/, Unit 47. Original papers tabled in the Legislative Assembly, transcripts of proceedings, Bowen transcript: 672–78.
PROV. Report and Evidence Osteopathy Committee (Pt.1–4), 27/11/975 (Pt. 2) 2261, VPRS 3253/P1, Unit 50. Original papers tabled in the Legislative Assembly, transcripts of proceedings, Hegyi transcript: 3284–96
Ward Inquiry Report – full title – Victoria Parliament, Osteopathy, Chiropractic and Naturopathy Committee, et al. *Report from the Osteopathy, Chiropractic and Naturopathy Committee: Together with Appendices*. Melbourne: C. H. Rixon, Government Printer, 1975. Accessed November 17, 2024. http://www6.austlii.edu.au/au/other/vic/VicLASelCPubInq/1975/1.pdf.

Secondary Sources

Capra, Frijov. *The Tao of Physics, an Exploration of the Parallels between Modern Physics and Eastern Mysticism*. Great Britain: Wildwood House, 1975.
Cerney, J. V. *Acupuncture Without Needles*. United States of America: Parker Publishing Company. 1974.
Chaitow, Leon with Judith Delaney. *Modern Neuromuscular Techniques*. New York: Churchill Livingstone, 1996.
Devereaux, Edwin, Brian O'Reilly, and John Cice. *History of the Sydney College of Chiropractic*. Sydney: Macquarie Lighthouse Press, 2012.
Dobkin, Gene. *The Bowen Companion*. Vol. 1 and 2. Perris, CA: US Bowen, 1998/99.
Dorsher, Peter. "Trigger Point Regions and Classical Acupoints." *Akapunktur. German Journal of Acupuncture and Related Techniques* (2001). https://doi.org/10.1016/J.DZA.2009.01.001. Republished at Anatomy Trains. Accessed November 17, 2024. https://www.anatomytrains.com/wp-content/uploads/2024/01/Trigger_Points_and_Classical_Acupuncture-1.pdf.
Dummer, Tom. *Tibetan Medicine and other Holistic Health Care Systems*. London: Routledge, 1988.
Govindan, S. V. *Massage Therapy for Diseases of Vital Areas: Marma Treatment*. New Delhi: Abhinav Publications, 2005. Accessed November 17, 2024. https://archive.org/details/massagetherapyfo0000govi/
Longhurst, John C. "Defining Meridians: A Modern Basis of Understanding." *Journal of Acupuncture and Meridian Studies* 3, no. 2 (2010): 67–74.

"Modern Acupuncture-Neuropathy." *Journal of the International Congress of Acupuncture and Moxibustion* (Tokyo: Japan Acupuncture and Moxibustion Society). The article is simply listed in *Natural Therapeutics*, under "Acupuncture" and is believed to relate to be collection of papers in the above journal published in 1965.
Murray, Col. *In Search of Tom Bowen and the Therapy he Inspired and Lots of Other Stuff* Armadale: Palmer Higgs, Booksonline, 2010.
Myers, Thomas. *Anatomy Trains.* 2nd ed. Edinburgh: Churchill Livingstone, Elsevier Australia, 2009.
Namikoshi, Tokijuro. *Shiatsu, Health and Vitality at your Fingertips.* San Francisco, CA: Japan Publications Inc, 1969.
Namikoshi, Tokijuro. *Shiatsu, Japanese Finger Pressure Therapy.* New York: Japan Publications, 1972.
Namikoshi, Toru. *The Complete Book of Shiatsu Therapy.* 11th Printing. Tokyo: Japan Publications Inc., 1981.
Pennington, Graham. *Fascial Therapy.* 2nd ed. Teaching Notes, 1993.
Pennington, Graham. *A Textbook of the Bowen Technique.* Barker Deane Publishing, Warrnambool, 2012.
Qian, Lin-xia et al. "Mechanism of the Acupoints of the Governor Vessel in Treatment of Post-stroke Depression on the Base of the Specificity of Meridian Points." *World Journal of Acupuncture – Moxibustion* 29, no. 3 (September 1, 2019): 244–48. Accessed November 17, 2024. https://doi.org/10.1016/j.wjam.2019.07.004.
Shah, J. P. N. Thaker, J. Heimur, J. V. Aredo, S. Sikdar, and L. Gerber. "Myofascial Trigger Points Then and Now: A Historical and Scientific Perspective." *PM* and *R: The Journal of Injury, Function, and Rehabilitation* 7, no. 7 (2015): 746–61. Accessed October 30, 2018. https://doi.org/10.1016/j.pmrj.2015.01.024.
Simons, David, Janet Travell, and Lois S. Simons. *Myofascial Pain and Dysfunction: The Trigger Point Manual, Volume 1. Upper Half of Body.* 2nd ed. Philadelphia: Lippincott Williams and Wilkins, 1999.
Smart, Brian. *Smart Bowen Therapy, the Practitioner's Guide.* Brian Smart, 2014. www.smartbowen.com
Su, Xuan et al. "'Governor Vessel-unblocking and Mind-regulating' Acupuncture Therapy Ameliorates Cognitive Dysfunction in a Rat Model of Middle Cerebral Artery Occlusion." *International Journal of Molecular Medicine* 43, no. 1 (2019): 221–32. https://doi.org/10.3892/ijmm.2018.3981.
Toguchi, Masura, and Frank Z. Warren. *Complete Guide to Acupuncture and Acupressure, Two Volumes.* New York: Gramercy Publishing Company, 1974.
Varma, Dewandchand. *The Human Machine and Its Forces.* London: Health for All Publishing, n.d. Reproduced in *Pranotherapy and the Origins of Polarity Therapy and European Neuromuscular Techniques, by Dewandchand Varma and Dr Randolph Stone, Pioneers of Manual Medicine, Volume 1,* edited by Phil Young. Great Britain: MWI Publishing, 2011.

Websites

"About Shiatsu Therapy." *Shiatsu College.* Accessed November 17, 2024. http://www.shiatsucollege.org/aboutshiatsu%20e.html.
"Advanced Diploma of Naturopathy." Accessed January 19, 2019. http://www.coss.com.au/govt.htm/ note this link is only workable via the link in the RTO (non-current) listing for COSS at https://training.gov.au.
"Bowen Methods." *Acupuncture 365.* Accessed November 17, 2024. http://www.acupuncture365.com.au/bowen-methods/.
"Overview." *Bowen Seminars.* http://bowenseminars.com.au/overview/.

"The Emmett Technique." *Emmett Technique*. Accessed November 17, 2024. http://www.emmett-technique-hq.com/about/about-the-emmett-technique.
"Tom Bowen's Therapy." *Emmett UK*. Accessed November 17, 2024. http://www.emmett-uk.co.uk/training-courses/tom-bowens-therapy-tbt/.
"VibroHarmonisation Technique History." *VHT World*. Accessed November 17, 2024. http://www.vhtworld.co.uk/vht-history/.
"What to Know about Shiatsu Massage." *Medical News Today*. Accessed November 17, 2024. https://www.medicalnewstoday.com/articles/shiatsu-massage#overview.
"Worsley Classical Five Element Acupuncture History." *Worsley Institute Website*. Accessed November 17, 2024. https://worsleyinstitute.com/pages/history-of-worsley-classical-five-element-acupuncture.

Video

Kevin Ryan. "Dr Kevin Ryan and Tom Bowen." *YouTube* Video, 51:31 minutes. Posted September 2024. Accessed November 17, 2024. https://www.youtube.com/watch?v=TLwKB4fu9p8.
Ryan, Kevin. "Practitioner Workshops Bowen Methods." *Acupuncture 365*. Accessed November 17, 2024. http://acupuncture.com.au/practitioner-workshops-bowen-methods.

6 Fluidity and Transformation

Bowen and His Peers in the South Pacific and Beyond

Introduction: The Broader Mission of the South Pacific Federation of Natural Therapeutics

The memoranda and articles of association for South Pacific Federation of Natural Therapeutics (SPFNT) were drawn up with the registered office as 228 Clarendon Street, South Melbourne and with Marcus Try as company director-agent in Victoria.[1] Try also served as a joint secretary the South Pacific for the Victorian subsidiary ACONPAL and represented the Victorian Branch as president at the Ward Inquiry.[2] Detailed in Chapter 7, Try was the practitioner who successfully sued the new Registration Board in the Supreme Court. The SPFNT paperwork addressed routine matters such as control of colleges, teaching, issuing certifications, publishing, research resources and providing insurances, as well as activities relating to improving laws and advocacy to the government. There were other standard items such as provision for contracts and the creation, acquisition and disposal of assets, such as schools, health centres, gymnasiums and hospitals.

In addition to serving as an umbrella body for a large number of sub-organisations with the aforementioned functions, the South Pacific articulated a much broader vision than Australia that was shattered with regulation. It was a regional vision for the wider South Pacific:

> Providing a central organisation for the several Federations and Associations of practitioners of natural healing in the South Pacific on order to ensure a full and efficient service in the field of public health generally in the various states and countries of such region of such natural methods of healing.[3]

The Australian Chiropractors, Osteopaths and Naturopathic Physicians Association Limited (ACONPAL) was a full organisational subsidiary of the South Pacific and the bodies had separate representation at the Ward Inquiry in 1973 and later on at the Webb Inquiry.[4] Individuals who were acting for the South Pacific /ACONPAL in Victoria appear closely connected with Bowen

DOI: 10.4324/9781003602125-7

by decade's end as they form a tiny eleven-member group called the Victorian Society of Specialist Osteopaths (VSSO) covered in Chapter 7. Other VSSO men are introduced in Chapter 7: Alan Wilkie as secretary and Richard Bennett as treasurer.[5] Beforehand they are placed in a leading role with ACONPAL. Wilkie's transcript of July 3, 1973, to the Ward Inquiry revealed the Victorian Branch of ACONPAL was only formed two years prior, so in 1971 which provides perspective for Bowen's involvement as a member in 1972.[6] Figure 6.1 shows Bowen's business card including his membership until the late 1970s.[7]

The driver for the Victorian presence was Ministerial press announcements about possible legislation.[8] On April 27, 1971, the secretary A.C. Hinks of NSW ACONPAL wrote to Vance Dickie, Victorian Minister for Health, asking the minister for a copy of the proposal underway to register chiropractors in Victoria and pointing out to the minister that ACONPAL had members in all states of the Commonwealth that could be affected. The letterhead shows Neville S Brittain was president and AC Hinks DO (and ND USA) as secretary of the NSW branch.[9]

The broader vision of the South Pacific is appreciated when seen in context of its membership of the International Federation of Practitioners of Natural Therapeutics (IFPNT) The IFPNT was established in 1965 from an initiative of Deutsche Heilpraktikeschaft (the German natural therapist organisation) with numerous objectives including to establish an international organisation to represent *bona fide* practitioners of natural therapeutics, a commitment to elevation of education and practice standards, stamping out diploma mills and protection of the public and freedom of choice in health.[10] The governance

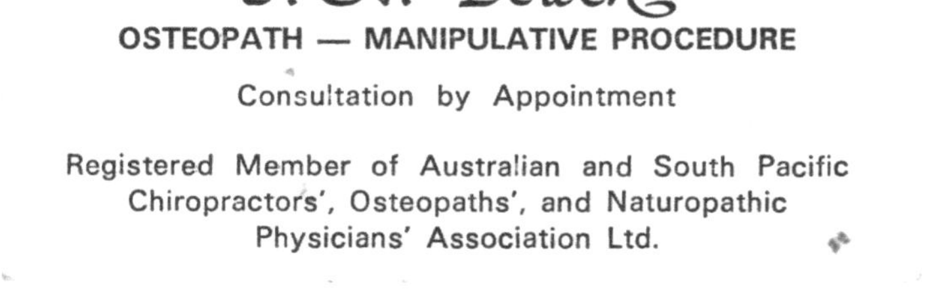

Phone: 21 3415

30 Villamanta Street
Geelong West 3218
P.O. Box 619

T. A. Bowen
OSTEOPATH — MANIPULATIVE PROCEDURE

Consultation by Appointment

Registered Member of Australian and South Pacific
Chiropractors', Osteopaths', and Naturopathic
Physicians' Association Ltd.

Figure 6.1 Bowen's business card for 30 Villamanta Street showing his continued membership of ACONPAL/South Pacific.

Source: Image courtesy Ron Phelan, Rene Horwood Collection.

reach of the IFPNT including Australia was described by Janssen, the president of the SPFNT and Australia's representative to the IFPNT:

> The IFPNT has a number of countries associated with it. In my term of office, Norway, Sweden and Denmark come in; before that, Great Britain and Northern Island has now come in; Holland, West Germany, France, South Africa, Israel, New Zealand and India. The Indian section has only come on over the last two years.[11]

Belgium had been suspended and a section of Canada refused.[12] In the UK, the IFPNT was concerned with changes as developments proceeded towards a European Common Market.[13] The honorary secretary, Thomas Dummer DO was Dean of the European School of Osteopathy (ESO) in Maidstone, Kent, where after establishment in Paris in 1951, it relocated in the 1960s.[14] Dummer and IFPNT personnel visited schools before accepting them as official members.[15] Dummer visited Australia around Christmas 1971 and early 1973 for inspections.[16] In 1969, the IFPNT had already accepted Gerritt Janssen's school (the National College of Osteopathy and Prescribing Chemists).[17] Gerritt Janssen was educated at the British College of Naturopathy in London in 1925 (deduced from the title to be Stanely Lief's School) and set up in business in New South Wales (NSW) in 1933. In 1936, he established the NSW branch of ACONPAL in response to threats of government regulation. The IFPNT accepted the Sydney College of Osteopathy (SCO) by 1973.

The focus on chiropractic during the Webb Inquiry is revealed by the fact that the IFPNT only received two mentions in the Webb Inquiry Report: one mentioning Janssen's role as an Australian representative and the other briefly relaying its educational role in standards' setting.[18] There was no mention of Tom Dummer nor connections to the ESO. The Webb Inquiry did not mention or visit the ESO in its report. The London School of Osteopathy (LSO) was visited and the British School of Osteopathy (BSO) was discussed as part of the visit.[19] These were solely the colleges where the members had graduated that formed the Australian Osteopathic Association (AOA).[20] Chiropractic schools dominated the Webb Inquiry itinerary. The European (and original American) universe of osteopathy seems to have been bypassed other than referring to graduates of Kirksville teaching at the elite schools and some publications. When the ESO first moved into the British College of Naturopathy and Osteopathy (BCNO) originally established as BCN by Stanley Lief before setting up at Maidstone, it enjoyed a strong collaboration with John Wernham, a specialist and leading practitioner in classical osteopathy.[21] According to Bloomfield, Dummer, as co-founder of the ESO, was able to 'impart some of the original essence of Andrew Taylor Still's Osteopathy, which had been subsequently misinterpreted, rightly or wrongly by his followers'.[22]

Membership Standards of ACONPAL/South Pacific

Bowen's ACONPAL/South Pacific membership dates to at least 1972 and was held throughout the 1970s, so he must have fulfilled the required standards for admission. The standards and processes of membership for the SPFNT are based on evidence to the 1973 Ward Inquiry provided by Federation President Gerritt Janssen, Bob Lucy (vice president) and Claire Goulsen (secretary and Janssen's business and life partner) present. A document produced by the Victorian Branch of ACONPAL (most likely for the government inquiries) outlines standards:

> The members of the Australian Chiropractors', Osteopaths', and Naturopathic Physicians Association Ltd., Victorian Branch, who specialise in the profession of osteopathy are practitioners who have received the best of training available, some having received their training overseas, others in Australia where in years past Victoria shared in the excellent training available in Australia. Most of our registered osteopaths have been in practice for many years, and because of their experience, are able to guide our younger members in the profession, and offer advice where considered necessary.[23]

It was Lucy who primarily gave evidence before the Victorian Parliamentary Inquiry about membership standards and gave insights into the processes involved:

> Each individual case is looked at on its merits. We realise that many people came to our profession long before there were colleges they could go to. If a man has been in practice for 20 years and displays to us that he had knowledge of his profession, we would like to accept him. Formal qualifications we would desire but not necessarily reject him because he does not have the qualifications. Such a case has not come up to my knowledge within the last four or five years.[24]

Barry Jones pressed Lucy on the point and asked, 'what about somebody who is in practice and has been in practice for six to seven years since the colleges were in operation?' Jones' question suggests he thinks colleges only came into being in the 1960s, but as described in Chapter 2, the Australian teaching concerns of Roberts and Doyle were operating much earlier as were overseas institutions. To this, Lucy replied:

> If he was in such a position that it was not easy for him to go to college, then we would probably accept him if he displayed competence and could write a thesis on the subject.[25]

Jones clarified with Lucy that a thesis would be submitted in every case in lieu of academic qualification for those who had not been to college and Lucy confirms this. This part of the transcript is interesting as it may explain why Lucy who was not a Victorian practitioner was remembered by Rene Horwood as visiting in his Kombi van from Canberra and an occasional attendee at Bowen's clinics.[26] Horwood does not mention Pruss, but his presence at the clinic was reportedly remarked on by Rentsch during his 1974–1976 contact period.[27] It seems clear that Bowen should be in the category of someone to have to write a thesis to become a member; however, the only mention of Bowen producing a manuscript was described in Chapter 2 and tied to a British organisation. The presence of Lucy and Pruss may initially have been as part of some accreditation process to observe Bowen's clinical standards for admission and developed into a genuine interest to learn from him.

Membership Quotas

There is a table of South Pacific membership quotas in the Ward Inquiry Report, a useful appendix three in the Webb Inquiry Report and an overview in Baer, but there are no histories about the personalities involved in the South Pacific and ACONPAL.[28] ACONPAL has left behind limited records. Though a long-standing NSW organisation established since 1936, ACONPAL does not have a media presence until cursory mention in 1973 and 1976 over regulation issues in the ACT and regarding Medicare cover for services provided by members.[29] The company appears in records of the Australian Securities and Investment Commission (ASIC) that reveal signatories from both the NSW and Victorian branches. The only other records are a monograph on *Natural Therapeutics* and submissions or transcripts by its presidents and secretaries to government inquiries.[30] No association records such as minutes appear to have survived.[31] In 1973, Marcus Try indicated there were thirty-nine to forty Victorian members.[32] These figures are similar to the Ward Inquiry Report where a selection of state association figures provides a comparison of membership numbers as follows: the American-trained members of the Australian Chiropractors Association (ACA) (78), the AOA representing graduates of the BSO and LSO (7), the United Chiropractors Association of Australasia (UCAA) representing those with Australian credentials from UCAA-endorsed colleges (83) and on the other side of the fence, the Australian Naturopathic Practitioners Association Limited (ANPAL) (previously ACONPAL) (38), the National Association of Naturopaths, Osteopaths and Chiropractors (NAN/NANOC) (40) and the VSSO (3).[33] Given these small numbers, it is obvious that Bowen would have become quickly acquainted with colleague osteopaths and be personally known within the overall Victorian ACONPAL group which helps explain the ease of introductions to him when he attended meetings.

The Webb Inquiry report documented the national memberships in January 1977.[34] These show the growth of the UCAA after the exodus from ACONPAL and NSW leading with 109 members, Victoria (VIC) 84, South Australia (SA) (46), Western Australia (WA) (9) and Tasmania (TAS) (5). Victoria was the stronghold for ACA (87) followed by NSW (69), WA (20),

Queensland (QLD) 18, SA (17) and Australian Capital Territory (ACT) (6). The AOA spread was limited to VIC (9), SA (3) and QLD (2). Regardless of the exodus, ACONPAL maintained strong numbers of 114 nationally alongside ACA (222), AOA (14), UCAA (319) NAN (ex NANOC) (82), South Australian Chiropractors Association (SACA) (35) and VSSO (5). The Webb report showed an ACONPAL breakdown of 51 each in NSW and VIC (so Victoria had increased by some 11–13 members), 2 each in QLD and SA, 3 in TAS and 5 in WA, totalling 114 ACONPAL members nationally.[35] It appears Bowen had very recently joined ACONPAL when interviewed on the afternoon of July 8, 1973. The Honourable Roy Ward chairing the Panel for the Victorian Ward Inquiry observed to Lucy as vice president that the SPFNT had engaged in a membership drive and referring to committee's morning visit to Geelong (Bowen was interviewed that morning) said:

> A gentleman in Geelong, for instance, said he wrote to you and he had a certificate hanging on the wall. The committee saw that this was numbered 112.[36]

Bowen is deduced to be the gentleman referred to. Others interviewed that morning are eliminated based on their credentials with the UCA or the AOA, including Nigel Love who became a Bowen observer. Love graduated from the Roberts' college in 1958 as ND/DC and confirmed at an interview he enjoyed dual memberships of the UCA and ACONPAL.[37]

The Ward Inquiry panel was curious about the surge in ACONPAL numbers and Lucy denied to Roy Ward that a membership drive had taken place but says he thinks that a large number of Victorian practitioners had become aware of South Pacific (and the related Victorian Branch of ACONPAL) in 1971 and left NANOC. Lucy added 'They all submitted qualifications and they all had been in practice for a considerable time'.[38] Regarding NANOC, Lucy was referring to the Blackmores group, formerly the NAN/NANC established in 1946, becoming NANOC in 1970 and returned to NAN again by 1977.[39] Wilkie said new ACONPAL members were dissatisfied with their existing associations and 'suddenly left'. Some antipathy towards NANOC and Blackmores existed in ACONPAL circles as NANOC was seen to be just a distribution vehicle for Blackmores remedies.[40] The politics were due to the dominance of business interests that required 80 per cent of remedies used by the NANC/NANOC practitioners to be the Blackmores brand.[41] Try was the first to rebel and left.[42] Alan Wilkie and later ACONPAL treasurer Richard Bennett also left.[43] According to Try, Jacka was a shareholder in Blackmores.[44] Wilkie, osteopathically oriented, was highly critical of NANOC and standards of Blackmores chiropractic training and said ACONPAL would not accept people graduated with Blackmores methods.[45]

In 1973 and referring to NANOC, President Jacka indicated the membership stood at forty-one for Victoria, 90 per cent were naturopaths who would be practising some chiropractic, three were practising 'pure osteopathy' and two chiropractic alone.[46] Wilkie, honorary secretary of the new Victorian branch of ACONPAL, said he was a former president of NANOC.[47] The transcript of Try, president of ACONPAL (VIC), revealed that over half the Victorian branch members of ACONPAL in 1973 were those departed from NANOC.[48] By 1973, NANOC was an association only and the former Blackmores school/association complex had come to an end. The NANOC major membership base was VIC, NSW and QLD. Though Victoria dominated in the south, NANOC was strong enough to have an SA Branch and was represented at the Ward Inquiry by Brian F Douglas and AE Stacey.[49] The SA NANOC branch outnumbered ACONPAL members by a ratio of 18:2 in 1977. Rene Horwood indicated that Bowen had presented to 'the chiropractors meeting in Adelaide'.[50] Though it cannot be confirmed, this statement by Horwood might suggest Bowen participated in NANOC before he joined ACONPAL. Bowen observers Davis DC/ND and Love DC/ND were NANOC before they joined ACONPAL. Bowen was a recent member of ACONPAL in 1973 and as an osteopath, belonged to a minority vocation. By 1976, Alfred Jacka the former Victorian branch president of NANC/NANOC held the role of federal deputy chairman of the South Pacific Council of Natural Therapeutics (SPCNT).[51] Marcus Try was the national chairman.[52] In a later report of April 14, 1978, by which time the current Australian Natural Therapists Association (ANTA) had formed with Jacka as president, Jacka gave the impression the majority of ANTA members were NANOC and largely graduates of his school (the Southern School of Natural Therapies (SSNT)).[53]

ACONPAL and the South Pacific Federation of Natural Therapeutists

ACONPAL was first established in 1936 in NSW a year after the threat of legislation there 'preventing nature healers, chiropractors, osteopaths, herbalists and the like' from practising.[54] NSW practitioners involved in ACONPAL also showed up in the SPFNT when formed in 1971 in Victoria.[55] These developments in 1971 show a concern by NSW interests to expand their influence into the Victorian scene in response to the rumours of legislation. ACONPAL was a subsidiary of the SPFNT. In the lead-up to regulation, a plethora of organisations nationally came under the South Pacific umbrella: nature cure colleges (some taught osteopathy and chiropractic) and their associations and colleges. The landscape of Bowen's regulatory decade before his death is confusing to navigate due to the intensely mercurial nature of partnerships and collaborations that saw rapid name changes, dissolutions and mergers of schools and bodies in response to rising pressure of imminent regulation. The leading soon-to-be government-recognised Australian colleges were no exception, dumping osteopathy from their titles to strategically align with chiropractic as the vehicle for successful registration. The behaviour appears frantic and haphazard but comes to life when attention is paid to the leading figures involved and viewing them through the lens of Bowen's standing as an actor in the shapeshifting political domain that eventually split into two broad camps – the SPCNT and the organisations that left to consolidate political power under the UCAA in a bid to secure registration for Australians educated in chiropractic and osteopathy at the prominent schools.

From Federation to Council, the Exodus to the UCAA

The Federation was reformed as a Council (SPCNT) in 1975 after a merger between the Federation and the Australian Council for Natural Therapeutics.[56] For simplicity, 'South Pacific' will be used to refer to both phases of the organisation and noting that in the second phase, an associated Australian college called the South Pacific also came into being and was regarded as the sister college to one similar-titled in New Zealand. The second phase coincided with the exodus of the graduates of the future government-prescribed colleges to the UCAA and their qualifications recognised under the Victorian *Chiropractors and Osteopaths Act 1978* and in New South Wales under the *Chiropractic Registration Act 1978*. Bolton provided an overview of the struggle for recognition of the leading Australian colleges in the lead-up to regulation, pitched against the Australian Associations representing overseas trained graduates that did not accept the standards of their Australian counterparts and termed them second-stream as they were mixers.[57] At the Sydney College of Chiropractic (formerly Osteopathy) (SCC/SCO since 1964, students had graduated with double DC/DO degrees. A SCC student in 1975–1981 John L Kelly (later CEO) confirmed students were exposed to the work of both Still and Palmer which reflects the entwined content that underpinned the dual DC/DO diplomas issued.[58] Kelly acknowledged the eclectic, diverse background of founder, Dr Kaufmann 'such as naturopathy, homeopathy, reform medicine, osteopathy and chiropractic' and his influence on the college foundations.[59] The Roberts' naturopathic college in Melbourne, entitled the College of Chiropractic and Osteopathy (COCA) from 1959 and the Chiropractic College of Australia from around 1977, started from similar beginnings with Roberts' overseas training as a naturopath.

Legislation in New South Wales and Victoria in 1978 led to the eventual successful registration of UCAA members who were Australian graduates of the SCC and CCA alongside the graduates of eminent overseas schools represented by their Australian associations – ACA and the AOA.[60] The South Australian Chiropractor Registration Board established under South Australia's early *Chiropractic Act* 1949 that catered to state graduates of the College of Chiropractic and Osteopathy South Australia (COCSA) supported portability and accepted UCAA members for registration. The UCAA strategy was a testament to the savvy of Edwin Devereaux a key figure at the SCC that ensured graduates of what came to be regarded as the traditional Australian colleges of chiropractic were successfully registered. Only the Western Australian Board continued to be dominated by overseas interests and refused to register the Australian UCAA chiropractors.[61] This national story is covered in detail by chiropractic historians of the SCC as well as Bolton earlier.[62]

Leading Members of the South Pacific Connected to Stanley Lief's London College of Naturopathy/Osteopathy

Below this stratum, another stratum of connections exists that sheds light on the operations of the South Pacific and relate to Bowen and his legacy. Connections begin with the theme of shared association with the British Naturopathic College concluded in Chapter 2 to be a reference to Stanley Lief's British College of Naturopathy (BCN) in London. The association is direct and indirect. According to Snider and Turner, Lief's college 'taught a slightly more eclectic naturopathy, although adhering closely to the Lindlahr model of dietary control, fasting, hydrotherapy, rest, and exercise, with osteopathy emphasizing the soft-tissue techniques that Lief had refined'.[63] The Nature Cure Association of Britain and Ireland was established in 1906 and Lief became president in 1932.[64] This evolved to become the British Naturopathic Association and graduates from the later BCNO are stated to have formed the core of the General Council and Register of Naturopaths and the British Naturopathic Association, the largest register and professional association of naturopaths in the UK.[65] The Association developed to include osteopathy and Lief held the position of President of the British Naturopathic and Osteopathic Association three times between 1945 and 1956.[66] In addition to the possibility identified in Chapter 2 that Bowen engaged in uncompleted studies with Lief's British College, based on their testimony in Government transcripts of the Ward Inquiry, individuals with a direct connection to Lief's college are Maurice Blackmore, Gerritt Janssen (President of the South Pacific) and Alfred (Alf) Jacka head of Blackmores NANOC association/school before making it his own with the SSNT in 1971. Only one other man by the name of McCulloch was active in Queensland in 1932 and claims also to have been educated at the 'British Naturopathic College' and a member of the British Association of Naturopaths.[67] Evidently, McCulloch operated his own Biochemic and Naturopathic Institute and was able to have diplomas from the British Naturopathic College issued and presented by the ex-Lord Mayor of Brisbane to two of his staff on the basis of correspondence studies and completing four years of clinical work with him.[68] McCulloch doesn't feature by name in the networks of this chapter, but his presence and activities confirm the availability of correspondence studies during the Great Depression with a college fitting the description of Lief's.[69]

Blackmore advertised in Australia that he obtained qualifications in London at the British Naturopathic College and the London-based British Chiropractic College and was also a member of the British Naturopathic Association described earlier.[70] Blackmore operated nature cure clinics in Queensland and developed his own system of prescribing based on his naturopathic education. Devereaux et al. describe Blackmore as 'one of Robert's most notable protégés.[71] This may be overstated, given Blackmores own claims in his advertising. He certainly would have been a strong competitor though the pioneers were collaborative too. By 1936, Blackmore had already set up the Health Society of Australia and was undertaking teaching activities and examining in naturopathy, chiropractic, massage and physio-therapeutics.[72] In his advertising, he tended to set chiropractic apart with advertisements showing the spine and nerve relationships to organs and placed osteopathy under naturopathic treatments.[73] Blackmore was revealed in Chapter 3 to be practising neuropathy.

Gerritt Janssen (1910–1974) also trained at the British Naturopathic College and started practice in NSW in 1933.[74] Janssen's legacy is intrinsic to the genesis of the ACONPAL and the South Pacific that followed as the umbrella body to a large number of associations and colleges, including both the NSW and later Victorian ACONPAL branches. Janssen was recognised as the founding president of the South Pacific.[75] The NSW South Pacific directors were also members of the Australian Association of Registered Osteopaths (AARO). AARO was established earlier in 1965 by Wallace Brown, second principal of the Sydney College of Osteopathy established by Alfred Kaufman in 1959. AARO had been set up to cater for SCO graduates.[76] The five founding South Pacific directors who were mid-1960s SCO graduates and also members of AARO in 1967 included William (Bill) Pruss, Arthur Hinks, Francis Gunter, Horace Lyttle and Alexander Taylor.[77] Others, not SCO-graduated included Gerritt Janssen and Neville Brittain who was secretary of ACONPAL. Janssen was a director too. Janssen represented the South Pacific at the Ward Inquiry as president, supported by vice-president Robert (Bob) Lucy (1929–1999), a new director in 1973. Janssen confirmed in his interview with the Ward Inquiry he was an NSW ACONPAL member as was Lucy.[78] As president of the South Pacific, Janssen was the Australian representative on the IFPNT.[79] The IFPNT and its connection to Thomas Dummer, dean of the ESO as IFPNT honorary secretary, was described earlier. Today, the ESO continues to enjoy a close collaboration with Lief's BCNO.

Subsidiaries and Recognised Schools of the South Pacific in 1973

Janssen's interview outlined the organisational memberships of the South Pacific which demonstrated the wide range of interests of those represented. They included both the NSW and Victorian branches of ACONPAL as full members, the SACA and the New Zealand Association of Naturopaths and Osteopaths (NZANO), AARO, the Australian Institute of Homeopathy, Dr Bach Society of NSW, Bernard Jensen Health Club, the SCO, the Youth Welfare Association (operated by Bailey of Hopewood House) and the National Health Federation, encompassing a total of 234 individual members nationally.[80] The South Pacific recognised three schools in 1973 – these included the SCO (Ashfield), New South Wales College of Osteopathy (Darlinghurst – this would have been Janssen's school though Wallace Brown set up a school there later) and Peter Derig's New South Wales College of Osteopathic and Naturopathic Sciences.[81] The articles of the South Pacific provided for three levels of organisational membership of subsidiaries – ordinary, associate and honorary.

Janssens' Death, Formation of the South Pacific Council and College

Janssen died in 1974 and in the aftermath, the Federation morphed into a Council in 1975 with a modified member base revealed in the Federal Webb Inquiry Report.[82] Regarding Janssen's school; the Webb Inquiry Report described the National College of Osteopathy and Prescribing Chemists as founded by Gerritt Janssen in 1974.[83] However, evidence from Janssen's own transcript indicates his school was submitted for acceptance by the IFPNT in 1968 (successful in 1969) suggesting it existed much earlier.[84] The Webb Inquiry Report confirmed that in 1974, this College of Osteopathy ceased to exist. Though the owner is not named, this is due to Janssen's death in 1974. Subsequently, the South Pacific College in Sydney came into being in 1976 and took over the osteopathy portion of Janssen's college.[85] The South Pacific College was formed by the amalgamation with the NSW College of Naturopathic Sciences at Doubleday owned by SCO graduate and NAN representative Dr Peter Derig DC/DO. It then was forced to change name to form the Natural Therapies Institute of NSW. Regardless, the college maintained an identity in the 1970s to students as the 'South Pacific' and is described as the sister college to the South Pacific College in New Zealand established in 1967.[86] When the Webb Inquiry attended the college on July 8, 1975, they were greeted by Mr Wilmot chair of the faculty board and among the others present were Mr W Pruss, Mrs CN Gulson, Mr C Paton (described in Webb Report as 'who built the place and was a practising chiropractor on the premises').[87] Pruss is reference to William (Bill) Pruss and Gulsen (Goulson) was the partner of Geritt Janssen, recently deceased. The New Zealand sister college arose from the NZANO being a subsidiary of the South Pacific pre-1975. Rumours exist of Bowen's work being taught in New Zealand.[88] If these are true, this would have been facilitated by these connections in the networks to which Bowen belonged.

At the Ward Inquiry, it was suggested Bowen had a membership with the Australian College of Osteopathy (Janssen's college and later partly integrated into South Pacific College). This seems a mistaken reference to ACONPAL as Bowen mentioned to the government panel his membership was by subscription and gave him automatic membership of the South Pacific. Bowen's work was also demonstrated at the South Pacific College in Sydney in the later 1970s by two South Pacific organisation directors, Lucy and Pruss.[89] This was recalled by Russell Sturgess, a 1970s graduate of osteopathic massage at the South Pacific College in Sydney and assistant to Dean Griffiths. Sturgess remembered the men were teaching ideas that he later recognised as Bowen-style from his training after Bowen's death. Sturgess later established his own Bowen School, 'Fascial Kinetics'.[90]

The ethos of the South Pacific College evolved from naturopathic schools teaching osteopathy and remained aligned to Still's original tenets. Alan Griffiths, the Dean of the South Pacific College in the mid-1970s, also owned the

AT Still College. In addition to owning AT Still College, Griffiths owned several other osteopathy business concerns while dean of the South Pacific College.[91] The college offered subjects in osteopathy and natural therapies. According to Sturgess, Griffiths was 'strongly aligned with the spiritual healing philosophy of the Father of Osteopathy, Andrew Taylor Still'.[92] Sturgess was also aware of Peter Derig being involved with the college.[93] Griffith's orientation to Still is reflected in various pieces of college correspondence dating to the late 1970s housed in the collection of the Kirksville Museum in Missouri.[94] Some of the correspondence is with prospective students. Griffiths' letters are from his business Hopewood Healing Centre in Kingswood, Sydney and the AT Still College shared the same registered address.[95] All were operating around the same time Griffiths was remembered as dean of the South Pacific.[96] With Griffiths as dean of the South Pacific, together with the presence of Brown as consultant for the AT Still College, Bowen's work was demonstrated at in a college culture keen to foster the original philosophy of Andrew Taylor Still.

Less is known about the teaching ethos of the SSNT which had formed in 1971 and its position with respect to osteopathy and Still, but it can be expected to be equally traditional. Marcus Try who later sued the Registration Board, trained with Jacka at the SSNT in naturopathy, chiropractic and osteopathy and chiropractors Feeley and Hanson were the tutors imparting gentle techniques. An expert witness to Try's case opined these were more osteopathic soft tissue techniques than chiropractic.[97] Ryan, a Bowen observer 1979–1982 and training in osteopathy at the SSNT, noted that Bowen was practicing craniosacral technique (CST).[98] CST was developed in 1937 by William Sutherland, one of Dr Still MD, DO's disciples.

Exodus of Federation Members to Join the UCAA

The SPCNT was formed when members of the South Pacific Federation left to join the UCAA and signalled their focus on the political chiropractic strategy of consolidation for registration. Affiliates that remained with the SPCNT were ACONPAL and its subsidiaries, the SACA and NANOC; those that held associate status included the Bach and Jensen group and as mentioned above, one school member, the South Pacific College of Natural Therapeutics was a merger of Janssen's and Derig's schools. The exodus included the UCAA-recognised affiliated organisations – the Sydney College of Chiropractic (SCC) (formerly Kaufmann's SCO in 1959, then Sydney College of Osteopathy and Chiropractic (SCOC) in 1964 then finally Sydney College of Chiropractic (SCC) in 1973, formalised in 1977 and led by Stavrou); AARO (since 1973, renamed Australian Association of Chiropractors and Osteopaths (AAC&O)); the Roberts' CCA (originally the British and Australian Institute of Naturopathy until 1959 then the Chiropractic and Osteopathy College of Australasia) and the Chiropractic, Osteopathic and Naturopathic College of South Australia established in 1963, which under Struthers at the time of the Webb Inquiry became the South Australian College of Chiropractic.[99] With reference to the SCC,

Wallace Brown, the second principal after Kaufmann, found himself squeezed out as head, resigning on October 7, 1973, the eve of the separate interviews of Bowen and Janssen and Lucy at the Ward Inquiry. Personality issues apart, it is interesting that Brown was later reported associated with a number of colleges with name changes related to naturopathy and osteopathy.[100] Earlier, Brown was found to be a consultant to the AT Still College in Sydney, registered to Griffiths who was dean of the South Pacific College formed in 1976. This suggests Brown's adherence to Still's original tenets which were no longer a fit for the SCC needing to embrace modern approaches and leading the politicised mainstream charge for registration under a chiropractic umbrella. The AT Still College is not mentioned in the Webb Inquiry Report, perhaps because it was used by Griffiths as his own business identity in relation to his South Pacific College dean role. The AT Still College published an article on osteopathy prepared by Wallace C Brown as their consultant.[101]

The Blackmores NANOC Network as Part of the South Pacific

Maurice Blackmore was also educated at Lief's college. Blackmores NAN-NANOC association/schools were focused on teaching chiropractic and distributing Blackmores naturopathic remedies. In Queensland, NANOC was operated by various chiropractors, in Sydney by Professor Mervyn T Judge (Sydney College of Chiropractic and Naturopathy) and in Victoria by Alf Jacka (Southern School of Natural Therapies). Peter Derig also straddled the NANOC camp; at the Webb Inquiry, Jacka represented the NANOC organisation, now returned to the NAN title, with Peter Derig and L McGrath in attendance.[102] The transcripts of Alf Jacka and Mervyn Judge confirmed their colleges were NANOC/Blackmores schools and operating dually as a national association.[103] Judge indicated he established the Sydney NANOC college in 1961/62.[104] Jacka's Melbourne NANOC school was also formed in 1961. According to Judge, the decision by NANOC to transition these schools to independent private ownership took place in 1971.[105] Later on, in 1971, Jacka transitioned the Victorian NANOC to his own private college, the SSNT and he as dean.[106] Judge indicated that his college had been operating for 'many years' and was based on the curriculum of the Bournemouth College that he considered the 'most recognised course of naturopathy training'.[107] Judge evidently took Blackmores Sydney training concern in a different direction than ongoing deference to the training at Lief's college which by the 1960s was moving in an osteopathic direction as the BCNO. Judge's reference may relate to the Bournemouth College which was chiropractic-focused: in June 1975, Professor Webb of the Webb Inquiry visited the 'Anglo European College of Chiropractic in Bournemouth' and found it to be providing a serious education but falling short of the standards of the counterpart mainstream North American colleges of chiropractic.[108] The course at Judge's college was evidently available by correspondence and presumably Jacka's early college offerings were too.[109] Judge indicated the course was theoretical only lasting eighteen months to three years depending on individual progress.[110] Matriculation was not required, instead, education to fourth year (the year below matriculation).[111] Clinic placements were required for the practical component to learn manipulation.[112] NANOC's major membership base was Victoria and Queensland by the time of the Ward Inquiry.[113] Clinic placements in Victoria appear to have been provided by Alister McAlister before McAlister completed formal studies with FG Roberts in 1958 and thereafter provided placements for Roberts' students too. Bowen is connected to Alister McAlister and may have had some involvement in attending NANOC gatherings before the ACONPAL branch was formed in Victoria in 1971 and before many left to join ACONPAL. In that same year, Blackmore retired from running schools to focus on remedies.

Another consumer of Blackmores NANOC courses that combined remedy prescribing and chiropractic and part of the Bowen story is James Robert (Bob) Lucy (1929–1999). At the Ward Inquiry, Lucy stated he was a student in the 1950s and initially started his training with 'the Blackmores school'.[114] This detail confirmed that Lucy did his initial training with Mervyn T Judge. Lucy stated in a magazine article in 1992 that he had originally trained as a chiropractor 'thirty-five years earlier', so in 1957 when turned thirty years of age.[115] Lucy believed 'that people needed treatments beyond just chiropractic adjustments and undertook diploma courses in osteopathy, herbalism, homeopathy and many other modalities in the natural health field'. Nutritional biochemistry followed. Lucy stated that when he discovered the curriculum at the Blackmores school was 'fifty years old' and 'borrowed from the British School' he left and studied at Edward Boughen's Sydney College of Osteopathy at Parramatta.[116] Boughen's college is a different establishment from Kaufman's SCO and it had ceased operating by the time of the Ward Inquiry. Lucy's reference to the British School in the context of chiropractic would be a reference to the Chiropractic College of London rather than Lief's institution which was oriented to osteopathy and nature cure/naturopathy. Lucy had a major interest in formulating and manufacturing his own therapeutic preparations. He established Prescribing Chemists Proprietary Limited in 1969.[117] Registered in 1971, it was deregistered in 1994.[118] Lucy stated that in the interests of standards, Manucom Proprietary Limited followed.[119] The article outlines that he established the College of Somatic Studies (COSS) with Dr Keightley to assist a wide range of practitioners better understand and utilise his formulations including chiropractors, osteopaths, acupuncturists, naturopaths and homeopaths. COSS was established in 1984.[120]

NANOC and ACONPAL Cease, Formation of ANTA and ATMS

With regulation, the South Pacific and its association subsidiaries ACONPAL, NAN/NANC/NANOC and others disappeared. Rising out of the ashes in 1978 was ANTA under Alf Jacka ND as president in Melbourne. Lucy headed in his own direction and established the Counsellors for the Preventive Medicine Movement.[121] The Preventive Medicine Movement Proprietary Limited was formed in 1979.[122] This movement became the forerunner of the Complementary Medicine Association (CMA) which became a company in 2000 a year after Lucy died.[123] Glen Gillard who had studied under Lucy at COSS between 1980 and 1992 indicated he played a role with Lucy in setting up the Preventive Medicine Movement.[124] Lucy's independent direction is believed to be because he was adamant that herbalism not be subsumed by the existing new associations. These associations were now catering to members excluded from osteopath/chiropractor status under the new regulatory regime and who were mixers.[125] Lucy's direction may also have been motivated by the fact that ANTA was associated with the SSNT and graduate members were significant consumers of Blackmores products. Blackmores was a competitor company to Lucy's own Prescribing Chemists and Lucy pursued a different philosophy in his formulas. Gillard was involved in facilitating the first posthumous teachings by Oswald Rentsch of Bowen's work, stated to be in Perth in 1986.[126] Derig who had formerly represented NAN with Jacka became a founding member of the Australian Traditional Medicine Society (ATMS) in 1984.[127] The ATMS would have catered to graduates of Derig's school, the South Pacific College and graduates of Simon Schot's Queensland Institute of Natural Sciences. Schot had operated an academy of natural healing in Sydney and the premises were sold in 1963 to the SCO (later SCC).[128] Today, ANTA, ATMS and CMA continue to be multimodal and have registered osteopaths and chiropractors as members whose training included naturopathy and continue to engage in remedy prescribing. About 40 per cent of CMA members practise bodywork of some kind. All of these associations now accept therapists qualified in Bowen Techniques as taught through various schools.

Bowen's Cultural Fluidity

The fight of the UCAA for recognition was significant. Despite the professionally demarcated landscape between the elite registered and lesser not, Bowen was found moving across both domains and his work in demand in each. This set in train the future posthumous tangents and legacy of his work. Despite heading towards defeat and unjustly becoming a victim of regulation, Bowen's work was sought after. He was welcomed across organisational boundaries, attended ACONPAL conferences, and was invited to conferences of the UCAA and to present at a workshop of the SCC after legislation in 1979.[129] Bowen's business card in Figure 6.1 shows he passed ACONPAL's membership standards and gained full registered membership status and he attended conferences with other qualified professionals, including those aspiring; he was introduced to this audience of qualified and unqualified practitioners alike keen to learn from him and make his acquaintance.

Keith Davis DC and Oswald Rentsch a lay masseur and aspiring natural therapist met Bowen at an unidentified gathering of natural therapists around

1973/1974 and Bowen was announced to those present.[130] Davis DC/ND made himself known to Bowen as he had heard about him from a patient.[131] By report, Bowen had said to him 'I've been wanting you to come down and learn my work' and Davis took up the invite to do so.[132] Davis worked on the other side of the bay from Geelong but soon introduced to Bowen Nigel Love, his brother-in-law who operated a Geelong practice.[133] Neave was Melbourne-based and followed in 1976. Romney Smeeton had heard of Bowen first while a student at the Chiropractic College of Australia (CCA):

> I was doing my clinic rounds with Keith Davis and Kevin Neave when I first got my exposure to Tom's work. Keith would write on his card, 'TB this' and 'TB that'. And I learned a lot through watching Keith and Kevin work and then I moved to Colac and purchased a clinic there. Keith rang me and asked me, 'Would you like me to ring and to arrange for you to work with Tom?' To which I agreed wholeheartedly and Tom rang me one day and said, 'Do you want to come up?', and I said, 'I'd love to Tom' and he said, 'Be here on Monday morning'.[134]

Smeeton attended weekly until Bowen's death in October 1982. Davis also introduced Alistair McCarthur to Bowen, a CCA student and like all UCAA members became registered in 1979. McCarthur practised with Davis, but his presence at Bowen's clinic was not notable in terms of time spent.[135]

In the lead up to the Ward Inquiry and afterwards, Bowen straddled the tensions between the old master-apprentice world of lay skill and practitioners qualified through the primarily naturopathic colleges pre-regulation and the new world of educated talent in the UCAA. Prior to the Ward Inquiry, Bowen had invited a football masseur, Doug Sells to work with him in the evenings at Latrobe Terrace from the late 1960s to early 1970s. At the Ward Inquiry, Bowen's reputation had preceded him well before he was connected with college-qualified practitioners seeking to learn from him. Positive testimony by medical respondents is drawn together in Chapter 7 that favourably referred to Bowen with select others of high profiles, including in discussion between Jens, the medical advisor to the inquiry and the chairman Austin. In the years that followed, Bowen maintained a link between the old and the new and never ceased his involvement as a trainer to the young football teams in the region. Early on he personally solicited John Garner and Brian Anderson but to their later regret, family commitments prevented them from taking up the opportunity at the time.[136] Bowen considered that his nephew Gary Shaw, then only seventeen-year old and no doubt with other plans on his mind, 'had the hands for the work', but likewise the invitation was not taken up.[137] Many more are unaccounted for who assisted Bowen at his clinics, for instance Russell Quick also stated he had assisted Bowen when treating football masseurs at Autumn Street.[138] Terry Molloy DC came from a family that would host regional travellers who attended Bowen's clinics. As a nineteen-year-old Molloy sat in to observe Bowen and he said, 'Tom sent me to the International

College of Chiropractic in 1976. I used to observe him every Saturday morning during 1976'.[139] In addition to the increased presence of fully qualified college-trained observers, two of whom were leading students and won student year prizes at the CCA (Neave DC and Smeeton DC), Bowen continued to encourage younger potential protégés that he considered had ability: client Ann Mortelliti was looking after Michael – a boy who had lost his father and was being raised by the Mortelliti family, but Michael did not take up the offer of training in the late 1970s.[140] The number of observers influenced by Bowen will never be fully known as he was so generous with his time. When regulation finally arrived and he was forced to change his title to 'natural therapist', Bowen made an open invitation to his ANTA colleagues and from this is it known that at least Neil Skilbeck DC took up the invitation.[141] Within his clinic, Bowen enjoyed a huge exposure to a broad and diverse section of the community from politicians, leading athletes, workers from the woollen mills around Geelong and the sheep farms to the West, those afflicted with neurological conditions and incurable diseases and he treated doctors, maintaining a special weekend clinic where they could slip in by a back door away from public eyes.[142] Whether rich or poor was of no consequence, Bowen did his work out of an intense sense of community service and would often treat for free.

In addition to attendances at UCAA conferences before regulation in the 1970s, Bowen was invited to present at the SCC in 1979 – a UCAA-endorsed college. The objectives of these seminars were documented to 'continually raise the standard of chiropractic and osteopathic education and practice'.[143] Due to being unwell, his clinic observers Kevin Neave DC and Keith Davis DC presented his work on his behalf.[144] The workshop is mis-recorded in the official history of the college as the 'Muscle manipulation techniques of Ted [*sic*] Bowen' held over the weekend of April 30 to May 1, 1979.[145] Since Bowen could very well have attended, and if not already acquainted through former ACONPAL conferences, the opportunity would have existed for professional interaction with other speakers such as Horace Lyttle (a former South Pacific director), now inaugural college director on the SCC board and workshop presenter.[146] Other SCC board members who presented on various topics included Dr Bernard Lyle (on therapy localisation) and Dr Gary Stavrou, head of SCC (rib adjustments). Other UCAA presenters were John Mumford (management of acute disc injuries), Dr Arthur Wright – first vice principal of the original SCO and a Doyle Pax College graduate – (cervical muscle release for headache); Dr Malcolm Henningham (psoas release for lumbar and cervical problems); Dr Alex Momot (management of acute torticollis) and Des Donovan (shoulder and arm problems).[147] Revealing the overlaps with early Roberts and Blackmore naturopathic teachings, in 1971, Bernard Lyle was originally connected with NANC as NSW president while Mervyn Judge, the Blackmores/NANC Sydney school owner was federal president.[148] This invitation to Bowen is a clear indication of his stature and standing that continued into the post-regulatory world. Since 1971/1972, the SCC curriculum (then also catering to osteopathy) included 'muscle manipulation' and 'muscle manipulation soft tissue techniques'.[149] Neave DC's notes and diagrams of this workshop have survived in the possession of Romney Smeeton DC. They are useful because they show example positioning of the foundational movements that Bowen would make – including the pelvis which he always addressed first on the basis of the osteopathic importance placed on it as the platform of the body.

Bowen Joins ANTA

Bowen was accepted for membership of ANTA and he had certificate number 121 for 1979/80, dated August 31, 1979, and signed by Percy Alfred (Alf) Jacka as president which has survived in the possession of Bowen's family.[150] Bowen was a member earlier, as Jacka advocated to the health minister for Bowen, McAlister and Wilson on April 14, 1978, to be registered.[151] Names associated with Bowen, also members of ANTA, in addition to McAlister and Fraser, include professional newcomers Kevin Ryan DO (Bowen clinic observer for three years before Bowen's death) and Skilbeck DC.[152] Pruss DO/DC may also have been a member as a mixer, as he wrote an article for the ANTA journal.[153] Around the same time that ANTA was established in 1978, the *Physiotherapists Act* repealed both the *Masseurs Act 1958* and the *Masseurs Amendment Act 1967*. This removed legal impediments to practising massage without formal training and registration.

Summary

This retrospective on the South Pacific through the lens of Bowen's involvement plucks him out of his passive, lone wolf, posthumous portrayal and shows him to be an engaged actor in professional domains pre- and post-regulation. He was engaged with the political process of the Ward Inquiry and due to his strong reputation was in demand and moved between the newly demarcated professional boundaries. The next chapter looks at Bowen's engagement with a small group holding out for osteopathic identity as the VSSO as the rest of the profession was swept into registration under a chiropractic wave and highlights his ultimate humiliation at the hands of the Victorian Registration Board in 1981, months before his death.

Notes

1 ASIC, Company Records, "Notice of Situation of Registered Office and of Office Hours and Particulars of Changes," August 26, 1971: 1; ASIC, "South Pacific Federation of Natural Therapeutics," Company Information.
2 PROV, Report and evidence Osteopathy Committee, Pt.1–4, 27/11/975 (Pt. 2) 2261, VPRS 3253/P1/, Unit 49, Original papers tabled in the Legislative Assembly, transcripts of proceedings, Try transcript, 2179.
3 ASIC, "Memorandum and Articles of Association," South Pacific Federation of Natural Therapeutists Ltd, August 26, 1971 drafted by Purves and Purves, William Street Melbourne.

4 PROV. Osteopathy, Chiropractic and Naturopath Joint Select Committee pp. 783–938, VPRS 241/P/, Unit 14, Transcripts of Committee, South Pacific Federation of Natural Therapeutics represented by Janssen, Lucy and Goulson, transcript: 891.
5 PROV. Report and evidence Osteopathy Committee (Pt.1–4), 27/11/1975 (Pt. 2) 2261, VPRS 3253/P1/, Unit 47. Original papers tabled in the Legislative Assembly, transcripts of proceedings, Wilkie transcript: 1–14; PROV. Report and evidence Osteopathy Committee (Pt.1–4), 27/11/975 (Pt. 2) 2261, VPRS 3253/P1/, Unit 49. Original papers tabled in the Legislative Assembly, transcripts of proceedings, Try transcript: 2198.
6 PROV, VPRS 3253/P1, Unit 47, Wilkie transcript, 2.
7 Bowen's Business Card for 30 Villamanta Street Showing Continued ACONPAL/ South Pacific Membership. Image Courtesy Ron Phelan, Custodian Rene Horwood Collection.
8 "PROV, Chiropractic Treatment and Reports Pt.1 VPRS 6345/P/, Unit 155, General Correspondence Files, press clipping, Osteopaths may be Registered," *Sun,* February 27, 1970.
9 "PROV, Chiropractic Treatment and Reports Pt.1 VPRS 6345/P/, Unit 155, General Correspondence Files, press clipping, Osteopaths may be Registered."
10 Marjery Bloomfield, *Tree of Life, a History of the European School of Osteopathy, The First Fifty Years* (Brighton, United Kingdom: Indepenpress, 2009), 21.
11 PROV, VPRS 241/P/, Unit 14 South Pacific Federation transcript (Janssen), 910.
12 PROV, VPRS 241/P/, Unit 14 South Pacific Federation transcript (Janssen), 894.
13 Bloomfield, *Tree of Life*, 20.
14 "About the ESO," European School of Osteopathy website states the School was founded in Paris in 1951 as Ecole Française d'Ostéopathie (EFO) and moved to England in 1965. Initially based in London, the EFO relocated to Kent in 1971 where it first operated from premises close to Maidstone town centre. In 1974, due to student demand in the UK, a new full-time, English speaking programme was created. The School was incorporated as a registered charity trading as the European School of Osteopathy/Ecole Européenne d'Ostéopathie and on October 1, 1974 its first four-year full-time diploma began.
15 PROV, VPRS 241/P/Unit 14, South Pacific Federation transcript (Janssen), 894.
16 PROV, VPRS 241/P/Unit 14, South Pacific Federation transcript (Janssen), 894A.
17 PROV, VPRS 241/P/Unit 14, South Pacific Federation transcript (Janssen), 894.
18 Webb Inquiry Report, 629, 673.
19 Webb Inquiry Report, Appendix 14, 756–62.
20 Webb Inquiry Report, 253.
21 Bloomfield, *Tree of Life*, vi.
22 Bloomfield, *Tree of Life*, vi.
23 "Osteopathy," in *Natural Therapeutics* (Melbourne: Australian Chiropractors' Osteopaths' and Naturopathic Association, 196-?), section 1, 1–3: 2. The State Library is uncertain of the date of the document.
24 PROV, VPRS 241/P/, Unit 14, South Pacific Federation transcript (Lucy), 893.
25 PROV, VPRS 241/P/, Unit 14, South Pacific Federation transcript (Lucy), 893.
26 Rene Horwood interview by Ron Phelan, July 15, 1998, transcript extract by Phelan in Shirley Strachan, *Healing Hands, Unsung Voices, Thomas Ambrose Bowen Osteopath (1916–1982)* (United Kingdom: Cloister House Press, 2016), 35.
27 Murray, *In Search*, 169.
28 Ward Inquiry Report, 9; Webb Inquiry Report, Appendix 3, "Brief History of Organisations," 261–75.
29 "Delay Likely ACT Moves for Chiropractors," *Canberra Times*, July 11, 1973: 12; "Error by Assessor," *Canberra Times*, January 20, 1976: 8.

30 *Natural Therapeutics* (Melbourne Australian Chiropractors' Osteopaths' and Naturopathic Association, 196-?).
31 Historical records on ASIC for ANTA do not include the former entities of ACONPAL and ANPA and no separate records for these are on the ASIC database.
32 PROV, VPRS 3253/P1, Unit 49, Try transcript, 2198.
33 Ward Inquiry Report, 9.
34 Webb Inquiry Report, 41.
35 Webb Inquiry Report, 41.
36 PROV, VPRS 241/P/, Unit 14, South Pacific Federation, transcript, 892.
37 PROV, Osteopathy, Chiropractic and Naturopath Joint Select Committee pp. 652–78, VPRS 241/P/, Unit 14, Transcripts of Committees, Love transcript: 652–59A, 652.
38 PROV, VPRS 241/P/, Unit 14, South Pacific Federation transcript (Lucy), 894.
39 Webb Inquiry Report, 263.
40 PROV, VPRS 3253/P1, Unit 49, Try transcript, 2198.
41 PROV, VPRS 3453/P1, Unit 49, Try transcript, 2198.
42 PROV, VPRS 3453/P1, Unit 49, Try transcript, 2198.
43 PROV, VPRS 3453/P1, Unit 49, Try transcript, 2198.
44 PROV, VPRS 3453/P1, Unit 49, Try transcript, 2198.
45 PROV, VPRS 3253/P1, Unit 47, Wilkie transcript, 14.
46 PROV, VPRS 3453/P1, Unit 47, Jacka transcript, 18.
47 PROV, VPRS 3453/P1, Unit 47, Wilkie transcript, 2.
48 PROV, VPRS 3453/P1, Unit 49, Try transcript, 2198.
49 Ward Inquiry Report, 70.
50 Rene Horwood interview July 15, 1998, notes by Ron Phelan.
51 PROV, Chiropractors and Osteopaths Registration Board VPRS 6345/P/, Unit 556, General Correspondence, Letter Jacka to Houghton, April 1, 1976.
52 PROV, Chiropractors and Osteopaths Registration Board VPRS 6345/P/, Unit 556, General Correspondence, Letter Jacka to Houghton, April 1, 1976.
53 PROV, Registration of Chiropractors and Oestopaths [sic] – New Act VPRS 6345/P/, Unit 545, General Correspondence, Jacka ANTA report April 14, 1978, to Digby Crozier, Member for Western Province April 19, 1978, forwarded to Minister Houghton May 4, 1978.
54 "Our Country as I See It," *Farmer and Settler (Sydney)*, September 5, 1935: 1.
55 PROV, Report and evidence Osteopathy Committee, Pt.1–4 27/11/975 (Pt. 2) 2261, VPRS 3253/P1, Unit 47, Wilkie transcript: 1–14, ASIC "Memorandum and Articles of Association."
56 Webb Inquiry Report, 265.
57 S. P. Bolton, "A Retrospective View of Historical Periods in Australian Chiropractic History," *Chiropractic Journal of Australia* 36, no. 1 (2006): 9–16.
58 John L. Kelly, "Philosophy of Chiropractic at the Sydney College of Chiropractic: 1975–2000," *Chiropractic Journal of Australia* 40, no. 4 (2010): 154–58.
59 Kelly, "Philosophy of Chiropractic," 154–58.
60 Edwin Devereaux, Brian O'Reilly, and John Cice, *History of the Sydney College of Chiropractic* (Sydney: Macquarie Lighthouse Press, 2012), 70.
61 Devereaux et al., *History of the Sydney College of Chiropractic.*
62 Devereaux et al., *History of the Sydney College of Chiropractic.* Bolton, "A Retrospective View of Historical Periods in Australian Chiropractic History."
63 Pamela Snider and Roger Newman Turner, "Nature Cure in Europe: The Transatlantic Journey from Pragmatism to Principles," *Naturopathic Doctors News and Reviews*, October 2, 2010.
64 P. S. Brown, "Nineteenth-Century American Health Reformers and the Early Nature Cure Movement in Britain," *Medical History* 32 (1988): 174–94.

65 Brown, "Nineteenth-Century American Health Reformers," 174–94.
66 "History of the British College of Osteopathic Medicine," *British College of Osteopathic Medicine*, accessed October 19, 2024.
67 "Naturopathic Diplomas Presented," *Telegraph (Brisbane, Qld): 1872 – 1947)* July 24, 1936: 18.
68 "Naturopathic Diplomas Presented."
69 Advertising," *Telegraph (Brisbane),* July 30, 1934: 19.
70 "Advertising," *Daily Mercury (Mackay),* November 14, 1935: 13; Advertising" *Maryborough Chronicle, Wide Bay and Burnett Advertiser (Qld)* May 5, 1937: 4.
71 Devereaux et al., *History of the Sydney College of Chiropractic*, 9.
72 "Advertising," *Townsville Daily Bulletin (Qld)*, September 15, 1936: 3.
73 "Advertising," *Maryborough Chronicle, Wide Bay and Burnett Advertiser (Qld),* May 25, 1937: 10.
74 PROV, VPRS 241/P/Unit 14, South Pacific Federation transcript (Janssen), 890.
75 Devereaux et al., *History of the Sydney College of Chiropractic*, 52 (information quoted from Bill Pruss).
76 Devereaux et al., *History of the Sydney College of Chiropractic*, 77.
77 Devereaux et al., *History of the Sydney College of Chiropractic*, 45, 76 and 84.
78 Ward Inquiry Report, 625; PROV, VPRS 241/P/, Unit 14, South Pacific Federation transcript (Janssen), 891.
79 PROV, VPRS 241/P/, Unit 14, South Pacific Federation transcript (Janssen), 891.
80 PROV, VPRS 241/P/, Unit 14, South Pacific Federation transcript (Janssen), 891, 910.
81 PROV, VPRS 241/P/, Unit 14, South Pacific Federation transcript (Janssen), 894.
82 ASIC, "South Pacific Federation of Natural Therapeutists," Changes to Directors; Ward Inquiry Report, 265.
83 Webb Inquiry Report, 274.
84 PROV, VPRS 241/P/, Unit 14 South Pacific Federation transcript (Janssen), 894A.
85 Webb Inquiry Report, 274.
86 Russell Sturgess personal communication to the author July 26, 2017; "Kia Ora Welcome," South Pacific College of Natural Medicine New Zealand.
87 Webb Inquiry Report, 672.
88 Murray, *In Search*, 169.
89 Sturgess personal communication to the author July 26, 2017.
90 Sturgess personal communication to the author July 26, 2017.
91 According to ASIC company records for Alan Raymond Griffiths, these included the Academy of Osteopathy, Osteopathic and Natural Health Care Centre, A.T. Still College of Osteopathy, the Australasian Academy of Cranial Osteopathy, Osteopathy House, Sit Right, the Back Pain Clinic, The Research Academy for Complementary Medicine, Naturally Good and Pain Busters.
92 Sturgess personal communication to the author July 26, 2017.
93 Sturgess personal communication to the author July 26, 2017.
94 Searchable online at Archives Museum of Osteopathic Medicine, A. T. Still University.
95 ASIC, "A.T. Still College of Osteopathy," and "NSW College of Osteopathy." Note both of these colleges have misreported registration dates of 1753. The former was cancelled in 1992, the latter in 2012. Another "A.T. Still College of Applied Osteopathy," BN146623, QLD was registered in 1980, later cancelled and date not recorded.
96 Letter from Alan Raymond Griffiths to Virginia Farnum dated January 24, 1978, confirms the connection via addresses and Griffiths' own advice about his role

establishing the A. T. Still College. Catalogue 2012.95.67, Museum of Osteopathic Medicine, AT Still University.

97 Marcus Try v Chiropractors and Osteopaths Registration Board of Victoria 1983/ November 18, Supreme Court Victoria, Action I5876, accessed November 17, 2024, http://aucc.sirsidynix.net.au/Judgments/Civil/289683.pdf.

98 Kevin Ryan, "Working alongside Tom Bowen," Presentation to the National Conference of Bowen Interest Groups, Geelong, 1999, transcribed by author, in Strachan, *Healing Hands, Unsung Voices*, 249.

99 Webb Inquiry, 276; UCAA colleges, Webb Inquiry Report, 266, 273; Devereaux et al., *History of the Sydney College of Chiropractic*, 187; Webb Inquiry, 640.

100 Devereaux et al., *History of the Sydney College of Chiropractic*, 94.

101 "What is osteopathy?"- A two-page pamphlet headed A.T. Still College of Osteopathy prepared by Professor Wallace Brown, Foundation Principal NSW College of Osteopathy and Osteopathic consultant to AT Still College. Held at Museum of Osteopathic Medicine, Kirksville Catalogue No. 2012.95.38

102 Ward Inquiry Report, 9.

103 PROV, Report and evidence Osteopathy Committee, Pt.1–4, VPRS 3253/P1, Unit 47, Original papers tabled in the Legislative Assembly, transcripts of proceedings, Jacka transcript 15–29; PROV. Report and evidence Osteopathy Committee (Pt.1–4), 27/11/975 (Pt. 2) 2261, VPRS 3253/P1, Unit 48. Original papers tabled in the Legislative Assembly, transcripts of proceedings, Judge transcript, 879–89.

104 Judge transcript, 879–89.

105 Judge transcript, 879–89.

106 Judy Jacka, *The Politics and the Passion* (Melbourne: Ringwood Natural Therapies Pty Ltd, 1998), 13.

107 PROV, VPRS 3253/P1 Unit 48, Judge transcript, 879–89.

108 Webb Inquiry Report, 140, 747–55.

109 Judge transcript, 885.

110 Judge transcript, 885.

111 Judge transcript, 885.

112 Judge transcript, 885.

113 Ward Inquiry Report, 9.

114 PROV, Osteopathy, Chiropractic and Naturopath Joint Select Committee pp. 783–938, VPRS 241/P/, Unit 14, Transcripts of Committee, South Pacific Federation of Natural Therapeutics represented by Janssen, Lucy and Goulson, transcript PROV, VPRS 241/P/, Unit 14, South Pacific Federation transcript, 896.

115 "Mr Robert Lucy," *Newsletter of the Hypoglycaemic Association* 8, no. 4 (December 1992): 1.

116 PROV, Osteopathy, Chiropractic and Naturopath Joint Select Committee pp. 783–938, VPRS 241/P/, Unit 14, Transcripts of Committee, South Pacific Federation of Natural Therapeutics, 897.

117 "Mr Robert Lucy."

118 ASIC, Prescribing Chemists Distributing Company, ACN 000 869 830, Registered NSW February 10, 1971, deregistered April 26, 1994.

119 "Mr Robert Lucy"; ASIC, Manucom Pty Ltd, ACN 001 450 228, Registered NSW April 22, 1977 deregistered September 14, 2015.

120 ASIC, "College of Somatic Studies Pty Ltd," (formerly Soguse Pty Ltd) ACN 002 828 275, registered September 5, 1984, deregistered February 2, 2015.

121 Clark personal communication to author.

122 ASIC, "Preventive Medicine Movement Pty Ltd," ACN 008 548 776, September 13, 1979, registered June 20, 2003.

123 "About," Complementary Medicine Association; ASIC ACN: 094 657 011 registered in Oxenford Queensland, October 4, 2000; Clark personal communication to author.
124 Information formerly on Glen Gillard's LinkedIn Profile – no longer online.
125 Janice Carless personal communication to author.
126 O. Rentsch, "The Bowen Story," *Bowens Hands, the Newsletter of the Bowen Therapy Academy of Australia* 19, no. 1 (1992): 3–4.
127 Stephen Eddey, et al., "Vale Peter Derig," *Journal of the Australian Traditional Medicine Society* 19, no. 2 (2013): 98–99.
128 Devereaux et al., *History of the Sydney College of Chiropractic*, 80; Webb Inquiry Report, 267.
129 UCAA conferences were mentioned by Romney Smeeton, interview by author, in Shirley Strachan, *Healing Hands*, 24 & 226.
130 Murray, *In Search*, 165.
131 Murray, *In Search*, 165.
132 Murray, *In Search*, 166.
133 PROV, VPRS 241/P/, Unit 14, Love transcript, 652, 653, 655.
134 Smeeton interview by author, in Strachan, *Healing Hands*, 226.
135 "Victorian Register of Chiropractors and Osteopaths as at 30 June 1980," Victorian Government Gazette No. 67, August 12, 1980, 2764; PROV, Osteopathy, Chiropractic and Naturopath Joint Select Committee pp. 1003–56 PROV, VPRS 241/P/, Unit 14, Davis transcript: 1037–46, 1038/1039.
136 John Garner interview by author in Strachan, *Healing Hands*, 46–47 and Brian Anderson personal communication.
137 Peter Harris email message to author April 3, 2015.
138 Russell Quick personal communication.
139 Verlie Molloy interview by author January 7 and June 25, 2015, including input from Terry Molloy and bearing in mind there was no osteopathic college then.
140 Ann Mortelliti interview by author.
141 Neil Skilbeck, "Typical Day Working with Tom Bowen," *Vic Bowen News* 1, no. 2 (May 1998): 3.
142 Rene Horwood interview by Ron Phelan, in Strachan, *Healing Hands*, 31.
143 Devereaux et al., *History of the Sydney College of Chiropractic*, 187.
144 Horwood interview by Ron Phelan October 8, 1998, transcript extract by Phelan in Strachan, *Healing Hands*, 35.
145 Devereaux et al., *History of the Sydney College of Chiropractic*, 187.
146 Devereaux et al., *History of the Sydney College of Chiropractic*, 187; Lyttle is listed in documents at ASIC, "South Pacific Federation of Natural Therapeutists."
147 Devereaux et al., *History of the Sydney College of Chiropractic*, 187.
148 PROV, Chiropractic Treatments and Reports, Pt.1, VPRS 6345/P/, Unit 485, General Correspondence Files, Letter January 22, 1971, Maurice Blackmore of NANC to Rossiter, Minister for Health with newsletter and NSW NANC report attached.
149 Devereaux et al., *History of the Sydney College of Chiropractic*, Appendix 6, 379.
150 A photograph of Bowen's youngest daughter Heather Edmonds holding the certificate appears in Murray, *In Search*, 153.
151 PROV, VPRS 6345/P/, Unit 545, Jacka ANTA Report April 14, 1978, 3.
152 PROV, VPRS 6345/P/, Unit 545, Jacka ANTA Report April 14, 1978, 3; "Victorian Register of Chiropractors and Osteopaths," Victorian Government Gazette, No. 84, October 9, 1986, Ryan with 'O' (osteopath) registration on 3.8.82, and Skilbeck 'C' (chiropractor) on 2.8.83, 3943.
153 W. Pruss, "Natural Therapies from the 1890s to the 1950s," *Journal of the Australian Natural Therapists Association* 21, no. 1 (2006): 31–33.

Bibliography

Newspapers

"Advertising." *Maryborough Chronicle, Wide Bay and Burnett Advertiser (Qld),* May 2, 1932: 3 (col.1). Accessed November 17, 2024. http://nla.gov.au/nla.news-article149075999.

"Advertising." *Telegraph (Brisbane)*, July 30, 1934: 19. Accessed November 17, 2024. http://nla.gov.au/nla.news-article17992543.

"Advertising." *Daily Mercury (Mackay),* November 14, 1935: 13 (col.1). Accessed November 17, 2024. http://nla.gov.au/nla.news-article173339866.

"Advertising." *Townsville Daily Bulletin (Qld)*, September 15, 1936: 3 (col.6). Accessed November 17, 2024. http://nla.gov.au/nla.news-article64083186.

"Advertising." *Maryborough Chronicle, Wide Bay and Burnett Advertiser (Qld),* May 5, 1937: 4. Accessed January 27, 2019. http://nla.gov.au/nla.news-article151235271.

"Advertising." *Maryborough Chronicle, Wide Bay and Burnett Advertiser (Qld),* May 25, 1937: 10. Accessed October 19, 2024, http://nla.gov.au/nla.news-article151256361.

"Delay Likely ACT Moves for Chiropractors." *Canberra Times,* July 11, 1973: 12 (col.3). Accessed November 17, 2024. http://nla.gov.au/nla.news-article110737278.

"Error by Assessor," *Canberra Times,* January 20, 1976: 8. Accessed November 17, 2024. http://nla.gov.au/nla.news-article110797897.

"Naturopathic Diplomas Presented." *Telegraph (Brisbane, Qld): 1872 – 1947),* July 24, 1936: 18. Accessed November 17, 2024. http://nla.gov.au/nla.news-article181916371.

"Our Country as I See It." *Farmer and Settler (Sydney),* September 5, 1935: 1. Accessed January 29, 2018. http://nla.gov.au/nla.news-article117208654.

Primary Sources

Anderson, Brian. Interview by author, December 10, 2014, check was January 14, 2015, transcript in Strachan, Shirley. *Healing Hands, Unsung Voices, Thomas Ambrose Bowen Osteopath (1916–1982).* United Kingdom: Cloister House Press, 2016.

ASIC. "Memorandum and Articles of Association, South Pacific Federation of Natural Therapeutists Ltd." August 26, 1971 drafted by Purves and Purves, William Street Melbourne.

ASIC. "South Pacific Federation and Natural Therapeutics, Notice of Situation of Registered Office and of Office Hours and Particulars of Changes." August 26, 1971: 1.

ASIC. "A.T. Still College of Applied Osteopathy." BN146623, QLD registered in 1980, later cancelled and date not recorded.

ASIC. "A.T. Still College of Osteopathy." E4009943, NSW; "NSW College of Osteopathy." F2200230. NSW.

ASIC. "Prescribing Chemists Distributing Company, CAN 000 869 830, Registered NSW February 10, 1971, deregistered April 26, 1994.

ASIC. "College of Somatic Studies Pty Ltd." (formerly Soguse Pty Ltd) ACN 002 828 275, registered September 5, 1984, deregistered February 2, 2015.

ASIC. Manucom Pty Ltd, ACN 001 450 228, Registered NSW April 22, 1977, deregistered September 14, 2015.

ASIC. "Preventive Medicine Movement Pty Ltd." ACN: 008 548 776, Registered ACT 1979.

ASIC. "South Pacific Federation of Natural Therapeutists." Changes to Directors.

Garner, John. Interview by author June 22, 2015, Transcript in Strachan, Shirley. *Healing Hands, Unsung Voices, Thomas Ambrose Bowen 1916–1982 Osteopath.* United Kingdom: Cloister House Press, 2016.

Griffiths, Alan. Correspondence in Kirkville Museum Collection, searchable. http://momicoh.pastperfectonline.com/archive/18C8026A-936A-4A12-8695-521468389971.

Horwood, Rene. Interview by Ron Phelan, July 15, 1998, transcribed by author November 15–30, 2018.

Horwood, Rene. Interview by Ron Phelan, October 8, 1998, transcribed by author November 15–30, 2018.

Molloy, Verlie. Interview by author January 7 and June 25, 2015. Transcript in Strachan, Shirley. *Healing Hands, Unsung Voices, Thomas Ambrose Bowen 1916–1982, Osteopath.* United Kingdom: Cloister House Press, 2016.

Natural Therapeutics. Melbourne: Australian Chiropractors' Osteopaths' and Naturopathic Association of Australia Limited, 196-?.

"Osteopathy." In *Natural Therapeutics.* Melbourne: Australian Chiropractors' Osteopaths' and Naturopathic Physicians Association Limited, 196-?, 1–3, 1–5.

PROV. Chiropractic Treatment and Reports Pt.1. VPRS 6345/P/, Unit 155, General Correspondence Files, Press Clipping. "Osteopaths may be Registered." Sun, February 27, 1970.

PROV. Chiropractic Treatments and Reports, Pt.1. VPRS 6345/P/, Unit 485. General Correspondence Files, Letter January 22, 1971, Maurice Blackmore of NANC to Rossiter, Minister for Health with newsletter and NSW NANC report attached.

PROV. Osteopathy, Chiropractic and Naturopath Joint Select Committee pp. 1003–56, VPRS 241/P/, Unit 14. Transcripts of Committee, Davis transcript: 1037–46.

PROV. Osteopathy, Chiropractic and Naturopath Joint Select Committee pp. 652–78, VPRS 241/P/, Unit 14. Transcripts of Committee, Love transcript: 652–9A.

PROV. Osteopathy, Chiropractic and Naturopath Joint Select Committee pp. 783–938, VPRS 241/P/, Unit 14, Transcripts of Committee, South Pacific Federation of Natural Therapeutics represented by Janssen, Lucy and Goulson, transcript: 890–914.

PROV. Registration of Chiropractors and Oestopaths [*sic*]– New Act VPRS 6345/P/, Unit 545. General Correspondence, Jacka ANTA report April 14, 1978, to Digby Crozier, Member for Western Province April 19, 1978, forwarded to Minister Houghton May 4, 1978.

PROV. Report and Evidence Osteopathy Committee (Pt.1–4), 27/11/975 (Pt. 2) 2261, VPRS 3253/P1 Unit 47. Report and evidence Osteopathy Committee, Original papers tabled in the Legislative Assembly, transcripts of proceedings, Jacka transcript: 15–29.

PROV. Report and Evidence Osteopathy Committee (Pt.1–4), 27/11/975 (Pt. 2) 2261, VPRS 3253/P1, Unit 48. Original papers tabled in the Legislative Assembly, transcripts of proceedings, Judge transcript: 879–89.

PROV. Report and Evidence Osteopathy Committee (Pt.1–4), 27/11/975 (Pt. 2) 2261, VPRS 3253/P1/, Unit 49. Original papers tabled in the Legislative Assembly, transcripts of proceedings, Try transcript: 2179–98.

PROV. Report and evidence Osteopathy Committee (Pt.1–4), 27/11/1975 (Pt. 2) 2261, VPRS 3253/P1/, Unit 47. Original papers tabled in the Legislative Assembly, transcripts of proceedings, Wilkie transcript: 1–14.

"Register of Chiropractors and Osteopaths as at 30 June 1980." *Victorian Government Gazette*, No. 67, August 12, 1980.

"Register of Chiropractors and Osteopaths as at September 8, 1986." *Victorian Government Gazette*, No. 84, October 9, 1986.

Ryan, Kevin. "Working alongside Tom Bowen." Presentation to National Conference of Bowen Interest Groups, August 21, 1999. Transcript in Strachan, Shirley. *Healing Hands, Unsung Voices, Thomas Ambrose Bowen 1916–1982, Osteopath.* United Kingdom: Cloister House Press, 2016.

Try, Marcus v Chiropractors and Osteopaths Registration Board of Victoria 1983 / November 18, Supreme Court Victoria, Action I5876. Accessed November 17, 2024. http://aucc.sirsidynix.net.au/Judgments/Civil/289683.pdf.

"Victorian Register of Chiropractors and Osteopaths as at 30 June, 1980." *Victoria Government Gazette*, No. 67, August 12, 1980, 2764.
"Victorian Register of Chiropractors and Osteopaths as at 8 September, 1986." *Victoria Government Gazette*, No. 84, October 9, 1986, 3939, 3943, 3945.
Ward Inquiry Report – full title – Victoria Parliament, Osteopathy, Chiropractic and Naturopathy Committee, et al. *Report from the Osteopathy, Chiropractic and Naturopathy Committee: Together with Appendices*. Melbourne: C. H. Rixon, Government Printer, 1975. Accessed November 17, 2024. http://www6.austlii.edu.au/au/other/vic/VicLASelCPubInq/1975/1.pdf.
"Webb Inquiry Report" – full title – *Report of the Committee of Inquiry into Chiropractic, Osteopathy, Homoeopathy [sic] and Naturopathy*. Canberra: Australian Government Publishing Service, 1977. Accessed November 17, 2024. https://www6.austlii.edu.au/au/other/cth/AUBCPubInq/1977/6.pdf.
"What Is Osteopathy?"- A two-page pamphlet headed A.T. Still College of Osteopathy prepared by Professor Wallace Brown, Foundation Principal NSW College of Osteopathy and Osteopathic consultant to A.T. Still College of University. Catalogue number, 2012.95.38. http://momicoh.pastperfectonline.com/library/B94E846E-EA61-4D9A-80EB-468774521418.

Secondary Sources

Bloomfield, Marjery. *Tree of Life, a History of the European School of Osteopathy, The First Fifty Years*. Brighton, United Kingdom: Indepenpress, 2009.
Bolton, S. P. "A Retrospective View of Historical Periods in Australian Chiropractic History." *Chiropractic Journal of Australia* 36, no. 1 (2006): 9–16. Accessed November 17, 2024. https://search.informit.org/doi/10.3316/informit.530550519029873.
Ceballos-Laita, Luis et al. "Is Craniosacral Therapy Effective? A Systematic Review and Meta-Analysis." *Healthcare (Basel, Switzerland)* 12, no. 6 (March 18, 2024): 679. https://doi.org/10.3390/healthcare12060679
Devereaux, Edwin, Brian O'Reilly, and John Cice. *History of the Sydney College of Chiropractic*. Sydney: Macquarie Lighthouse Press, 2012.
Eddey, Stephen et al. "Vale Peter Derig." *Journal of the Australian Traditional Medicine Society* 19, no. 1 (2013): 98–99.
Hartman, Steve E. "Cranial Osteopathy: Its Fate Seems Clear." *Chiropractic & Osteopathy* 4, no. 1 (2006): 10. https://doi.org/10.1186/1746-1340-14-10
Jacka, Judy. *The Politics and the Passion*. Melbourne: Ringwood Natural Therapies Pty Ltd, 1998.
Kelly, John L. "Philosophy of Chiropractic at the Sydney College of Chiropractic: 1975–2000." *Chiropractic Journal of Australia* 40, no. 4 (2010): 154–58.
Murray, Col. *In Search of Tom Bowen and the Therapy He Inspired and Lots of Other Stuff*. Armadale: Palmer Higgs, Booksonline, 2010.
Pruss, W. "Natural Therapies from the 1890s to the 1950s." *Journal of the Australian Natural Therapists Association* 21, no. 1 (2006): 31–33.
Rentsch, O. (Ossie). "The Bowen Story." *Bowens Hands, the Newsletter of the Bowen Therapy Academy of Australia* 1, no. 1 (1992): 3–4.
Rentsch, O. (Ossie). "The Challenge, The Choice, The Change." *Bowen Hands, the Official Journal of the Bowen Therapy Academy of Australia* 9 (2), no. 33 (June 2000): 5–6.
Rentsch, O. (Ossie). "Bowen Chose Me!" *Bowen Hands, the Official Journal of the Bowen Therapy Academy of Australia* 21 (4), no. 83 (December 2012): 1.
Skilbeck, Neil. "Typical Day Working with Tom Bowen." *Vic Bowen News* 1, no. 2 (May 1998): 3.

Websites

"About CMA." *Complementary Medicine Association.* Accessed November 17, 2024. https://cma.asn.au/about-cma/.

"Archives Museum of Osteopathic Medicine." *A T Still University.* Accessed November 17, 2024. https://momicoh.pastperfectonline.com//archive/.

"History of the British College of Osteopathic Medicine." *The British College of Osteopathic Medicine.* Accessed November 17, 2024. https://bcnogroup.ac.uk/about-us/the-bcno-group/history-of-bcom/.

"Kia Ora Welcome." *South Pacific College of Natural Medicine New Zealand.* Accessed November 17, 2024. http://www.spcnm.ac.nz/.

Video

Kevin, Ryan. "Dr Kevin Ryan and Tom Bowen." *YouTube* Video, 51:31 minutes. Posted September 2024. Accessed November 18, 2024. https://www.youtube.com/watch?v=TLwKB4fu9p8.

7 The VSSO and Bowen

A Victim of Regulation

> 'The Chiropractors and Osteopaths Registration should be sacked', Mr Mackenzie said. 'Their treatment of Geelong's best known and successful osteopath Tom Bowen, is a disgrace'.[1]
>
> Rod Mackenzie, Labour MP, Geelong Province, 1982

Introduction: Osteopaths a Minority

Representing the Victorian branch of the Australian Chiropractors, Osteopaths and Naturopathic Practitioners Association Proprietary Limited (ACONPAL), future Victorian Society of Specialist Osteopaths (VSSO) President Alan Wilkie's transcript to the Ward Inquiry provides useful background on the numbers of osteopaths in Victoria in the early 1970s. He said, there were thirty-eight members of ACONPAL, with only seven osteopaths in Victoria and three chiropractors, one herbalist, the rest naturopaths.[2] He estimated there were only twenty osteopaths in Victoria overall.[3] This confirms that within ACONPAL, Bowen was a member to a tiny cohort of osteopaths in the Victorian branch and one of only twenty statewide. Bowen appears in the Ward Inquiry report under 'leading group of osteopathic practitioners'.[4] The group included Benes, Bowen, Gardini, McAlister, Peters, Woodley and Wright and they all self-reported data on patient visits over a seventeen-week period (see Table 7.1 with data adapted from Ward Inquiry Report and ranked by patient visits and noting whether formally credentialled or not).[5]

Benes and Woodley were British-qualified osteopaths and both later immediately registered on January 1, 1979, as 'DO UK'.[6] Peters is thought to be Maxwell Clifford Peters registered under Section 8 (4) on July 28, 1979, of unknown training. McAlister was qualified with Roberts' BAIN in 1958. Bowen, Gardini and McAlister were members of ACONPAL and joined the VSSO. Wright is considered to be DE Wright of Boronia who is listed in the Webb report but never registered and a likely candidate for the VSSO but who failed to be registered like Bowen. At the time of the Inquiry, Bowen was practising at 283 Latrobe Terrace and his business card was simply 'Osteopath' (see Figure 7.1).[7]

DOI: 10.4324/9781003602125-8

Table 7.1 Figures Sourced from Ward Inquiry Report, 'Leading Osteopathic Practitioners'

One clinic, one practitioner	*Total patient visits*	*Average visits per week*	*Hours worked*	*Average number of patients per hour*	*Average number of patients per day*	*Approximate number of patients in 40-hour week*	*Formal credentials in osteopathy*
Bowen	13000	270	32	8.5	60	320	
Benes	10625	125	40	3	24	125	LSO
Gardini	2360	139	33	4	44	160	? credentialled in UK
Peters	1946	23	50	0.5	4	20	Yes, nk
Wright	1320	78	37	2	10	80	
McAlister	952	56	40	1.5	12	56	Roberts BAIN
Woodley	873	51	34	1.5	11	60	BSO

Note: Rearranged by patient volumes and qualifications added.

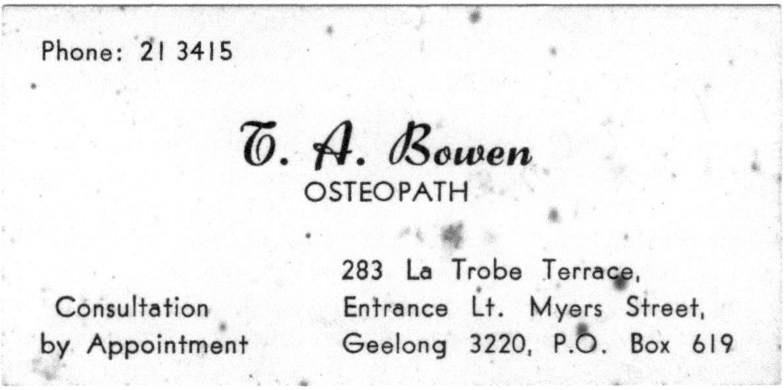

Figure 7.1 Bowen's business card for 283 Latrobe Terrace where his Ward Inquiry interview was held.

Source: Image courtesy of Ron Phelan, Custodian Rene Horwood Collection.

Formation of the VSSO

In 1975, the Victorian Society of Specialist Osteopaths (VSSO) was established and Bowen joined this tight group of 'straight' osteopaths. There are no records with ASIC that suggest the VSSO was ever formally established as an entity. President Wilkie's letter transcribed next gives valuable insights into characteristics of the members; other information is restricted to comments in Government Inquiry reports and the Victorian Parliamentary Hansard. This group makes an important statement about the marginalisation of a talented osteopathic minority and Bowen's connection to a rare community of osteopathic practitioners and his views about his identity. It was not until much later that osteopathy achieved demarcation and separate legislation for registration in 1996.[8] In 1973, Bowen had signalled his concerns to the Ward Inquiry when questioning moved to possible government registration and examinations. Bowen was supportive of both and stated his opinion that the examination should involve 'a great deal of practical work set into it' and said, 'There are too many of us with different methods. Mr Roberts has a chiropractic school in Melbourne, has he not? There is a college there at the present time. Which way are you going? Their way or another way? That is the only thing that is worrying me'.[9] The Panel advised their role was to make recommendations and for the government to work it out and Bowen replied, 'I brought this up in Melbourne a few months ago. Where are all these doctors coming from? One day you see a person is a homeopath and next day, he is a DC. This is also one of the things I am concerned about'.[10] The panel thought Bowen was being critical of Roberts but he replied, 'I have no criticism at all of Mr Roberts. When you start this college, what system is to be used. Are you going to use the chiropractic theory or are you going to use another theory? There are many branches of this profession'.[11] It does appear from Bowen's transcript he had some concerns with the proliferation of chiropractors and chiropractic theory having the upper hand. The views of other VSSO members become relevant in this regard.

Growth and Membership of the VSSO

It is not known when Bowen was invited to join the VSSO, a select group of long-standing practitioners. The VSSO first appears referenced in the Ward Inquiry Report numbering three in 1975.[12] In the later Webb Inquiry Report, they are recorded as lobbying as 'straight' osteopaths and then numbering five.[13] The VSSO was formed in the same year the exodus to the UCAA took place from the South Pacific Federation of Natural Therapists (SPFNT), so the formation was a protest against osteopathy being subsumed under the UCAA chiropractic identity. The government Inquiry reports do not identify the VSSO members by name, only the quantum of members. Former Parliamentarian Rod Mackenzie OAM named some of them in parliament in late 1981 when they then numbered eleven.[14] Among them are key figures introduced in Chapters 2 and 6 and involved with ACONPAL/South Pacific. Including Bowen, the named others were of his generation including President Alan Robinson Wilkie (1918 – death date unknown but post-1988), Secretary Richard (Ritchie) Charles Bennett (1918–1981), Alister McAlister (1915–2011) and the slightly younger Robin Gardini (1925–1995). Others are considered possible members. Similar in age to Gardini, Marcus Try (1926 whose death date not known but post-1983) could be expected to be a member due to his close working relationship with Wilkie; Try had represented the Victorian branch of ACONPAL at the 1973 Ward Inquiry.[15] The Webb

Inquiry Report described the VSSO established in 1975 and member formerly of ACONPAL. The report represented the specialist issues to be distinguishing themselves as not selling remedies which seems to be a detraction of the key issue around 'specialist' identity, 'these osteopaths who offer osteopathic treatment only are the nucleus of this Society. This Society has remained affiliated with the South Pacific Council for Natural Therapies'.[16]

The Webb report suggested the VSSO enjoyed ongoing affiliation with the renamed South Pacific Council for Natural Therapies (SPCNT), yet that is not the impression given by VSSO president Wilkie in his letter to Houghton, Victorian Minister for Health on April 5, 1978. The timing is after the Webb Inquiry and during the drafting of the Victorian bill to register chiropractors and osteopaths. Wilkie, identifying as an osteopath, wrote from Phillip Island and said to the minister that he was 'authorised to offer the congratulations of the of VSSO on the proposed Bill to register osteopaths and chiropractors'. This suggests positive support for registration and formal representative process of some sort based on the mandate of the members. His letter is stamped 'Registered Member'. Wilkie wrote advising that VSSO members had fully assisted with the Ward and Webb Inquiries and further professional support was offered through a representative for the pending Registration Board and to meet with the Minister at any time to provide more information about the VSSO and its members. Wilkie advised that the VSSO was independent of any other group or association and said its members 'are chosen by invitation only, due regard being given to professional qualifications and standards in practice'.[17]

Unfortunately, there is no record at the Public Records Office of Victoria (PROV) of a response by the Minister.[18] A highlighted feature by Mackenzie in parliament was the decades of experience of the individual practitioners; 175 years' experience between them, reinforcing Wilkie's advice that seasoned and talented practitioners formed the group.[19] Between eleven members, 175 years' averages to nearly 16 years of practice each. The VSSO men all shared one thing in common – they held out for a 'straight' osteopathic identity and refused to gain registration by joining those who were comfortable being registered under a chiropractic banner with the UCAA. Through evidence in Hansard and drawing on relevant sources, the following personalities were confirmed as involved or very likely candidates to be members of the VSSO (see Table 7.2).[20] Those in bold are confirmed from Mackenzie's statement in Hansard and Wilkie's letter, the others are among the few osteopaths practising at the time with a longstanding professional presence either never registered or eventually registered under Section s8(4) with non-prescribed qualifications. The records at PROV have not retained minutes of the Registration Board and how applicants were assessed. Excepting Gardini, the osteopaths assigned a double asterisk in Table 7.2 are those trained at the Southern School of Natural Therapies (SSNT) (not prescribed qualifications) and were registered under the relevant part of Section 8 (4).

Table 7.2 Known and Potential Members of the VSSO

Name	*Profile*
Alan Wilkie	Noted in Hansard, President, involved in Government Enquiries. Roberts BAIN trained 1954. Never Registered
Alister McAlister	Hansard, involved in Ward Inquiry, 'Leading osteopath', ANTA nominee. Strathmore, Robert's BAIN trained 1958. Registered 5.7.83
Robin Gardini**	Noted in Hansard, Ward Inquiry – 'Leading osteopath', letters to Government, most popular ANTA nominee, Leader Freedom of Practices organisation. Believed trained in manipulative therapies at Northern Institute of Massage (UK). Never registered.
Thomas Bowen	Noted in Hansard, involved in Ward Inquiry, 'Leading osteopath', representations to Mackenzie MP. Never registered
Richard Bennett	Secretary of VSSO, involved in Inquiries with Wilkie. Never registered in Victoria.
Graham Rhodes**	Close associate of McAlister, Ascot Vale, Melbourne Registered 2.8.83 SSNT
Andrew Fraser**	Close associate of McAlister, Geelong, Registered 3.8.82 Blackmores then SSNT
CJ McKenzie	ANTA nominee for Board Never Registered in Victoria.
Bill Wilson	Age and high reputation with McAlister and Bowen within ANTA. Shepparton, Never Registered in Victoria.
DE Wright	Ward Inquiry – 'leading osteopath', Boronia, Melbourne, Never Registered in Victoria
Neville Brittain	Respondent to Ward Inquiry, ACONPAL director. Never registered in Victoria.
Marcus Try – possible	Represented ACONPAL at Ward Inquiry, took action against the Victorian Registration Board in the Supreme Court and won. Trained as a naturopath and chiropractor with SSNT and the only person registered both DO and DC in Victoria.

Backgrounds of Select VSSO Practitioners

What is known about the VSSO men? The following information is gleaned primarily from their transcripts and other sources about Wilkie, Bennett, McAlister and Gardini who were named VSSO members. Of the possible VSSO identities, backgrounds on Andrew Fraser DO and Marcus Try DO/DC are also provided. Details follow on their treatment by the Registration Board after the introduction of a grandfather clause in May 1981 intended to register experienced longstanding practitioners and applicable to the VSSO men most of who were not credentialled.[21] Common themes are their similar ages, born between 1915 and 1926, their attention to the whole body and not just the spine, their reliance on tactile ability, feeling with their hands and forgoing x-rays, the use of language such as 'releasing nerve pressure' (except Try who naturopathically talks of 'vital force'), pursuing a limited number of treatments, aspiring to greater finesse and more precise positioning in manipulation of the neck vertebrae, lack of force and bone cracking, gentler more nuanced approaches than chiropractic, critical of teaching at the FG Roberts school which had swung to chiropractic, self-study, auto-didactic, intuitive style, tactile acuity and considered painful areas as sites of compensation and not the source of the problem.

Alan Wilkie

VSSO President Alan Wilkie was born in 1915 in Pascoe Vale, Melbourne. He had an engineering background and there is evidence of his role as a clergyman for a period.[22] His eldest son suffered brain damage thanks to an accident. Recommendations to see an unnamed osteopath in Shepparton were not taken up at the time but inspired Wilkie's own future career in osteopathy.[23] Wilkie indicated to the Ward Inquiry he graduated from Roberts' college in 1954 as an osteopath; his study had taken place over a four-and-a-half-year period that included 4,400 hours and clinical work and a two-year part-time component of three nights a week and Saturday mornings amounting to sixteen hours per week.[24] Other employment is mentioned and it was not until 1972 that Wilkie first appeared in the electoral rolls carrying the designation of osteopath. Throughout the 1970s, Wilkie was living at Pall Mall, Ventnor, on Phillip Island and working as an osteopath. On the island, his client base comprised the permanent locals and tourists. Wilkie was a former President of the 'Blackmores Group' (NANOC).[25] He considered this a 'nice group for a while, enough said' and was critical of the Blackmores' training which was limited to an eight-week chiropractic training course.[26] At the time of the Ward Inquiry, Wilkie was honorary secretary of ACONPAL.[27] Soon after, Wilkie appeared in correspondence as president of the VSSO.[28] Wilkie was critical of correspondence training in the USA especially since he doubted the credentials of American-trained chiropractors and wished them to be checked to see that they had actually passed examinations.[29]

As a VSSO member, Wilkie belonged to a minority of osteopaths who worked by tactile feel alone and avoided use of x-rays.[30] Wilkie defined osteopathy as involving the whole body, every joint and that it was not massage.[31] Wilkie said, 'The spine serves the whole body and poor supply leads to malfunctioning of joints or muscles creating nerve pressure which upsets the system'.[32] He considered osteopathy to be 'applied neurology'.[33] Barry Jones of the Victorian Ward Inquiry sought to imply to Wilkie as secretary of ACONPAL that in comparison to orthodox medicine, chiropractic and osteopathy had not developed since the time of their founders.[34] Wilkie proceeded to give some interesting insights into how osteopathy had been changing which would have been topical in the VSSO and ACONPAL group. In particular, Wilkie distinguished osteopathy over chiropractic on the basis of involving very precise positioning – such as the neck – which could involve twenty-nine points for adjusting. Osteopathy was more nuanced with multiple positions and involved 'safety stops' 'so one cannot go too far'.[35] He criticised chiropractic treatments as being based on a short number of moves and forceful.[36] He said chiropractic relied on force.[37] An osteopath could have twenty nine ways to influence the neck for example, whereas chiropractors concerned themselves with just nerve impingement in the spine and relied on force and adjusted in one swoop.[38] In Wilkie's view, the greater care and detail in osteopathic positioning was more demanding and a factor in the popularity of chiropractic which was less involved. Wilkie outlined that considerable research and change was going on with leveraging movements and positioning and the association was conducting its own research on posture and lumbar five and its facets on the sacrum. He said, 'We are finding many things now that we did not know even two or three years ago'.[39] Bowen was known to be an experimenter and in the lead-up to his death and observed by Ryan to develop a double-handed way of addressing an anterior (forward positioned) fifth lumbar which is a difficult joint to put back in place.[40] While credit for any successful implementation of innovations is entirely owed to Bowen, it must be born in mind that his Victorian ACONPAL/VSSO peers since 1971 had been specifically researching positioning in this area to specifically alleviate chronic posture problems. Resonating with Bowen's language on nerve pressure, Wilkie distinguished osteopathy from chiropractic on the grounds that osteopaths worked on releasing nerve pressure from joints or muscles and used quite technical positioning with leverage and safety stops.

Wilkie was critical of chiropractic and considered it was dangerous if the practitioner was not adequately trained and stated 'Chiropractic will take the head and by the time it is finished, you may be looking back the other way'.[41] Wilkie was also opposed to the chiropractic approach of each patient getting the same treatment and the multiple treatment approach 'a patient should be well in weeks', not in 'years' with chiropractic.[42] Wilkie said, 'in my temerity', he questioned this with Roberts as student and recalled, 'I was told to mind my own business'.[43] McAlister apparently was likewise questioning at training wanting to know more than what was accessible in books but was likewise resisted.[44] Wilkie was critical of osteopathic teaching at the Roberts school, he considered himself an auto-didact pursuing his own research 'to bring myself up to world standard'.[45] This self-perception of autodidact shows up in Bowen's transcript too, yet it is clear in Wilkie's case, he was a product of formal learning. Though Wilkie was more articulate and elaborative in his transcript than Bowen, both men shared use of similar terminology of 'nerve pressure, a concept applied in osteopathy that was discussed in Chapter 3. Wilkie's description 'the release of nerve pressure would then stimulate or free the nerve flow to the particular organ' is entirely consistent with the discussion on this topic.[46] Wilkie distinguished Palmer chiropractors as focusing solely on the neck and adjusting the vagus nerve on the basis of its systemic influence and Canadian College chiropractors who adjusted each bone in the spine.[47]

Richard Bennett

Contact was made with John Stewart, a relative of VSSO secretary Richard (Ritchie) Bennett. Stewart remembered when the VSSO numbered eight and they were connected by having had the same kind of training and shared similar ideas.[48] Secretary Richard (Ritchie) Charles Bennett (1918–1981) was born in Kew, Melbourne, and held a managerial role until 1980 as a printer's representative.[49] According to Stewart, Bennett had trained with a small group of osteopaths which involved more hands-on practical training with study compared to those with American qualifications. Bennett's orientation was osteopathy because it addressed more of the body than chiropractic which focused only on the spine.[50] Bennett also spoke of removing [nerve] pressure too.[51] Apparently, Bennett also started to take a great interest in iridology and 'although he did not claim to be expertly proficient in this, would sometimes do some iris analysis as part of his consultation'. Fraser, a close colleague of McAlister also studied iridology but later in 1972 at the SSNT.[52] Stewart considered that Bennett's 'practical intuitive style gave him a good feel for osteopathy' and he had an 'excellent feel for problems people brought to him'.[53] Bennett was not aggressive in his work and did not do bony adjustments, his style involved doing deep tissue massaging and stretching. Some cracking might occur at the end of a session to 'relieve pressure' with a particularly stubborn problem, but any click was elicited by 'a gradual and prolonged stretch then a slight tweak at the end', rather than sudden actions almost straight off [like chiropractic]. Like Bowen, Bennett did not keep people coming back for treatments. A stubborn problem might involve two or three visits but that was all.[54] Unlike Bowen, Bennett did use liniment and later on a powered massager for deeper work that may have utilised ultrasound. Bennett rejected the chiropractic notion that all problems came from the spine and considered that many could be muscular in origin. Painful areas were thought of as sites of compensation. From the description given, Bennett's work was not minimalist as massage was a substantial part of the treatment and remembered as relatively continuous contact.[55] Stewart remembered his relative talking about the period around the introduction of the regulation period and time, 'The feeling was very much of him and those few colleagues being squeezed out'. Wilkie lived and worked on Phillip Island and Bennett holidayed there too so it is very possible the men were friends as well as colleagues.

Alister (Lal) McAlister

Alister Lal McAlister's community profile was a highly respected, well-known osteopath who was generous with his time and in encouraging others.[56] In addition to fragmentary information in the Ward Inquiry, what has survived in oral history about McAlister's style of working? These range from Professor Murtagh's memories of the 1960s when Murtagh was a teenager to the 2000s by clinic associates working with him before his death in 2011.

Murtagh reflecting later in 2015 considered McAlister more a manipulator of joints than muscles.[57] According to Murtagh, McAlister worked with liniment and massage before doing adjustments.[58] McAlister had suggested work to Murtagh's back was in order and Murtagh recalled McAlister did a thoracic adjustment that was a firm manipulation which relieved back pain from kyphotic scoliosis believed due to childhood poliomyelitis.[59] Murtagh mentioned McAlister's expertise in a paper where he took a retrospective view of the development of musculoskeletal medicine in Australia.[60] Murtagh had attended McAlister for a badly sprained ankle and associated sciatica, sent to him by his football club at Coleraine.[61] McAlister had a strong reputation and football clubs sent players to him for their musculoskeletal injuries.[62] Murtagh considered that McAlister was 'very thorough and good at his work'.[63] It was recalled McAlister was operating out of private rooms and was not carrying titles such as osteopath.[64] Murtagh was inspired to pursue a specialist career in musculoskeletal medicine and commented on his experiences from the 1960s. He reported the dramatic benefit his relative and sporting associates would gain from treatments by Mitchell, Saunders and McAlister who were household names. As a GP registrar, he was acutely aware of the need for spinal therapy services and said, he 'felt frustrated by my inability to deliver relief to the extent achieved by some chiropractors and self-taught therapists'.[65]

McAlister worked only with his hands and did not use x-rays.[66] Later clinic associate Heather Hay who worked at his clinic before his death in the 2000s described his work as gentle with treatments lasting about thirty minutes. He utilised massage not limited to cross-fibre techniques working only with fingers and thumbs.[67] Hay said McAlister did not like skin polished (oiled) which suggests a preference for tactile awareness than the glide provided by lubrication.[68] Heat in tissues was a potential red flag for cancer and in the bone a breakage. According to Hay, McAlister spoke to patients in terms of tissues being tense or tight.[69] Hay recalled McAlister would have a chart of the spine that he would print off for patients.[70] He was old-fashioned in his style and emphasised 'seeing and feeling' issues in clients and was fascinated by how the body moved.[71] Younger osteopaths considered McAlister to be 'old school'.[72] Otherwise, McAlister's work style was considered gentle and he paid attention to details, it was important to be thorough and 'observe the body', McAlister had a dictum of 'don't miss anything'. Tactile feedback was important and he considered that many practitioners had 'their eyes open but their pupils shut'.[73] Along with palpatory sensitivity and detailed observation of the patient, from McAlister's own testimony to the Ward Inquiry, he shared approaches adopted by Bowen. He espoused the osteopathic dictum of the pelvic base being the foundation of the body and it must be levelled first.[74] He too used pressure approaches and discussed putting pressure on the fifth and sixth cervicals to alleviate migraine.[75] Chapter 5 highlighted that in other parts of his testimony to the Ward Inquiry, he discusses reflex points on the feet suggesting he was versed in the pressure techniques of reflexology.[76] The Inquiry report did not understand what he was saying as he was described as believing all diseases originate in the feet which is a misunderstanding of the theory of zone therapy.

The presence of McAlister among the VSSO men is interesting as he is the only one with any track record in mentoring others and providing clinic placements and can be expected to have been a central figure among the aspiring osteopaths when training. Protégés and close associates of McAlister who fit the profile to have joined the VSSO are Andrew Fraser and Graham Rhodes. McAlister also offered placements to Roberts College students after he qualified there in 1959.[77] According to Jacka, diplomas were only awarded after time spent at endorsed clinics.[78] No records of other practitioners among the individuals researched so far have been found performing this clinic placement role. McAlister promoted a strong political position at his clinic; around 1972, he is recalled having a logo on his wall recalled as an umbrella with COCA underneath. This is throwback to an earlier iteration of the Roberts College when it left behind its earlier identity as the British and Australian Institute of Naturopathy (BAIN) in 1959 and became the College of Osteopathy and Chiropractic Australia (COCA).[79] By the later 1970s, it was the Chiropractic College of Australia (CCA) and then by 1979 became the Preston Institute of Technology, simultaneously the International College of Chiropractic (the forerunner of the Royal Melbourne Institute of Technology (now RMIT)).[80]

Robin Gardini

Robin Gardini (1925–1995) was born in Penrith NSW.[81] In the electoral rolls, he was living in Queensland in the 1960s. There is quite a gap in census records until 1963 when he appeared as a manager of a health centre in Bundaberg with his wife Louise as receptionist.[82] By 1968, Gardini was living in Nambour and entered as an osteopath and this continued when he moved to Ringwood in Melbourne by 1977 and was maintained throughout to 1980 which is the last available digitised record.[83] Some indications of Gardini's background and educational background in manual therapies are indicated by the initials LCSP FBRA (London) next to his name as a certified 'osteopath and manipulative therapist' in a letter to Rossiter, minister for health on June 22, 1971.[84] LCSP represents the London and Counties Society of Physiologists, an organisation established in 1919 in the UK on massage and chiropody and has a branch in Canada.[85] According to the current registrar at the LCSP, it was not a training body and primarily provides insurance services for those qualified in the professions within its remit, such as osteopath and usually the relevant initials appear next to the organisation.[86] The British organisation since 2002 is now retitled the LCSP Register of Remedial Masseurs and Manipulative Therapists.[87] Though the LCSP registrar was not familiar with the initials FBRA, it has been established that Gardini was also qualified in reflexology as the FBRA represents 'Fellow of the British Reflexology Association'.[88] To be a member of the LCSP, Gardini would have required formal qualifications, and the registrar followed up with further information that Gardini had been a member since 1965.[89]

The formally recognised college of the LCSP was the Northern Institute of Massage (founded in 1924) which among other things offered diplomas in Swedish Massage and Manipulative Therapies. Training was available full-time, part-time or by correspondence with the latter accredited by the Council for Accreditation of Correspondences Courses.[90] Given the gap in Gardini's presence in the current digitised Australian electoral rolls between his birth year of 1925 in NSW and appearing next in 1960 in Queensland, it seems most likely that Gardini may have lived and/or studied in the UK before then.

The purpose of Gardini's letter to Rossiter was in response to lobbying for registration in the lead-up to the Ward Inquiry and to support the public need for protection against unscrupulous individuals holding out to be practitioners of chiropractic and osteopathy. Gardini was also advocating for registration to support ethical and reputed practitioners and the establishment of the registration board similar to what had been achieved in Western Australia. Gardini forwarded a copy of the West Australian *Chiropractors Act 1964* with his letter.[91] He was Chairman of the Council for Freedom of Practitioners, a body concerned about militarism and advocating for the less vocal practitioners.[92] As shown in Table 7.1, Gardini is included with Bowen as one of the seven 'leading osteopaths' in the Ward Inquiry Report.[93]

Gardini also became a member of the VSSO along with leading practitioners such as Bowen, McAlister, Wilkie and Bennett. Later on, Gardini also became a member of ANTA, suggesting a prior membership of ACONPAL or NANOC and was the clear favourite nominee of ANTA's then ninety-five members to represent the organisation on the proposed Registration Board under the new Act.[94] In 1976, Jeanette Patrick MP also supported Gardini's nomination to represent ANTA on the new registration board in the lead-up to the proclamation of the act.[95] Other nominations had included McAlister and CJ Mckenzie.

Information about Gardini is focused on his political leadership, no specific descriptive information exists about Gardini's style but like Bowen, Gardini's practice flourished despite his lack of registration.[96] Gardini was evidently highly regarded among practitioners of his time and invited to demonstrate techniques at the Preston Institute and mentioned in Parliament by Mackenzie to that effect in 1992.[97] It is not clear whether Gardini did not seek to become registered or was failed by the Board even though he would have held non-prescribed qualifications to attract LCSP insurance since 1965.

In the late 1970s, Gardini was a board member of the Footman Foundation Association and is recognised in memoriam as a founding Life Member of the Association, a charitable trust set up involving businesses supporting those in need. In the late 1970s and the 1980s, Gardini was serving in local government roles and in 1982 stood as an unsuccessful independent for Ringwood in the Victorian Government State Election.[98] Several photographs are online of Gardini in his councillor role and media coverage of his retirement.[99] In 1991, Gardini was awarded a Medal of Order in the General Division (OAM) for services to the community and to local government.[100]

Potential Members Andrew Fraser and Marcus Try

Table 7.2 gives a brief overview of other potential members. The following are summaries of two individuals – Andrew Fraser and Marcus Try. Fraser was a close associate of McAlister. Fraser's style of work also involved 'lifting pressure off nerves' suggesting his exposure to neuropathy through Blackmore under his chiropractic focus. Fraser gave a specific example in his book of nerves to kidneys being pinched at the level of the tenth dorsal vertebra. Fraser had an engineering approach to the body and structural alignment all important and diseases due to imbalances in the musculoskeletal framework.[101] Inflammation caused by misalignments caused tissues to dry up and tendons to shrink so it was necessary they be restored back to their correct position.[102] A sacroiliac joint that was misaligned in the pelvis caused lower back muscles to harden, and realigning the joint softened the muscles but if inflammation had set in, massage was necessary to restore blood flow to the area.[103] Schmidt said Fraser had three rules: always check, reset and check torsion, stand up and check movement.[104] These are echoed in Bowen's approach too. Fraser practised iridology and Blackmores remedy prescribing which illustrates his traditional naturopathic education under Blackmore and with Jacka, a Blackmores shareholder. According to Schmidt who helped Fraser publish his book, Fraser also practised craniosacral therapy and fascial techniques.[105] Fraser and Bowen were acquainted and Bowen apparently treated Fraser.[106] Fraser's training with McAlister was evidently derived from Blackmores NANOC and this explains why he advocated for NANOC and its members in a protest letter to the minister for health when the minister indicated on a Four Corner's program only American-trained chiropractors would be registered.[107] Oddly, given his political participation in the lead-up, Fraser was not a respondent to the Ward Inquiry.

Try was trained as a naturopath and chiropractor but with a non-prescribed school – namely Alf Jacka's SSNT. The Ward Inquiry recognised the overlaps between chiropractic and osteopathy at this time and it's very possible that due to his close working relationship with Wilkie and Bennett that Try would have joined the VSSO in protest against the only mechanism for registration being via membership of the UCAA and having credentials from a prescribed UCAA-endorsed school. Marcus Ian Try (1926–death date not established but post-1983) was introduced to natural therapies and around 1958/1959 as a consequence of finding relief for his wife's health.[108] Try trained with Alf Jacka for four years emerging with a naturopathic qualification.[109] Try was a Seventh-Day Adventist.[110] Judy Jacka mentioned in her book that most naturopaths-in-training at the same time as her in 1969 at the SSNT were Adventists and the Warburton Sanatorium illustrated the strong role that the Adventists played in promoting nature cure at this time.[111] Try first appeared on electoral rolls as a naturopath in 1968 and continued in this profession until 1977 when chiropractor appears in the rolls until at least until 1980.[112] Evidently, he undertook further training through the SSNT to train in chiropractic. As a natural therapist of the period, Try's treatment style encompassed chiropractic, manipulative therapies and vitamins, herb and minerals. He also used iridology or iris diagnosis in conjunction with other assessments to decide a treatment strategy that could involve chiropractic adjusting.[113] Unlike the osteopaths trained through the FG Roberts School, Try did not talk of 'nerve pressure' but rather more naturopathically of 'vital force' and typical for chiropractic work was largely focused on the spine which he assessed through palpation.[114] Try was also opposed to x-rays, more on account of health risks and in his opinion overuse then by chiropractors generally.[115] Try did not treat other areas of the body such as tennis elbow.[116] Try distinguished his work from massage on the basis that 'a masseur only releases muscle tension or loosens soft tissue. A manipulator does more than that, he moves specific areas'.[117] Like Wilkie, Try had formerly been involved with NANOC and brought into the Blackmores system of prescribing as Jacka was a shareholder and representative of Blackmores products.[118] Try was one of the first to object to the system of utilising 80 per cent of Blackmores remedies and made himself unpopular before he left.[119] Try became president of the new Victorian branch of ACONPAL formed in 1971 and mentioned that 50 per cent of its members were former NANOC members.[120] As ACONPAL president he expressed his view on the thirty-day timeline set by the Ward Inquiry to produce scientific evidence, 'I feel this is pretty irregular'.[121] Within ACONPAL, Try was supported by Alan Wilkie as secretary and Mr Bennett as treasurer.[122] By 1976, Try was assisting Alf Jacka as Federal Deputy Chairman of the SPCNT as Victorian state chairman.[123] By 1976, the SFPNT had transitioned to a Council and Try's role was a progression of his earlier representation of ACONPAL, a SPFNT subsidiary. Try's successful action against the Victorian Registration Board in the Supreme Court is described later.

Legislation Proclaimed

Legislation was finally rolled out in New South Wales and Victoria in 1978 followed by Queensland in 1979. This saw the eclipse and ultimate dissolution of the umbrella South Pacific organisation that accommodated the plethora of subsidiary organisations that existed beforehand, including those Bowen was involved with prior to regulation. ANTA led by Alfred (Alf) Jacka as president was formed and accommodated the former members of NANOC, ACONPAL and the VSSO. In the lead-up to the proclamation of the *Chiropractors and Osteopaths Act 1978* (Vic), Gardini had lobbied the government about a grandfather clause but the legislation overlooked a provision in Victoria. The NSW Act allowed registration solely as a chiropractor or osteopath or a dual registration with both. The act did not define chiropractic nor osteopathy and this was a recommendation of the Webb Inquiry Report, but it is clear chiropractic subsumed osteopathy in the Act. The original Section 8 subsection (4) subparagraphs (i)–(iii) of the act in 1978 only provided for registration if:

(i) the practitioner had obtained a suitable degree, diplomat or other qualification in chiropractic or osteopathy or undergone suitable training in chiropractic or osteopathy, whether in Victoria or in a place outside Victoria,

(ii) obtained any other degree, diploma or other qualification or undergone any training in chiropractic or osteopathy whether in Victoria or a place outside Victoria and obtained any further degree, diploma or other qualification or undergone any further training required by the Board in the particular case or

(iii) carried on the practice of chiropractic and osteopathy under circumstances and for a period approved by the Board.[124]

The subparagraph (iii) did not go far enough to be useful as a grandfather clause for uncredentialled practitioners with strong reputations. Victorian legislators were guilty of an oversight in drafting the *Chiropractor and Osteopaths Act 1978 (Vic)* and omitted a legacy provision in the form of a grandfather clause. Then opposition Labor ministers Tom Roper and Rod Mackenzie OAM ensured a similar provision was introduced in May 1981 under s8(4) iii. It differed from NSW only to the extent that five years were specified instead of four. The *Chiropractors and Osteopaths Amendment Bill* substituted paragraph (iii) below for Section 8 (4) (a) which became law on May 5, 1981.[125] It was constructed to provide clear timeframes of practice as the criteria for registration for those with long experience but no formal credentials:

> (iii) carried on the practice of chiropractic and osteopathy *at any time during the period of ten years before the commencement of this Act, either for a continuous period of five years or for any periods the aggregate of which is five years.* [emphasis added]

Bowen and the VSSO practitioners that had no formal qualifications were clearly eligible under this change and Bowen's years in practice amounted to nineteen years in formal business. According to Mackenzie Bowen was 'pretty excited' about the introduction of the grandfather clause.[126] Bowen applied in 1981 to be registered but unfortunately, the Board had other ideas and instituted an examination process that was not designed to accommodate those elder practitioners whose diagnosis relied entirely upon palpation and without x-rays. Ultimately, Bowen's fate seems to have been set by the peculiar differences in the composition of the Victorian Registration Board compared to the New South Wales Board and its weighting towards biomedical expertise. The NSW registration board comprised a representative from the Health Commission, one from chiropractic education, one a ministerial nomination, one a medical practitioner and one a barrister. In contrast, the Victorian board was statutorily set up under Section 8 (2) (a)–(d) to comprise seven – three who were registered chiropractors and osteopaths, a specialist medical practitioner in orthopaedics, a medical practitioner teaching medicine (neither a chiropractor nor osteopath), one teaching medicine and one a member of the Royal Australian College of Physicians. The Victorian legislation was silent on specifying institutions to be represented on its Board, but it is clear that there was no intention of allowing access to Board membership to those who would represent the relevant constituencies of the Australian Natural Therapists Association (ANTA) and whose education was at the SSNT or equivalent lifelong experience and self-study. Contrary to the recommendations of the Webb Inquiry Report, the Victorian Act did include a definition of chiropractic.

Bowen Fails Clinical Competency Test

The Victorian Registration Board flexed its biomedical muscle alongside representatives of the newly legitimated professions and demonstrated an excessive show of power and biomedical dominance in its implementation of the grandfather clause. The Board would have been well appraised of the fact that those eligible under s8(4) iii had been discussed at government inquiries (some like Bowen personally by name) and could show long years of strong and successful clinical practice but lacked formal credentials in the biomedical sciences and medical diagnosis. Despite this, the Board gave applicants like Bowen, a list of some thirty-two medical books to acquire and answer questions on a range of topics such as anatomy and physiology, pathology, diagnosis and principles and practice of osteopathy and chiropractic. Radiography was included.[127] Purchase and sourcing the readings were onerous and the parliamentarian Mackenzie noted many of the books were hard to source and out of print.[128] Smeeton DC had a patient who remembered assisting Bowen with medical questions and they would go for a drive while she tested him.[129]

These readings were required in preparation for an examination on clinical competency, yet as the section on Marcus Try confirms, the Board did not have the power to summon practitioners to present for examination. In a draconian move biased to biomedical standards rather than Bowen's evident skills in demand by many thousands in the community and championed by parliamentarian Rod Mackenzie, Bowen not only failed outright but also was denied any opportunity to retry after further training. Bowen died within seven months of the publicity. The Webb Inquiry Report had recommended the provision of a grandfather clause but subject to a test of competency prescribed by the Registration Board.[130] This recommendation was not enacted in NSW and the spirit of the Victorian amendment was not followed resulting in Bowen and several of his peers suffering the humiliation of being stripped of their long-standing professional identities as osteopaths.

The records at the Public Record Office have not retained any minutes of the Victorian Boards' deliberations, nor their record of examinations of individuals forced to present. The file is reduced to some annual reports to parliament and some briefings to the minister for health. Showing preservation of biomedical power, allied with the newly legitimated professions, no evidence exists of uncredentialed talented candidates being grandfathered by the Victorian Board. On the first gazetted register of chiropractors and osteopaths in 1980, there was a code that revealed whether registration was based on qualifications from the elite overseas schools or the UCAA-endorsed schools or given double asterisks to show status otherwise. Instead, the Board shifted to admitting to registration with a double asterisk (but no code) for those holding diplomas from naturopathic colleges such as the SSNT whose dean was also president of ANTA. Also registered were the VSSO such as McAlister who had refused to join the UCAA and be registered under the chiropractic umbrella but had prescribed credentials from a UCCA-endorsed institution. In the medical landscape, they represent the fledgling push for demarcation and unique identity in a chiropractic-dominated profession. By 1992, the grandfather clause was removed in favour of setting up a provisional practising status. The world had moved on to accommodate arrangements for overseas graduates to work twelve months with an Australian practitioner, yet parliamentarians including Mackenzie remained concerned that some twenty or so practitioners who had been in practice before the Victorian Act were still in abeyance regarding their professional status. Retrospectively, Victorian practitioners were treated in a discriminatory fashion compared to their NSW counterparts. In 1992, the membership of the board was amended to nine reducing the biomedicine weighting and specifically providing for osteopathic representation.[131] It allowed for three chiropractors and one osteopath (voted in from among the profession), one teaching osteopathy or chiropractic, one a member of the Royal Academy of Practising Surgeons and engaged in orthopaedic surgery, one a barrister and one a chiropractor, osteopath or medical practitioner with knowledge in the general public interest. Demarcation was finally achieved in 1996 with the proclamation of the *Osteopaths Registration Act 1996* Act No. 75/1996.[132] It provided for a board of seven, four being osteopaths, one a lawyer and two not osteopaths.

The tragedy for Bowen who relied so much on his tactile sensitivity and high sensitivity overall to achieve the results he did was that the examination process for clinical competency was conducted over several hours. In Bowen's case, he was presented with an empty chair as his client. Others were given patients as subjects who did not have any clinical issues and ANTA protested about this to the government.[133] Bowen's discontent at the session was reportedly expressed by addressing each member of the Board regarding what was wrong with them before walking out the door.[134]

Bowen failed the examination and a spokesperson for the Board said Bowen failed on the professional clinical competency.[135] This was a power the board had under Section 8 (3) 'The Board may refuse to register an applicant who is otherwise qualified to be registered under this section . . . if the Board is not satisfied that the applicant is professionally competent to practise as a chiropractor and osteopath in Victoria'. Bowen was failed outright and denied the opportunity to seek training or mentorship and re-test.[136] Otherwise, the original Act provided for retraining under Section 8 (4) (ii).[137] As friend and patient Barry Tattersall said, 'If he had a body to put hands on at those examinations, he would have left everybody else in the dust of his feet'.[138] As Davis DC said too, 'He could have had more talent in the tip of his little pinkie than the whole lot put together but it wouldn't have made any difference to being registered'.[139] It was no compensation to Bowen that he enjoyed an immensely successful track record and successes and this was covered in the press. The thing that affected him most was that his rejection meant his patients could not claim Medicare rebates and this was the most significant blow for him.[140]

Though Bowen had dutifully presented for examination, many of his ANTA colleagues had not. In the Legislative Council, Mackenzie referred to a letter from ANTA dated November 16, 1981, that outlined why its members were unable to comply with the procedures of the Registration Board (some then were refusing to attend for examination). Mackenzie highlighted ANTA's concerns that many of the practitioners can only 'make a diagnosis by feel and touch' by considering temperature and aberrations in tissues, and that they need a sick person to diagnose not someone with no issues as proposed by the Board.[141]

The VSSO's interest in representation on the Registration Board to be established under the act was ignored, and post-implementation in a repeat of the disregard for the marginalised, ANTA was also denied representation and this was an issue that was taken up by Mackenzie in parliament.[142] In retrospect, the stark contrast between pre-act expectations and positive support of regulation and what transpired must have come as a shock to the stakeholders negatively impacted. This sort of undemocratic behaviour on the part of the government would have received scathing criticism today when the size and reach of this constituency nationally is considered.

Outcome

The issue for the VSSO men, especially those with formal qualifications from earlier iterations of Roberts' college, was that they had refused to join the UCAA and therefore could not be automatically registered and so had to apply within three years under s8 (4) of the Act. Many of the older uncredentialled VSSO members named by Mackenzie, like Bowen, failed to be registered: Bennett died in 1981, Wilkie and Gardini were never registered. Unfortunately, the names of applicants for registration are not on the government files inspected, nor minutes of the Registration Board's deliberations. The only records are their reports for parliament and some formal correspondence between the secretary and the minister for health. The Chiropractors and Osteopaths Registration Board indicated in their third Annual Report for the year 1981 that nine individuals had presented for clinical competency examination on December 9, but no other details given.[143] Bowen is deduced to be one of these and his failed examination was reported soon after in the *Geelong Advertiser* on March 31, 1982.[144] The article mentioned another man failed outright. This could be a reference to Marcus Try who exercised his rights under Section 15 of the Act and on March 17, 1982, lodged his appeal against the Board's decision which was within the three months prescribed under the act.[145] Try had presented for interview but refused to present for examination and instead, invited the Board to observe him at work in his clinic but this was declined by the Board. Bowen publicly echoed Try's key grievance that the Board did not assess him in-clinic.[146] He highlights the unfairness in having no physical contact with a patient for his assessment and said, 'I only use my ten fingers in my work'.[147] In the article, Bowen said, 'Osteopathic, [*sic*] in contrast to chiropractic which involves manipulation of the spinal column, is a system of diagnosis and treatment of disorders by manipulation of muscle and nerve tissue'.[148]

Marcus Try's Successful Action Against the Registration Board in the Supreme Court

Try filed his successful action against the Board in the Supreme Court on March 17, 1982.[149] Neither Bennett nor Bowen lived to see Try's victory on November 18, 1983.[150] Bennett had died in 1981 and Bowen died on October 27, 1982. The judgement included that the Board did not have the power to compel practitioners to present for examination and using the definition of chiropractic in the Act, paved the way for the plaintiff Marcus Try to be registered in Victoria as DC/DO.[151] Try became the only practitioner to carry a dual registration of osteopath and chiropractor though the NSW Act had express provision for dual titles.[152] The Board mentioned three appeals in its 1983 report and, without naming Try, stated that only one was successful. However, Try was not the only person to have made a successful appeal in the Supreme Court. Kenneth Lloyd had been successful in 1980 on the basis of his physiotherapy training which involved manipulation complying with the definition of chiropractic and osteopathy under the Act.[153] Lloyd was registered as a chiropractor on September 9, 1980.[154] McAlister was also known to have resisted presenting for an examination.[155] In the lead-up to the Supreme Court finding on November 18, and the registration of Try on November 29, 1983, the Board evidently registered McAlister and Fraser without examinations.[156] This would have been due to their possessing non-prescribed qualifications but eligible to apply under the s8 provisions.

The Board justified its handling of the examinations of those without prescribed qualifications and started inserting a section in its report to the Parliament titled 'Examinations' to explain its handling of those 'not possessing the prescribed qualifications'. It was claimed that the tests and appraisal of candidates were intended to demonstrate existing skills, pitched at practitioner rather than academic level. The Board was looking for safety and clinical proficiency and language used was aimed at lay-person language to demonstrate the techniques they would use to assess and treat common conditions seen in an osteopath/chiropractic practice.[157]

This statement was made ahead of the Supreme Court's findings of Try's action against the Board. A month after, and a week after the Court's findings, on November 25, 1982, Tom Roper, then health minister and former champion with Rod Mackenzie of the grandfather clause, was terse when he wrote to the Board finding its annual report 'deficient' and seeking further information on those nine assessed before he was willing to table their report in parliament.[158] Brian Cusack, registrar for the Board, responded on December 7, 1982, indicating that the unnamed nine were examined on December 6, 1981 (oddly, a Sunday): five had passed, two were failed but would be passed without examination on completion of further seminars and two were failed outright.[159] Since Marcus Try was failed, it should be expected he must be accounted for with Bowen as the two failed outright. Logically, only a complete rejection could have allowed an appeal under Section 15. However, according to his court papers, Try had actually refused to submit for either written examination or the clinical competency and had presented instead for interview on December 2.[160] Try had invited the Board to attend his clinic to examine him at work, an invitation that was not taken up before his rejection. Roper would have taken an interest in the process due to his earlier advocacy for the grandfather clause. The sole osteopath on the Board at the time of the clinical competency assessments of Bowen and Try was Alan Woodley a BSO graduate and on the executive of the ASO. The examinations were not designed to accommodate those elder practitioners whose diagnosis relied entirely upon palpation and without x-rays. If Bowen had lived, would he have had a case for legal action against the Board to reinstate him as an osteopath as the judgment found the Board did not have the power to enforce examinations to therefore fail Bowen and deprive him of a retest? If he had lived and chosen to challenge the Board, the legal argument would have been interesting. How, apart from the illegal examination, would the Board be able to find Bowen incompetent to practise in Victoria? The grandfather provision only substituted original Section 8 (4) (a) iii. The existing Section 8 (4) (b) allowed registration if an individual was deemed professionally competent to practise in Victoria, was of good character (c) and had paid the prescribed fee for registration (d). Under (b), it is difficult to see how the Board could decide Bowen was professionally incompetent as his track record said otherwise. In retrospect, is it unjust that this judgement is held against his name for posterity? If not registered, Section 21 of the 1978 Act made it an offence to use the title or initials designating osteopath or chiropractor.[161] Today these vocations continue as protected titles under Section 113 of the National Law.[162] Bowen obeyed the law and his earlier business card was replaced to state, 'Natural Therapist' (see Figure 7.2).[163] The New South Wales *Chiropractic Act* (1978) also included a grandfather clause, and without any powers given to the Board to examine practitioners first. They could only be denied if there was some failure of good character. During this period, Bowen reduced his business card identity to 'natural therapist' reflecting his new organisational

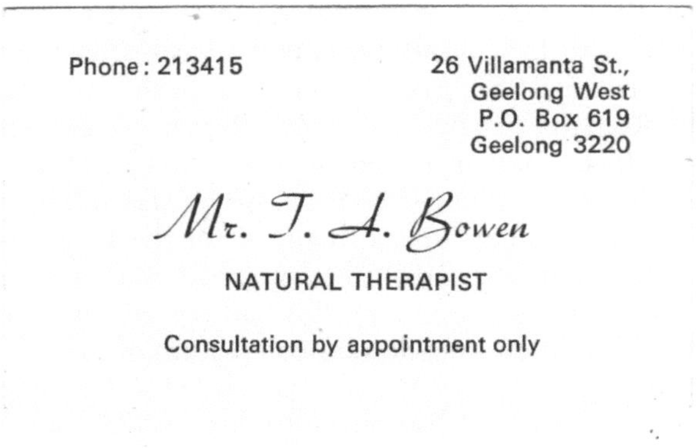
Phone: 213415

26 Villamanta St.,
Geelong West
P.O. Box 619
Geelong 3220

Mr. T. A. Bowen

NATURAL THERAPIST

Consultation by appointment only

Figure 7.2 Bowen's last business card, 26 Villamanta Street, 'Natural Therapist'.

membership and was stripped of the right to call himself an osteopath, which became a protected title under the new legislation.

There is no indication in the registrations gazetted after Try's success that any were the result of the implementation of the grandfather clause. The first June 30, 1980, gazette notice pre-grandfather clause had a legend that explained the double asterisk as 'registered pursuant to the provisions of Section 8 (4) of the Act'. This legend does not appear in subsequent gazettes, only the asterisks.

Post-regulation, the premier bodies and prescribed institutions prevailed. These were the national UCAA representing Australian practitioners with formal training (chiropractors as well osteopaths who submitted to chiropractic politics and joined), and the ACA and the AOA representing overseas-trained chiropractors and osteopaths respectively.[164] The UCAA-affiliated colleges were the SCC (founded as SCO in 1959 – becoming the Sydney College of Osteopathy and Chiropractic (SCOC) in 1964 then the Sydney College of Chiropractic (SCC) by 1973 (formalised in 1977*)* and the Roberts' CCA and the South Australian College of Chiropractic completed the three.[165] By the time of regulation, Roberts CCA was known as the Preston Institute (the forerunner of today's RMIT and formally recognised as producing graduates with the prescribed qualifications accepted by the Registration Board. Bowen's clinic associates and members of the UCAA namely Davis, Love, Neave and Smeeton were all automatically registered on January 1, 1979.[166] Kevin Ryan DO was registered before Bowen died.

In 1992, moves were successfully made to remove the grandfather clause altogether. Bowen was by then ten years deceased. Mackenzie spoke of the Board as a 'gentleman's club' that had 'gone against the spirit of the legislation'; and Mackenzie mentions Bowen again as 'the Geelong man' in parliament and, especially given the successful Try case, shows continued misgivings over the felt discriminatory behaviour of the Board that still rankled years after the introduction of the grandfather clause in 1981.[167] In 1992, a new Section 8A removed the grandfather clause from the act. Along with McKenzie, ministers such as Weideman of Frankston South remained concerned for some twenty-nine individuals remaining disenfranchised as twenty-four had been practising before the 1978 Act.[168] Mackenzie highlighted that Gardini who was never registered was in demand with the Director of the Preston Institute to observe his work.[169] With the removal of the grandfather clause, the requirement for apprenticeships was introduced including for those overseas trained, a prerequisite before they could work in Australia. The once beleaguered McAlister enjoyed a strong reputation and was in demand to provide apprenticeships and placements and did so for BSO graduates in the 1990s: BSO graduates who took up the opportunity included David Meeks now practising in Bunbury Western Australia who spent three years with McAlister from 1989.[170] Others believed to have done so include Australians Sylvia Tucker and John Baker of Albury.[171] In 2019, an article titled 'Good Osteopath in Melbourne CBD?' appeared on a bicycle network website and mentioned Bruce Duncan DO as working under McAlister in the 1990s. Duncan went on to establish North Carlton Osteopathy and acts as an osteopath to the Australian Open Tournament and Hawthorn Football Club.[172] Duncan also lectured at the RMIT.[173] According to a later clinic colleague Hay, osteopathy-trained clinic associates of McAlister included Graham Rhodes who was a respondent to the Ward Inquiry in 1973 and registered on August 2, 1983, and Glen Bales who established Moonee Valley Osteopathy in 1996.[174]

Summary

This chapter has highlighted that osteopaths formed a very small group compared to chiropractors in the 1970s. Part of this may have been due to practitioners adopting the chiropractic identity as part of the strategy of the UCAA to achieve registration in the face of strong opposition from medical and overseas trained interests. The VSSO represented the practitioners born in the early 1900s who had long successful careers as osteopaths and provided treatment services to the community without controversy. They set themselves apart from chiropractic by reliance on tactile acuity, no use of x-rays and treating the whole body, not just the spine. For those in the group that performed joint adjustments, their approach featured more nuanced gradations. The government considered they regarded themselves as specialists because they did not mix osteopathy with remedy prescribing, but it was rather the case, including for those with prescribed qualifications that they did not wish their identity subsumed by a chiropractic one for registration. The need for legacy provisions in legislation through a grandfather clause had been raised in government inquiries to accommodate the successful and talented but uncredentialled practitioners. While New South Wales included one, Victoria did not and despite a special amendment to create one, the weighting of medical interests on the Registration Board alongside those representing elite mainstream overseas schools thwarted its implementation. Instead, Bowen and others like him became a victim of regulation and were subjected to an illegal examination process to determine clinical competency skewed to a biomedical perspective. The final chapter brings the Bowen story together under various themes related to the topic of Medical Pluralism and Beyond.

Notes

1 Jan Breen, "Red Tape Ties Healing Man's Hands," *Geelong Advertiser*, March 31, 1982: 22.
2 PROV. Report and evidence Osteopathy Committee (Pt.1–4), 27/11/1975 (Pt. 2) 2261, VPRS 3253/P1/, Unit 47. Original papers tabled in the Legislative Assembly, transcripts of proceedings, Wilkie transcript: 14.
3 PROV. Report and evidence Osteopathy Committee (Pt.1–4), 27/11/1975 (Pt. 2) 2261, VPRS 3253/P1/, Unit 47. Original papers tabled in the Legislative Assembly, transcripts of proceedings, Wilkie transcript: 14.
4 Ward Inquiry Report, Appendix T, 81.
5 Ward Inquiry Report, Appendix T, 81.
6 "Victorian Register of Chiropractors and Osteopaths as at 30 June 1980," *Victorian Government Gazette*, No. 67, August 12, 1980, 2760, 2767.
7 Bowen's Business Card for 283 Latrobe Terrace. Image, Ron Phelan, Custodian Rene Horwood Collection.
8 *Osteopaths Registration Act 1996* (Vic).
9 PROV. Report and evidence Osteopathy Committee (Pt.1–4), 27/11/975 (Pt. 2) 2261, VPRS 3253/P1/, Unit 47. Original papers tabled in the Legislative Assembly, transcripts of proceedings, Bowen transcript: 676.
10 PROV. Report and evidence Osteopathy Committee (Pt.1–4), 27/11/975 (Pt. 2) 2261, VPRS 3253/P1/, Unit 47. Original papers tabled in the Legislative Assembly, transcripts of proceedings, Bowen transcript: 676.
11 PROV. Report and evidence Osteopathy Committee (Pt.1–4), 27/11/975 (Pt. 2) 2261, VPRS 3253/P1/, Unit 47. Original papers tabled in the Legislative Assembly, transcripts of proceedings, Bowen transcript: 676.
12 Ward Inquiry Report, 9.
13 'Straight' was a term with the opposite meaning to 'mixer' which designated practitioners who were multi-modal and prescribed or mixed therapeutic approaches like naturopaths.
14 VIC, Parliamentary Debates, Legislative Council, Vol. 362, December 9, 1981: 4497.
15 Ward Inquiry Report, Appendix A, 67.
16 Webb Inquiry Report, 266.
17 PROV, of Chiropractors and Oesteopaths [sic]- New Act 1977, VPRS 6435/P/, Unit 556, Correspondence Alan Wilkie President of VSSO to Minister Houghton, April 5, 1978.
18 VIC, Parliamentary Debates, Legislative Council, Vol. 362, December 9, 1981: 4497.
19 VIC, Parliamentary Debates, Legislative Council, Vol. 362, December 9, 1981: 4497.
20 VIC, Parliamentary Debates, Legislative Council, Vol. 362, December 9, 1981: 4497.; The Webb Inquiry Report identified A. Wilkie and R. Bennett as representatives; Ward Inquiry Report, 10.
21 PROV. Report and evidence Osteopathy Committee (Pt.1–4), 27/11/1975 (Pt. 2) 2261, VPRS 3253/P1/, Unit 47, Wilkie transcript: 2, 4–5.

22 PROV. Report and evidence Osteopathy Committee (Pt.1–4), 27/11/1975 (Pt. 2) 2261, VPRS 3253/P1/, Unit 47, Wilkie transcript: 2, 4–5.
23 PROV. Report and evidence Osteopathy Committee (Pt.1–4), 27/11/1975 (Pt. 2) 2261, VPRS 3253/P1/, Unit 47, Wilkie transcript: 2, 4–5.
24 PROV. Report and evidence Osteopathy Committee (Pt.1–4), 27/11/1975 (Pt. 2) 2261, VPRS 3253/P1/, Unit 47, Wilkie transcript: 2, 4–5.
25 PROV. Report and evidence Osteopathy Committee (Pt.1–4), 27/11/1975 (Pt. 2) 2261, VPRS 3253/P1/, Unit 47, Wilkie transcript: 2, 4–5.
26 PROV. Report and evidence Osteopathy Committee (Pt.1–4), 27/11/1975 (Pt. 2) 2261, VPRS 3253/P1/, Unit 47, Wilkie transcript: 2–3.
27 PROV. Report and evidence Osteopathy Committee (Pt.1–4), 27/11/1975 (Pt. 2) 2261, VPRS 3253/P1/, Unit 47, Wilkie transcript: 2.
28 PROV, of Chiropractors and Oesteopaths [sic]- New Act 1977, VPRS 6435/P/, Unit 556, Correspondence Alan Wilkie President of VSSO to Minister Houghton, April 5, 1978.
29 PROV, VPRS 3253/P1/, Unit 47, Alan Wilkie transcript, 7A.
30 PROV, VPRS 3253/P1/, Unit 47, Alan Wilkie transcript, 7A, 10.
31 PROV, VPRS 3253/P1/, Unit 47, Alan Wilkie transcript, 7A, 5.
32 PROV, VPRS 3253/P1/, Unit 47, Alan Wilkie transcript, 7A, 5.
33 PROV, VPRS 3253/P1/, Unit 47, Alan Wilkie transcript, 7A, 9.
34 PROV, VPRS 3253/P1/, Unit 47, Alan Wilkie transcript, 7A, 7.
35 PROV, VPRS 3253/P1/, Unit 47, Alan Wilkie transcript, 7A, 7.
36 PROV, VPRS 3253/P1/, Unit 47, Alan Wilkie transcript, 7A, 7.
37 PROV, VPRS 3253/P1/, Unit 47, Alan Wilkie transcript, 7A, 7.
38 PROV, VPRS 3253/P1/, Unit 47, Alan Wilkie transcript, 7A, 7.
39 PROV, VPRS 3253/P1/, Unit 47, Alan Wilkie transcript, 7A, 13–14.
40 Kevin Ryan, "Working alongside Tom Bowen," Presentation to National Conference of Bowen Interest Groups, August 21, 1999, transcript in Shirley Strachan, *Healing Hands, Unsung Voices, Thomas Ambrose Bowen 1916–1982, Osteopath* (United Kingdom: Cloister House Press, 2016), 248.
41 PROV, VPRS 3253/P1/, Unit 47, Wilkie transcript, 13–14.
42 PROV, VPRS 3253/P1/, Unit 47, Wilkie transcript, 7A, 11.
43 PROV, VPRS 3253/P1/, Unit 47, Wilkie transcript, 11–12.
44 Heather Hay personal communication to author July 29, 2017. (Hay was a clinic associate of McAlister in the decade before his death in 2011).
45 PROV, VPRS 3253/P1/, Unit 47, Wilkie transcript, 13.
46 PROV, VPRS 3253/P1/, Unit 47, Wilkie transcript, 9.
47 PROV, VPRS 3253/P1/, Unit 47, Wilkie transcript, 7–7A.
48 John Stewart personal communication to the author February 26, 2019.
49 Stewart email messages to author February 25 and February 28, 2019.
50 Stewart email messages to author February 25 and February 28, 2019.
51 Stewart email messages to author February 25 and February 28, 2019.
52 Andrew Fraser, *Osteopathic Natural Treatments* (Geelong: Deakin University Press, 1994), 93.
53 Stewart emails to author, February 25 and February 28, 2019.
54 Stewart emails to author, February 25 and February 28, 2019.
55 Stewart emails to author, February 25 and February 28, 2019.
56 Hay personal communication to author July 29, 2017.
57 Professor John Murtagh personal communication to author, October 13, 2015.
58 Murtagh personal communication to author, October 13, 2015.
59 Murtagh personal communication to author, October 13, 2015.
60 John Murtagh, "Musculoskeletal Medicine in Australia, a 50 Year Journey and Perspective," *Australasian Musculoskeletal Medicine* 18, no. 1 (2013): 8–10.

61 Murtagh, "Musculoskeletal Medicine in Australia," 8–10.
62 Murtagh, "Musculoskeletal Medicine in Australia," 8–10.
63 Murtagh, "Musculoskeletal Medicine in Australia," 8–10.
64 Murtagh, "Musculoskeletal Medicine in Australia," 8–10.
65 Murtagh, "Musculoskeletal Medicine in Australia."
66 PROV. Report and evidence Osteopathy Committee (Pt.1–4), 27/11/975 (Pt. 2) 2261, VPRS 3253/P1/, Unit 50, Original papers tabled in the Legislative Assembly, transcripts of proceedings, McAlister transcript: 3429.
67 Hay personal communication.
68 Hay personal communication.
69 Hay personal communication.
70 Hay personal communication.
71 Hay personal communication.
72 Paul Schmidt personal communication to author.
73 Hay personal communication.
74 PROV, VPRS 3253/P1/, Unit 50, McAlister transcript, 3441.
75 PROV, VPRS 3253/P1/, Unit 50, McAlister transcript, 3446.
76 PROV, VPRS 3253/P1/, Unit 50, McAlister transcript, 3433.
77 Michael Quinlivan email message to the author July 21, 2017.
78 PROV. Report and evidence Osteopathy Committee (Pt.1–4), 27/11/975 (Pt. 2) 2261, VPRS 3253/P1 Unit 47. Report and evidence Osteopathy Committee, Original papers tabled in the Legislative Assembly, transcripts of proceedings, Jacka transcript: 19.
79 Quinlivan email message to the author July 21, 2017.
80 Edwin Devereaux, Brian O'Reilly, and John Cice. *History of the Sydney College of Chiropractic* (Sydney: Macquarie Lighthouse Press, 2012), 195.
81 PROV, Registrar of Probates Supreme court, VPRS 28/P0025, 1105654, Probate and Administration Files (CourtView) (17379), Box 317, S PRB 2011 12670, Robin Gardini.
82 *Australia, Electoral Rolls 1903–1980*, available on Ancestry.com.
83 *Australia, Electoral Rolls 1903–1980*, available on Ancestry.com.
84 PROV, Registration of Chiropractors and Oestopaths [*sic*], VPRS6345/P/, Unit 545, General Correspondence Files, Letter Gardini to Health Minister June 22, 1971.
85 "London and Counties Society of Physiologists."
86 Steven Foster email message to author February 23, 2019.
87 "LCSP Register of Masseurs and Manipulative Therapists."
88 Margot McCarthy, ed., *Natural Therapies, The Complete A-Z of Complementary Health* (London and San Fransico: Thorsons, Harper and Collins, 1994), 297.
89 Foster email to author March 1, 2019.
90 Barbara Priestley, *British Qualifications: A Comprehensive Guide to Educational, Technical, Professional and Academic Qualifications in Britain*, 8th ed. (London: Kogan Page, 1977), 590.
91 Priestley, *British Qualifications.*
92 PROV, VPRS 6345/P/, Unit 545, Letter Robin Gardini to Minister, April 14, 1978.
93 Ward Inquiry Report, appendix T: 81.
94 Nomination forms in PROV, Registration of Chiropractors and Osteopaths – New Act. VPRS 6345/P/, Unit 545, Jeanette Patrick MD nomination of Gardini to Houghton, Minister for Health, July 5, 1976; PROV, Chiropractors and Osteopaths Registration Board VPRS 6345/P/, Unit 556, General Correspondence – circa 10 ANTA member nominations of Robin Gardini to Houghton Minster for Health, period June 20 1978 to November 21, 1978.
95 PROV, Registration of Chiropractors and Oestopaths [sic] – New Act 1977, VPRS 6345/P/, Unit 545, General Correspondence Files, Jeanette Patrick MP, nomination of Robin Gardini for Registration Board to Minister for Health, July 5, 1976.

96 Peter Hawkins and Arthur O'Neill, *Osteopathy in Australia* (Bundoora: Preston Institute of Technology Press, 1990), 31.
97 Hawkins and O'Neill, *Osteopathy in Australia*, 31; VIC, Parliamentary Debates Legislative Council, 221.
98 Robin Gardini, Australian Politicians Database (AuspolDB), Candidates.
99 "Photograph of Council, 1986," Ringwood and District Historical Society, Victorian Collections; "Cr Gardini Retires", Newspaper Scrapbook Ringwood Library, Victorian Collections.
100 *Commonwealth of Australia Gazette. Special (National: 1977 – 2012)* June 10, 1991: 13.
101 Fraser, *Osteopathic Natural Treatments*, 1.
102 Fraser, *Osteopathic Natural Treatments*, 24.
103 Fraser, *Osteopathic Natural Treatments*, 24.
104 Schmidt personal communication to author.
105 Schmidt personal communication to the author.
106 Schmidt personal communication to the author.
107 PROV, Chiropractic treatments – Letters and Reports, Pt 1, VPRS 6345/P/, Unit 155, Andrew Fraser letter to Minister for Health, November 22, 1972,
108 PROV, VPRS 3253/P1/, Unit 49, Try transcript, 2181.
109 PROV, VPRS 3253/P1/, Unit 49, Try transcript, 2179, 2193.
110 PROV, VPRS 3253/P1/, Try transcript, 2181.
111 Jacka, *The Politics and the Passion*, 14–15.
112 *Australia, Electoral Rolls 1903–1980.*
113 PROV, Try Transcript, 2181.
114 PROV, Try transcript, 2183–84.
115 PROV, Try transcript, 2183–84.
116 PROV, Try transcript, 2187.
117 PROV, Try transcript, 2184.
118 PROV, VPRS 3253/P1/, Try transcript, 2193.
119 PROV, VPRS 3253/P1/, Try transcript, 2198.
120 PROV, VPRS 3253/P1/, Try transcript, 2198.
121 PROV, VPRS 3253/P1/, Try transcript, 2196.
122 PROV, VPRS 3253/P1/, Try transcript, 2196.
123 PROV, Registration of Chiropractors and Oestopaths [sic] – New Act, VPRS 6345/P, Unit 545, General Correspondence Files, ANTA report April 14, 1978.
124 *Chiropractors and Osteopaths Act, 1978* (Vic).
125 *Chiropractors and Osteopaths Registration Act, 1981* (Vic).
126 Mackenzie interview by author March 18, 2015, transcript in Strachan, *Healing Hands*, 187–90, 188.
127 VIC, Parliamentary Debates, Legislative Council, Vol. 362, December 9, 1981, 4495.
128 VIC, Parliamentary Debates, Legislative Council, Vol. 362, December 9, 1981, 4495.
129 Romney Smeeton personal communication to author.
130 Webb Inquiry Report, 131.
131 *Chiropractors and Osteopaths (Amendment) Act* (Vic) 1992.
132 *Osteopaths Registration Act 1996* Act No. 75/1996.
133 VIC, Parliamentary Debates, Legislative Council Vol. 362, December 9, 1981, 4496.
134 Kevin Neave letter to Ron Phelan, May 9, 2002 personal communication to author.
135 Breen, "Red Tape Ties Healing Man's Hands."
136 Breen, "Red Tape Ties Healing Man's Hands."
137 Breen, "Red Tape Ties Healing Man's Hands."; The statistics are confirmed in PROV, VPRS 16432/P1/, Unit 1, Chiropractors and Osteopaths Registration Board, Annual Reports.

138 Tattersall interview by author, 8.
139 Keith Davis personal communication to author.
140 Karen Matthews, "Healing Hands," *Geelong Advertiser*, April 3, 1999: 37.
141 VIC, Parliamentary Debates, Legislative Council, 4496.
142 VIC, Parliamentary Debates, Legislative Council, Vol. 353, October 22, 1980, 1452–53.
143 PROV, Chiropractors and Osteopaths Registration Board VPRS 16432/P1/, Unit1, Annual Reports and Papers: 1979–1987, Third Annual Report.
144 Breen, "Red Tape Ties Healing Man's Hands."
145 *Try, Marcus v Chiropractors and Osteopaths Registration Board of Victoria* (1983 / November 18), Supreme Court Victoria, Action I5876.
146 Breen, "Red Tape Ties Healing Man's Hands."
147 Breen, "Red Tape Ties Healing Man's Hands."
148 Breen, "Red Tape Ties Healing Man's Hands."
149 "*Try, Marcus v Chiropractors & Osteopaths Registration Board of Victoria*," Supreme Court Victoria, Action I5876, November 18, 1983.
150 "*Try, Marcus v Chiropractors & Osteopaths Registration Board of Victoria*."
151 "Register of Chiropractors and Osteopaths as at September 8, 1986," Victorian Government Gazette, no. 84, October 9, 1986, 3945.
152 *Chiropractic Act* 1978 (NSW).
153 Kenneth Herbert Lloyd vs Chiropractors and Osteopaths Registration Board (1980/August 13), Supreme Court Victoria, Action M116/1980, Law Library of Victoria.
154 Kenneth Herbert Lloyd vs Chiropractors and Osteopaths Registration Board (1980/August 13), Supreme Court Victoria, Action M116/1980, Law Library of Victoria.
155 Hay personal communication to the author February 9, 2019.
156 Ryan personal communication to the author, February 13, 2019.
157 PROV, Chiropractors and Osteopaths Registration Board VPRS 16432/P1/Unit 1, Annual Reports and Papers: 1979–1987, Draft notes for the Fourth Annual Report 1982.
158 PROV, Chiropractors and Osteopaths Registration Board VPRS 16432/P1/ Unit 1, Annual Reports and Papers: 1979–1987, Ministerial Memorandum Roper to Cusack, Registrar Registration Board. November 25, 1982.
159 PROV, Chiropractors and Osteopaths Registration Board VPRS 16432/P1/ Unit 1, Annual Reports and Papers: 1979–1987, Memorandum Brian Cusack Registration Board to Minister for Health Tom Roper, December 7, 1982.
160 "Try, Marcus v Chiropractors & Osteopaths Registration Board of Victoria."
161 *Chiropractors and Osteopaths Act 1978.*
162 *Health Practitioner Regulation National Law (Victoria) Act 2009.*
163 Bowen business card as 'Natural Therapist', image courtesy Ron Phelan, Custodian Rene Horwood Collection.
164 Section 9(6) of the *Chiropractors and Osteopaths Act* 1978 gave the Registration Board the power to approve 'teaching and research institutions'. In practice, these were limited to institutions recognised by the peak associations – the UCAA, ACA and AOA. The ACA only recognised American Schools, there were no specifically osteopathic colleges recognized at the time. Politically, the emphasis was on chiropractic to secure registration given the antipathy of the American interests towards Australian training standards.
165 UCAA colleges, Ward Inquiry Report, 266, 273; Devereaux et al., *History of the Sydney College of Chiropractic*, 187.
166 "Register of Chiropractors and Osteopaths as at 30 June 1980," *Victorian Government Gazette*, No. 67, August 12, 1980.
167 VIC, Parliamentary Debates, Legislative Council, Vol. 406, April 7, 1992, 219, 220.

168 VIC, Parliamentary Debates, Legislative Assembly, Vol. 406, March 17, 1992, 45; VIC, Parliamentary Debates, Legislative Council, Vol. 406, April 7, 1992, 221.
169 VIC, Parliamentary Debates Legislative Council, 221.
170 "About Us," Bunbury Osteopathy Clinic.
171 Michael Quinlivan personal communication and by email July 21, 2017.
172 "Bruce Duncan," North Carlton Osteopathy.
173 "Bruce Duncan," North Carlton Osteopathy.
174 Heather Hay personal communication July 29, 2018 and February 9, 2019; "Moonee Valley Osteopathy."

Bibliography

Newspapers

Breen, Jan. "Red Tape ties Healing Man's Hands." *Geelong Advertiser*, March 31, 1982: 22.

Primary Sources

Chiropractic Registration Act (NSW). 1978. Accessed November 17, 2024. https://legislation.nsw.gov.au/view/pdf/asmade/act-1978-132.

Chiropractors and Osteopaths Act (VIC). 1978. Accessed November 17, 2024 http://www.austlii.edu.au/au/legis/vic/hist_act/caoa1978315.pdf.

Chiropractors and Osteopaths (Registration) Act (VIC). 1981. Accessed November 17, 2024. http://www6.austlii.edu.au/cgi-in/viewdb//au/legis/vic/hist_act/caoa1981458/.

Chiropractors and Osteopaths (Amendment) Act (VIC). 1992. Accessed November 17, 2024. https://classic.austlii.edu.au/au/legis/vic/hist_act/caoa1992395/.

Commonwealth of Australia Gazette. Special (National: 1977 – 2012). June 10, 1991: 13. accessed November 17, 2024. http://nla.gov.au/nla.news-page25896809.

"Cr Gardini Retires." Photograph of Council, 1986, Ringwood and District Historical Society. Victorian Collections. Accessed November 17, 2024. Victorian Collections. https://victoriancollections.net.au/items/5c1838d26b785e0ebc9c7f1b.

"Cr Gardini Retires." Newspaper Scrapbook Ringwood Library. Accessed November 17, 2024. Victorian Collections. https://victoriancollections.net.au/items/650173c020282ca43c53401d.

Health Practitioner Regulation National Law (Victoria) Act. 2009. Accessed November 17, 2024. https://www.legislation.vic.gov.au/as-made/acts/health-practitioner-regulation-national-law-victoria-act-2009.

Lloyd, Kenneth Herbert vs Chiropractors and Osteopaths Registration Board, 1980/August 13. Supreme Court Victoria, Action M116/1980. Law Library of Victoria. Accessed November 17, 2024. http://aucc.sirsidynix.net.au/Judgments/Civil/224819.pdf.

Neave, Kevin. Letter to Ron Phelan, May 9, 2002.

Osteopaths Registration Act 1996 (VIC). Accessed November 17, 2024. https://www.legislation.vic.gov.au/as-made/acts/osteopaths-registration-act–1996.

PROV. Chiropractic Treatment – Letters and Reports, Pt 1. VPRS 6345/P/, Unit 155. General Correspondence Files, Letter, Andrew Fraser letter to Sir (Minister for Health), November 22, 1972.

PROV. Chiropractic and Osteopaths Registration Board, VPRS 6345/P/, Unit 556. General Correspondence, Alan Wilkie President of VSSO to Minister Houghton, April 5, 1978.

PROV. Chiropractors and Osteopaths Registration Board. VPRS 16432/P1/ Unit 1. Annual Reports and Papers: 1979–1987, Third Annual Report.

PROV. Chiropractors and Osteopaths Registration Board. VPRS 16432/P1 Annual Reports and Papers: 1979–1987 Unit 1, Draft notes for the Fourth Annual Report 1982.

PROV. Chiropractors and Osteopaths Registration Board. VPRS 16432/P1, Unit 1. Annual Reports and Papers: 1979–1987, Ministerial Memorandum Roper to Cusack, Registrar Registration Board. November 25, 1982.

PROV. Chiropractors and Osteopaths Registration Board. VPRS 16432/P1, Unit 1. Annual Reports and Papers: 1979–1987, Memorandum Brian Cusack Registration Board to Minister for Health Tom Roper, December 7, 1982.

PROV. Registrar of Probates Supreme court. VPRS 28/P0025, 1105654. Probate and Administration Files (CourtView) (17379). Box 317. Item S PRB 2011 12670, Robin Gardini.

PROV. Registration of Chiropractors and Oestopaths [*sic*]– New Act VPRS 6345/P/, Unit 545. General Correspondence, Jacka ANTA report April 14, 1978 to Digby Crozier, Member for Western Province April 19, 1978 forwarded to.

PROV. Report and Evidence Osteopathy Committee (Pt.1–4), 27/11/975 (Pt. 2) 2261, VPRS 3253/P1/, Unit 47. Original papers tabled in the Legislative Assembly, transcripts of proceedings, Bowen transcript: 672–678.

PROV. Report and Evidence Osteopathy Committee (Pt.1–4), 27/11/975 (Pt. 2) 2261, VPRS 3253/P1/, Unit 50, Original papers tabled in the Legislative Assembly, transcripts of proceedings, McAlister transcript: 3424–60.

PROV. Report and Evidence Osteopathy Committee (Pt.1–4), 27/11/975 (Pt. 2) 2261, VPRS 3253/P1/, Unit 49. Original papers tabled in the Legislative Assembly, transcripts of proceedings, Try transcript: 2179–98.

PROV. Report and Evidence Osteopathy Committee (Pt.1–4), 27/11/1975 (Pt. 2) 2261, VPRS 3253/P1/, Unit 47. Original papers tabled in the Legislative Assembly, transcripts of proceedings, Wilkie transcript: 1–14.

PROV. VPRS 16432/P1/, Unit 1, Chiropractors and Osteopaths Registration Board, Annual Reports.

"Register of Chiropractors and Osteopaths as at 30 June 1980." *Victorian Government Gazette*, No. 67, August 12, 1980.

"Register of Chiropractors and Osteopaths as at September 8, 1986." *Victorian Government Gazette*, No. 84, October 9, 1986.

Ryan, Kevin. "Working alongside Tom Bowen." Presentation to National Conference of Bowen Interest Groups, August 21, 1999. Transcript in Strachan, Shirley. *Healing Hands, Unsung Voices, Thomas Ambrose Bowen 1916–1982, Osteopath.* United Kingdom: Cloister House Press, 2016.

Tattersall, Barry. Interview by author, January 9, 2015. Transcript in Strachan, Shirley. *Healing Hands, Unsung Voices, Thomas Ambrose Bowen 1916–1982, Osteopath.* United Kingdom: Cloister House Press, 2016.

Try, Marcus v Chiropractors and Osteopaths Registration Board of Victoria 1983 / November 18, Supreme Court Victoria, Action I5876. Accessed November 17, 2024. http://aucc.sirsidynix.net.au/Judgments/Civil/289683.pdf.

VIC. Parliamentary Debates. Legislative Council. Vol. 353, October 22, 1980.

VIC Parliamentary Debates. Legislative Council. Vol. 362. December 9, 1981.

VIC. Parliamentary Debates. Legislative Assembly. Vol. 406, March 17, 1992.

VIC. Parliamentary Debates, Legislative Council. Vol. 406, April 7, 1992.

"Victorian Register of Chiropractors and Osteopaths as at 8 September, 1986." *Victoria Government Gazette*, No. 84, October 9, 1986, 3939, 3943, 3945.

Ward Inquiry Report – full title – Victoria Parliament, Osteopathy, Chiropractic and Naturopathy Committee, et al. *Report from the Osteopathy, Chiropractic and*

Naturopathy Committee: Together with Appendices. Melbourne: C. H. Rixon, Government Printer, 1975. Accessed November 17, 2024. http://www6.austlii.edu.au/au/other/vic/VicLASelCPubInq/1975/1.pdf.

"Webb Inquiry Report" – full title – *Report of the Committee of Inquiry into Chiropractic, Osteopathy, Homoeopathy [sic] and Naturopathy*. Canberra: Australian Government Publishing Service, 1977. Accessed November 17, 2024. https://www6.austlii.edu.au/au/other/cth/AUBCPubInq/1977/6.pdf

Secondary Sources

Devereaux, Edwin, Brian O'Reilly, and John Cice. *History of the Sydney College of Chiropractic*. Sydney: Macquarie Lighthouse Press, 2012.

Fraser, Andrew. *Osteopathic Natural Treatments*. Geelong: Deakin University Press, 1994.

McCarthy, Margot, ed. *Natural Therapies, The Complete A-Z of Complementary Health*. London and San Francisco: Thorsons, Harper and Collins, 1994.

Murtagh, John. "Musculoskeletal Medicine in Australia, a 50 Year Journey and Perspective." *Australasian Musculoskeletal Medicine* 18, no. 1 (2013): 8–9. Accessed November 17, 2024. https://search.informit.org/doi/10.3316/informit.354643897972196.

Priestley, Barbara. *British Qualifications: A Comprehensive Guide to Educational, Technical, Professional and Academic Qualifications in Britain*. 8th ed. London: Kogan Page, 1977. Accessed November 17, 2024. https://archive.org/details/britishqualifica0000prie/.

Websites

"About Us." *Bunbury Osteopathy Clinic*. Accessed November 17, 2024. http://bunburyosteopathicclinic.com.au/about-us/.

"Bruce Duncan." *North Carlton Osteopathy*. Accessed November 17, 2024. http://northcarltonosteopathy.com.au/about-nco/

"LCSP Register of Masseurs and Manipulative Therapists." Accessed November 17, 2024. http://www.lcsp.uk.com/about-us/.

"London and Counties Society of Physiologists." Accessed November 17, 2024. https://lcsp.uk.com/.

"Moonee Valley Osteopathy." Accessed November 17, 2024, https://mvosteopathy.com.au/."Robin Gardini." *Australian Politicians Database (AuspolDB)*. Accessed November 17, 2024. https://auspoldb.org/candidates/view/22322.

8 The Bowen Story Medical Pluralism and Beyond

Medical Pluralism

Medical pluralism is the availability of different medical approaches, treatments, and institutions that people can choose from while pursuing health: for example, combining biomedicine with so-called traditional medicine or alternative medicine.[1] Stereotypically, biomedicine focuses on purely biological factors such as the germ theory of disease and its objective is to treat diseases with chemical therapy through pharmaceutical drugs and where needed remove diseased parts with surgical intervention. The randomised controlled trial (RCT) is held up as the gold standard of scientific rigour in biomedicine. Biomedicine enjoys great power attributed to globalisation and enjoys greater homogeneity as a result.[2] In comparison, traditional and alternative medicine within the field of complementary and alternative medicine (CAM) is a biopsychosocial model.[3] It relies on healing arts that sit apart from biomedicine and includes different medical approaches that share distinct knowledge systems and worldviews. Because of the power of biomedicine, discussion of medical pluralism can tend to portray the landscape as polarised between the powerbase of biomedicine and its subjugation of CAM. In practice, the lines are blurred with the increase of integrative practitioners who have medical degrees and prescribe natural remedies. CAM has a strong constituency and within CAM, there is great diversity which is a perceived threat to biomedicine.

Within this diversity are CAM modalities engaged in the struggle for legitimation and mainstream acceptance too. Regardless, consumers have individual rights of choice in the landscape of medical pluralism and there is a shift towards integrative approaches.[4] Uibu and Koppel highlight that medical pluralism does not only mean the presence of multiple therapies, they look at how societies are communicating health information and observe,

> Meanings offered by CAM-related health approaches are increasingly visible and influential as unlicensed health workers and laypeople contribute more to public communication due to the openness of social media. On the other hand, critics of CAM and proponents of scientific

DOI: 10.4324/9781003602125-9

thinking have mobilized to set boundaries to defend the authoritative position of scientific medicine.[5]

They refer to other writers such as Cant and Sharma who identify that 'resurgence' of the medical pluralism concept has happened because of the growing popularity of CAM and the public health care funding crisis that is putting pressure on governments to change their health care policies.[6]

Medical pluralism can suggest types of medicine coexisting and insulated from each other but diversity or superdiversity brought about by immigration, multiculturalism and globalisation involves interrelatedness and borrowing of ideas. Instead, medical landscapes are more fluid. They capture movement and connections across boundaries.[7] The writers are interested in the behaviours of patients in search of cure and the Estonian study looks at communities that have a distrust of biomedicine and favour the use of traditional herbs and practices; these give them a sense of agency and sovereignty to have power over their own health and choices.

Bowen: A Victim in the Historical Grand Narrative of Legitimation of Osteopathy

The Bowen story historically is a microhistory of victimisation within the grander narrative of legitimation of osteopathy and chiropractic. Baer identified that through the eighteenth century, the Australian medical system and its various subsystems were on a relative equal footing; however, in the twentieth century, it became a plural one, whereby biomedicine came to dominate other medical subsystems.[8] Baer has also written on the legitimation of mainstream osteopathy and chiropractic in Australia.[9] Bolton provided an overview of the difficulties that mainstream chiropractic faced in the journey to legitimation.[10] Nothing comparable has been written from within the Australian osteopathy profession on the historical trajectory of osteopathy towards legitimation, reflecting that the story is dominated by the chiropractic narrative. Instead, like chiropractors, osteopathy writers tend to focus on research and education and clarifying the role of osteopathy in modern healthcare.[11] Baer's views are reflected in the historical backdrop to the Bowen story and how the events of legitimation moved forward.

Chapter 1 described the historical long view and the issues osteopathy's pioneer Dr Still MD, DO faced in his own lifetime against the power of the biomedical faction even though he too was medically trained. The impact of educational reform and the Flexner Report in America in 1910 set in train the tensions transposed by America on overseas colleges, including Australia as regulatory forces advanced a more scientifically rigorous pathway and a departure from the more spiritually holistic thinking of Dr Still MD, DO. The Bowen story should also have been one of legitimation of Bowen personally as a practitioner of osteopathy: Chapter 7 showed that the legal mechanism was put in place for this to happen, but Bowen's treatment at the hands of the

Victorian Registration Board was dramatically different to what he would have received had his nineteen years of successful practice occurred in New South Wales (NSW) instead of Victoria. In NSW, he would have been registered under Section 15 2(c) of the *Chiropractic Act 1978* (NSW), solely on the basis of having practised for four years continuously or in aggregate in the ten years prior to the act.

The travesty for Bowen's legacy played out in this medical landscape is amplified when it is considered that Bowen was practising a style of osteopathy that had its roots in older osteopathy more authentically aligned to the work of its pioneer Dr Still MD, DO. His work and that of his VSSO colleagues did not feature the risky manipulations adopted by mainstream practice in chiropractic and osteopathy – medical systems that were not demarcated in Australia at the time as they are now. If the government enquiries had within their remit a deeper understanding of the divergent historical evolution of osteopathy in the twentieth century, and not focused exclusively on standards of training of mainstream elite schools based on biomedical sciences and clinical work, they would have arrived at a category of practice like Bowen's that was a successful throwback to an older naturopathic osteopathy. Bowen could have been afforded recognition without the political drama of entrenched interests that conspired against his vocational identity. In the aftermath, consumers exercised choice and still flocked to the disenfranchised men of the VSSO and both Bowen's and Gardini's clinics were as busy as ever and their work was sought out by registered professionals. For Bowen who managed a large Saturday clinic for individuals – children, pensioners and workers physically challenged with a neurological condition or spinal trauma of some kind that affected mobility and daily functioning, his primary concern was they could no longer claim Medicare rebates for his services. The state-backed unyielding Victorian Registration Board did not succeed in putting these practitioners out of business, they simply dropped any use of the protected titles of DO or osteopath, but the consumers were penalised through losing Medicare support (see Bowen's amended business card from 'Osteopath' to 'Natural Therapist' at Figure 7.2 in Chapter 7). This was a huge issue for Bowen personally as his greatest concern was always the care of his patients and their ability to afford treatment. Undoubtedly, his diminished official standing and demotion from his chosen vocational status would have caused reputational harm and resulted in some turning away too.

Community Healers Among the Football Masseurs

Bowen's life's work rose out of the overlooked culture of senior VFL, later AFL football masseurs who provided community outreach services attended by all levels of society searching for relief from pain at a time when general medical practitioners were not versed in musculoskeletal medicine. This is borne out in the Bowen story in Chapters 2 and 4. Importantly, the football masseurs also played a significant role in charitable and humanist activities as well as providing healing service to the public at large. They represent a form of consumer choice in what would be called folk medicine in medical pluralism as advice would be accompanied by household remedies such as soda crystals for swelling. The Ward Inquiry noted that 'fringe' practitioners would be consulted after 'a collapse in confidence in an orthodox physician' when, for example, a back complaint was not addressed. People would reluctantly take the advice of workmate or friend and consult a chiropractor or osteopath reluctantly with a low expectations only to find rapid relief of symptoms, 'This would often produce a strong psychological reaction against the doctor in favour of the fringe practitioner'.[12] Football doctors were also part of this humanist culture. Dr McCarthy (1895–1938), long-time president of the Footscray Football Club (ten years standing in 1936), was a philanthropist committed to supporting the area's poor and his social conscience reflects the community spirit in the working-class echelons of the football culture.[13] Ernest (Ernie) Saunders described in Chapter 4 was senior to Bowen and in the generation of Bowen's father. Saunders and other VFL trainers became professionally organised in 1927 with an association and the culture fostered in humanist activities was influential, supported by both lay masseurs and others professionally registered. Early leaders of the Australian Massage Association (AMA) took part in charity work, including Teepoo Hall and Alfred Peters, Hugo Leschen and Henrich (Henry) Best.[14] Registered Victorian football masseurs in 1928 supported initiatives.[15] Saunders' associate Pleass was a driving force in organising fundraising carnivals for hospitals. In his leading role with the trainers, Pleass was an active organiser of the Veteran Fundraising events for the Children's Hospital that saw him declared a life governor in 1932.[16] Saunders is found regularly assisting Pleass and organising the trainers for the annual fund-raising event.[17] Pleass treated Casaly who retired to Tasmania to pursue a physiotherapy career and is heralded in the press as 'Tasmania's Ernie Saunders' and he too treated polio sufferers for free.[18] Regional trainers included Ernest (Ern) James Davie (1898 –1958) head trainer for Geelong Football Club between 1925–1941.[19] Leading city names and their clubs included H (Henry) Sampson (Carlton), J (Jack) Marshall and P (Peter) McColl (South Melbourne), Lindsay (Fitzroy) and B Wallace (Hawthorn) and registered masseurs G Haines and Henry Best. Registered masseurs supported other charities too.[20] Leveson, head trainer for Hawthorn, was a stunt diver and sought to undertake daring dives to raise funds for other causes such as the Lord Mayors Fund.[21] Aaron Beattie taught physical culture for twenty-two years and raised money for war orphans through Legacy.[22] In 1933, Pleass and other head trainers made visits to the Frankston Orthopaedic Hospital to assist crippled children.[23] The annual events organised by these masseurs have not made it to the history books despite their dedication.[24] The Frankston Hospital link is interesting because Bowen's family spent time in the Dandenongs during the war and Rene Horwood recalled Bowen had been introduced to sister Kenny's methods 'up in the Dandenongs' working with polio cases.[25] It seems the Bowen family may have known Kenny personally as Agnes Shaw was recorded in a video, saying Kenny was her godmother.[26] Shaw gave an account believed to be of this period, of her brother getting a crippled boy who had never walked out of his wheelchair.[27] Bowen established an early clinic for polio sufferers which evolved to accommodate a wide range of spinal and neurological conditions such as spina bifida, cerebral palsy and epilepsy.[28] These masseurs responded to the polio outbreaks, to those crippled by disease and treated the community-at-large working from the football grounds, local halls, their own homes if they had a dedicated practice room and for some their kitchens or a spare room that were effectively part-time makeshift cottage-industry 'clinics'. Bill Mitchell in Bowen's generation was famous for his donations tin and it is reported he gave this money away to charity.[29] Treatments were free or by donation as the *Masseurs Act* prohibited fees unless the masseur was registered. Within this community, there was also an overlapping community of Freemasons. Ernie Saunders was a brother of the Duke of Brunswick Lodge 132 which no longer exists and received a Mason's funeral.[30] A man with the same initials as Fred Pleass' father (John James) J Pleass was an Immediate Past Master (IPM) in 1885 for the Lodge of Emerald.[31] In 1904, Teepoo Hall was a brother of the Minerva Lodge of the International Order of Odd Fellows.[32] Alister McAlister's brother Ron Graham Henry McAlister (1922–1996) was a Freemason.[33] It was confirmed Alister McAlister was too.[34]

Saunders was legendary in his generosity for free treatments even after he could legally charge with registration.[35] When Saunders died, the papers ran a story with the headline 'He loved his fellow man':

> Ernie Saunders would have died a millionaire but for one thing. He loved his fellow man more than money. In a humble home in Brunswick, Saunders, whose death this week has been mourned by thousands of people, gave back to the cripple those precious things in life that count more than anything else. Globe writers here pay well deserved tributes to a worthy citizen.[36]

Until he turned professional in 1959, Bowen initially treated for free until Hugh Opperman, the champion cyclist and politician brought his wife to Bowen's clinic at the Horwood home and brought a donations box to help Rene with the wear and tear on her home and electricity bills.[37] Even when Bowen set up in professional business, he would treat for free and Horwood used to ensure clients were charged as monetary gain was not a motivator at all for his work. Horwood said he would 'turn in his grave' at profiteering in his name.[38] Bowen had a framed saying of unconfirmed attribution to a Quaker of mid-nineteenth-century origin and would publish the words on calendars for patients:

> I pass through this world but once. Any good therefore I may do, any kindness that I may show to any fellow creature let me do it now. Let me not defer nor neglect it, for I may not pass this way again.[39]

Despite his professional successes, Bowen never left his association with football and looking after football teams. As a group, the men described next are a small community known to each and well-remembered for their expertise in attending to physical ailments of the community, even though the services of qualified massage therapists, osteopaths and chiropractors were available and long before GPs ever decided to train in musculoskeletal medicine. Part of the appeal was affordability too. These football masseurs are an overlooked group in the landscape of medical pluralism last century. Despite the power structure of the dominant biomedical sector, boundaries were fluid and these football masseurs were visited by politicians and doctors alike as their services were so much in demand. The culture of the football masseur-healer has died out due to the impact of the professionalisation of physical therapies enforced by government regulation later last century.

In transcripts to the Ward Inquiry, Bowen was also aligned by reputation with masseurs of his own generation, including Ernie's son George Saunders (1918–1981), Robert William (Bill) Anderson Mitchell (1904/5–1980) (attached to South Melbourne Football Club) and in northeast Victoria, the Shepparton-based farmer, William (Bill) Edmund Wilson (1916–1990). The Ward Inquiry panel was interested in Bowen's background in football massage and his views on other leading masseurs connected to football clubs. Bowen said he was involved with 'the little clubs and junior leagues'.[40] Pressing for more detail, Jones asked 'How did you come to do massage in the clubs?' to which Bowen replied, 'I joined the clubs and watched the other fellows doing it'.[41] Bowen indicates his awareness of the legal situation when he registered his business as an osteopath in 1959. He said, 'They [the Department of Health] did not care what I called myself as long as it was not a physiotherapist'. Ivor Trayling MP, commenting on massage training, said to Bowen:

> That is one of the reasons we are inquiring into these professions. We are looking at the overall situation. I believe Mr Mitchell would be in the same category as Mr Saunders. Would you bracket yourself in the same category as Mitchell and Saunders?[42]

'Yes' was Bowen's reply. Bill Mitchell and George Saunders were both in the same generation as Bowen and well known. This is born out in the testimony of other respondents to the Ward Inquiry including Mr Jens, a Ballarat Orthopaedic Surgeon and medical advisor to the Ward Inquiry. At Jens' interview, the Panel raised the names of osteopaths Tom Bowen and Alan Goldby (Ballarat) who had huge practices. Jens acknowledged some doctors had a fairly high opinion of them save their lack of training in [medical] diagnosis, he thought they had 'good hands and good commonsense and do a lot of good' and there was 'little evidence of doing damage' as they 'refer on early' if required.[43] Jens added Bill Mitchell of South Melbourne and Bill Wilson of Shepparton to the discussion.[44] Dr Shiels, a colleague of Jens at Ballarat Base Hospital, was treated by Bowen when dying of painful kidney cancer.[45] Eric Edward Allchin was also a respondent and a well-known manual therapist in Melbourne and for a period in the 1950s was doctor at the Footscray Football Club. At the Ward Inquiry, Allchin also mentioned Saunders, [Tom] McKay and Mitchell.[46] No information has surfaced so far in local history, either oral, documented or digitised referring to a male called Tom with the surname McKay having any reputation as a gifted therapist in the football or general community. A Tom McKay without this reputation is mentioned as a trainer for Geelong West before becoming Head Trainer for the Geelong Cats.[47] Given Bowen's contact with Footscray, it is possible Allchin confused the names of Tom McKay and Tom Bowen who was known to be associated with Alister McAlister who worked from Footscray Football Club and mentored others?

The reputation of these men was widespread among medical practitioners. Dr James (Jim) Dudley Rose of Ballarat (1940–2017) attended medical school the year after Professor Murtagh and was well aware of Saunders and Mitchell and the reputation of Bowen in the Ballarat region. Rose recalled a patient's account of waiting in a 'row of contorted shapes' waiting to see a masseur who just sat on a chair with a donation bowl by the door. The knee problem was fixed in thirty seconds.[48] Rose recalled this was Saunders and similar accounts of Saunders' philanthropy were shared in the press.[49] When Frank Harrison told a top Geelong orthopaedic surgeon (believed to be Huffam) that he was seeing Bowen, the reply was 'Well, what are you doing wasting your time here, that man has healing hands!'.[50] Bill Mitchell is remembered as having a robust style of working in the 1960s yet some 1970s accounts record gentle treatment. Like the Saunders men and Bowen, Mitchell had a knack at quickly rectifying painful complaints. Mitchell's ability was viewed in mystical terms, 'Bill was a modern-day shaman, with a mystic air and always smiling and happy'.[51] Both men clearly were swift, intuitive and effective in their practice and awareness of correcting pressure on nerves was a common theme. Mitchell trained others, including Wally Zunneberg the 'bush chiropractor' who was masseur and trainer to the famous Cliff Young.[52] Zunneberg said, 'I put my fingers on people and I can feel where the work needs doin'. It's like electricity underneath my hands'.[53] Jameson described Mitchell's work as 'chiropractoring'.[54] Mitchell also trained another Western District man by the name of Norman (Norm) Williams at the South Melbourne football grounds.[55] Williams had 'healing in his hands' and worked with his fingertips.[56] Mitchell also trained Kevin Cleaver who followed in Saunders' footsteps as a head trainer at Richmond Football Club from 1955, the same role Ernie Saunders held from 1924 to 1936.[57] According to press accounts, Mitchell was involved with training famous footballer Bob Skilton who held him in high regard, 'He had magic fingers' Skilton said.[58] Through Bob Skilton, there is a connection between Mitchell and Les Dettman (source of the Eastern medicine narrative described in Chapter 5) as both men treated him. There is minimal information about Bill Mitchell's style, but he was clearly very effective with an ability to quickly rectify ligament issues like Saunders and Bowen and worked with an awareness of nerves like Bowen and Albert (Bert) Donald (1915–1991). Posts no longer available on Melbourne Football Club's Demonland site described Mitchell as 'a genius', 'a legend', 'a sports doctor miles ahead of his time', 'completely untrained but with magic fingers' and 'a master with manipulation'. Other posts on the Sydney Swans Fans site confirmed his ability to run out and put ligaments quickly back in place and that 'he could feel ligaments and muscles through a telephone book'. The Premier Henry Bolte suffered a sore neck and was recommended to see Mitchell but was initially reluctant because of the police raids as they were practising without a licence, but as the story goes 'eventually he went to see Bill, weeks later when he was fixed they were granted a licence'. More detail about Mitchell's style is evident in the account of Professor John Murtagh who took his aunt to see Mitchell around 1962/1963, Mitchell then was in his fifties. In his recollections of Mitchell, Murtagh stated words to the effect that Mitchell was a very fast worker and no massage or use of liniment is recalled. Mitchell operated out of a hall in South Melbourne and had dozens queuing to see him. Each would take their turn and when exhausted, he would just stop for the day. He accepted donations. Mitchell had a knack of getting footballers quickly back on the field.[59]

Recalling the treatment of his aunt for sciatica, Murtagh remembered a 'resounding crack'. Murtagh's description of Mitchell's treatment for sciatica is different from the talent that Bowen brought to this condition.[60] Other accounts also confirm that Mitchell's style was quite robust compared to Bowen.[61] However, in the 1970s, Davis DC thought that Mitchell and Bowen's techniques looked similar when he took a daughter to Mitchell to be treated at the sports shop at Heidelberg where Mitchell had relocated.[62] A blog owner Sue Bell described her experience with Mitchell (pre-1966 given the imperial currency).[63] The complaint was a chronic frozen shoulder and Mitchell got to work without questions. Bells could remember the muscles being freed after she felt nerve impulses between her shoulder and elbow. One visit and five shillings donation was involved.[64]

Gentleness in Mitchell's approach too is confirmed by another 1970s' account by Leonie Appelt who was a young teenager when her mother took her to see Mitchell in sparse room with just a massage table and chair. Appelt had ligament damage and significant scarring from surgery in a leg that would not straighten. Mitchell warned her that she would get a shooting pain down her leg to her big toe. He pushed finger behind her knee and she remembered feeling an electric shock. The treatment was less than five minutes and her leg straightened to by the time she was at her parents' car. Appelt considered Mitchell a shaman and working with chi energy. She said, 'The bend was quite significant and meant some kind of mobility device for a long time so, God bless Bill Mitchell'.[65]

A legendary northeast Victorian practitioner mentioned at the Ward Inquiry was Bill Wilson. Wilson was a member of Australian Natural Therapists Association (ANTA) in 1978; President Alf Jacka put forward to the government the names of Wilson, Bowen and McAlister as men of skill that should be registered.[66] Wilson was regarded as 'one of the ligament men' of the area and 'one of the old legends' and 'fix-it men' by sports clubs in the region with his reputation extending as far as Echuca to the west.[67] His approach is also remembered as a cross-fibre technique but not regarded as someone who had a systemic approach like Bowen. He would treat areas that were symptomatic rather than considering compensatory patterns or considering sources of pain remote to the symptomatic site as Bowen would.[68]

Throughout his clinic years, Bowen kept up his role of trainer with regional under-eighteens and junior league football clubs in Geelong and throughout the Western District. With Garner, he was teaching VFL trainers in the 1970s.[69] When Bowen died, there were many sympathy notices in the press thanking him and including from local football clubs that included Bannockburn, Bell Post Hill, Geelong West Cricket and Football Club, Hamlyn Rangers and Soccer, Portarlington and Belmont Football Clubs.[70] Today, among those who remember Bowen continue to refer to him as the 'football masseur down on Villamanta Street' even though Bowen had two osteopathic clinic addresses there from 1976 to 1982 with signage. McAlister likewise was considered a masseur by Murtagh even though his role with Footscray Football Club in 1962 was as a Roberts' college-trained osteopath.

An immediate example close to Bowen is Ronald (Ron) Charles Garner (1924–1985) who worked with Bowen at Autumn Street in the mid-1950s and was associated with Newport West, Sorrento and the Geelong Cats Football Clubs.[71] Garner worked from the kitchen at his home in Norlane, and in addition to his role supporting the Olympian cyclist John Hine, tended to a wide range of patients from Geelong and the wider western district region for free and many would pay him in kind.[72] One of the values instilled in Garner was not to charge for his work as he would lose his gift.[73] These talented football masseurs proved a strong culture of humanism. They worked by donation, for free, or asking minimal fees when professionalised. They were revered by their communities enjoying strong 'belonging' and connectedness afforded by the significant role that football clubs played in community life, both metro and regional. They all shared the idea they had 'a gift'.

Biopsychosocial Mystique: The Non-heterodox and Esoteric

A less visible part of the cultural landscape of medical pluralism was the attraction of the community to individuals with odd abilities and insight and who performed treatments with a unique symbolic interaction and practice. This attraction defied the biomedical science-based standards imposed by governments on training to provide health services considered legitimate or not. Despite his demonstrable grasp and development of traditional osteopathic ideas, Bowen's giftedness did not solely lie in this knowledge in how he applied the pressure movements with neurological and anatomical precision to achieve therapeutic effect. Bowen's grasp of osteopathy and his rare sensory abilities allowed him to masterfully, as Ryan said, 'take the ordinary and make it extraordinary'.[74] Bowen undoubtedly had an uncanny intuition that allowed him to appraise what was wrong with his patients without history-taking coupled with an unusual tactile sensitivity. As Graham Webber Martin said, 'He had an active intuition that was weird'.[75] Bowen's abilities as a manual therapist were so remarkable that he was seen by the general community as a 'miracle maker', a 'wonder man' whose work was 'woo woo'. Police officer Phil Dower had been treated by Bowen when a young man injured in sport and saw him one day at a pub near his last practice at Villamanta Street in 1981/1982. He looked much older and the barman confirmed, 'oh yes, I've heard all about him you know, he does this some fan-dangled sort of practice that's strange'. When Dower introduced himself to Bowen those years later, he said to him, 'I must admit when I first went to you, I thought you were a witch doctor', to which Bowen replied 'Yes, I've been told that many a time'.[76] Bowen had already lost his first leg by then and the impacts of regulation were in full swing and Dower recalled that Bowen never said anything critical or bitter at all. Dower had first seen Bowen with a rolled ankle around 1966/67 when he was thirteen/fourteen years of age. He remembered being puzzled why Bowen worked on his back, left the room, came back, tweaked his back some more, worked down the leg and did something to his ankle and told him he should be right to train on Tuesday. This was a very short time as Dower expected to be out of the game for two weeks. The treatment was not painful and in his description he said:

> Tom never seemed invasive. It was more like giving in, intuitive to the body. He seemed more like it was within his hands. It was like, – it might be stupid when I say this – but it was like a miracle happening to me you know. The body was being calmed by him and that seemed really strange particularly for a young person who's never had anything like that before.[77]

When asked about Bowen's touch, Kevin Neave DC said, 'Really soft, really soft to point you feel something radiating from the touch you know'. Referring to Bowen's instructions about pressure when working on client, 'He'd like, he'd put your hand on, on there and you'd wait, and just gradually put a little bit more pressure on . . . and he'd say, "You've got it"'. Anytime he'd say, 'I'd "got it", with Tommy I knew I didn't have to go beyond that point'.[78]

Bowen's community considered him a genius and there is an elusive element that even Bowen himself could not fathom; his hairdresser said, 'he did not know how it worked and didn't want to either'.[79] These attributes place Bowen in a different realm as an actor in the field of medical pluralism altogether though it is worth remembering that Dr AT Still MD, DO was also known to espouse more spiritual and esoteric ideas that were abandoned as the mainstream schools evolved on a more scientific pathway. Though Bowen never overtly practised clairvoyance like Still, nor communicated ideas about spirituality to those around him, he had an uncanny giftedness and deep commitment to service of humankind and healing that led to this kind of aura developing around his abilities and aligns him with high-profile osteopaths who included esoteric adjuncts in their osteopathic practice.[80]

The non-heterodox and esoteric elements in Bowen's practice contributed to the biopsychosocial mystique of his abilities that saw him akin to a witch doctor. Those of prominent ability were often quite humble and described their natural talent in terms of a gift, or a gift of God. Donald surprised his family by appearing in the press as 'Mr Donald attributes his gift to God' as he was not religious.[81] Saunders too was on record saying simply it was 'a gift', 'Saunders was without a university degree but had a wonderful gift which he himself could not explain'.[82] The same is true of Bowen, he too just said his ability was a 'gift of God'. From Bowen's hairdresser Doug Griffiths:

> I said to him once, 'what was your secret, Tom?' and he said, 'I don't know'. I thought he was a bit devious, but he wasn't, and I don't think he really knew what talent he had, well that was ridiculous to say that, he had this gift and I suppose he thought it was a privilege to have that gift, I suppose that's the way I thought about Tom. But Tommy Bowen was, you'd never know he was, he had this genius in him. People often spoke about that. Well, he was a genius in his own right, but a more humble man you'd never meet, he was so, just an everyday country man.[83]

Bowen said to one of his apprentices Kevin Neave 'I don't know what I'm doing'.[84] Bert Donald reflected 'I don't know what I did'.[85] Another attribute assigned to masseurs of talent was magnetism or electricity. Saunders was described in parliament by Mr Prendergast:

> This man whose name has been mentioned in the course of the debate appears to have the faculty of transferring some magnetic power from himself to those on whom he lays is manipulative hands, and that way he is able to improve their bodily system and overcome their complaints.[86]

On this, Fay who was scientifically inclined, said, 'this kind of talk leads nowhere' and emphasised the benefits of massage by plain and systematic means.[87]

Bowen conceptualised healing and sensitivity to bodies he was treating in electrical terms and perceived himself to have 'too much electricity' in his body.[88] Bowen laid great store by people's hands whether they were 'positive' or 'negative'.[89] To some, he explained he was taking the pain out of their body and taking it into his own so that those suffering could have a rest.[90] Sensing bio-electricity or having electricity or magnetism in the hands was a cultural hallmark of the gifted masseurs. When the young John Garner witnessed his father Ron and Bowen meet, he said,

> I remember him and Dad shaking hands or trying to shake hands and the sparks fly and they sort of went, bang! One went to one end of the bar and the other to the other end and, 'Wow', they said, 'That's magic',

so instead of shaking hands they hugged and the barman made comment 'There's got to be magic in those hands'.[91]

John recounted the ability of both Tom and his father to 'feel a nerve working'.[92] Important to John's understanding of his father and Ron's giftedness was the pulsation or energy current that could be felt during a treatment, especially if both laid hands on him and this was a unique experience; other than one rare occasion, he never felt this again in treatments he had sought out after their deaths, from those trained posthumously in Bowen's techniques, including osteopaths. Bowen would receive shocks from patients; one incident he swore about and Smeeton DC knew of one account where Bowen said he would not be able to work for a week.[93] Skilbeck DC/ND too recounted an occasion when Bowen said, 'I burned my fingers'.[94] Sensing a shock when treating was not necessarily unusual. Heather Hay, a clinic associate of Alister McAlister DO, recalled his mention of experiencing a shock when adjusting a patient's joint.[95] Bert Donald's fingers were so sensitive he would feel they were inflamed or burning when he touched bodies, he worked through a barrier and found it hard to treat people as he got older.[96]

One of the most unusual areas of Bowen's sensitivity was his cognisance of cycles of the moon when scheduling patient attendances at his disability clinic. The determinant was the effect on him personally as it controlled which days he would treat all his clients who suffered palsies or other neurological conditions that affected the spine and their functioning; it was not customised to his patients, but rather himself. On one occasion, Bowen sent all of his patients home as they had 'got the day wrong for the moon'.[97] Analysis of surviving patient cards has failed to produce an explanation other than he personally experienced a change in with lunar cycles that helped his work with clients with neurological issues.

Bowen was not a superhuman and was not always successful, but he did not mislead with false claims: if he could not help he said so and referred on. Not all patients sang his praises and current therapists attest to receiving remarks from former Bowen patients, 'he did nothing for me'.[98] Bowen's exoteric practice of osteopathy sits at the non-biomedical end of the spectrum of medical pluralism, but on the esoteric aspect, he was possessed of other attributes that place him in another realm of ability altogether. These contributed to the reasons why he was so sought out by the community as a practitioner and contributed to his legendary status and aura that motivated others to teach his work when he died. Others have written about prominent osteopaths such as Robert Fulford whose practice and ideas included ideas about energy healing and esoteric adjuncts such as magnets and crystals.[99]

Integration of Eastern Ideas

Historically, Chapter 5 contextualised the upsurge of interest in Eastern medicine after the visits of Whitlam and Nixon to China. Using the transcripts to the Ward Inquiry as a barometer, this was the major influence within the overall impact of globalisation in that period. Evidence of the effects of earlier phases of globalisation were evident in the personal testimony of the Austrian John Joseph Mik who had encountered acupuncture in 1918 through a Russian who had been to China and Mik spent five years learning from him before he emigrated to Australia in 1949.[100] Cant discusses the globalised health market of the 1970s and the importation of non-western therapeutics in the 1970s in the UK including 'Asian Knowledges'. Cant acknowledges that though globalisation has fostered biomedical homogeneity with knowledge, capital and labour flows, it has also fostered medical pluralism by allowing opportunities for exchanges between orthodox and non-orthodox medicines.[101] Despite the incorporation of the non-orthodox medicines, biomedicine continues to dominate due to capitalism, free market capitalism and the colonial legacies.[102] CAM is seen as new variant of medical pluralism, but hierarchies of power exist and the term CAM reflects a binary term which reinforces the dominance of biomedicine and it suffers from mainstream marginality.[103] In Australia, a Chinese Medicine Board is regulated by the government through the Australian Practitioner Health Regulation Agency (APHRA), so in principle, Chinese Medicine is recognised alongside biomedicine under allied health, however only general practitioners of biomedicine have the power to provide medical referrals for care plans under Medicare and prescribe pharmaceutical drugs.

Another viewpoint is possible when considering the integration of 'Asian knowledges' in the interpretive pluralisms around the legacy of Bowen's work and the shift in his own symbolism in the 1970s to an Eastern frame. Bowen's sensitivity to bioelectricity would have allowed him to detect acupoints even if he had no knowledge of Eastern Medicine. Acupoints are clinically palpable and are '*ah shi* points according to TCM, or myofascial trigger points according to Western medical acupuncture'.[104] Acupoints are described as having 'distinct electrical properties', and these include 'increased conductance, reduced impedance and resistance, increased capacitance, and elevated electrical potential compared to adjacent non acupuncture points'.[105] Bowen had the ability to sense nerve activity and knew how to trace the paths of nerves. Translating the Eastern system to Western physiology, Longhurst explained:

> Modern physiologists have put forward the 'neural hypothesis' stating that the clinical influence of acupuncture is transmitted primarily through stimulation of sensory nerves that provide signals to the brain, which processes this information and then causes clinical changes associated with treatment.[106]

Bowen's symbolism around nerve pressure and other protocols he followed aligned him with an osteopathic knowledge system traced to neuropathy and practised within the scope of Dr Still MD, DO's original osteopathic tenets. The shift to an Eastern frame in the 1970s was an effect of influence of the time but he never left the Western osteopathic context of his work. In his last press interview before he died and shortly after being failed by the Registration Board, he returned to the Western anatomy and said, 'I only use my ten fingers in my work'.[107] In the article, Bowen says, 'Osteopathic, [*sic*] in contrast to chiropractic which involves manipulation of the spinal column, is a system of diagnosis and treatment of disorders by manipulation of muscle and nerve tissue'.[108] Frijov Capra explored the parallels between modern physics and Eastern mysticism and quoted semanticist Alfred Korsybski's slogan 'the map is not the territory'.[109] Regardless of culture, human bodies share the same gross anatomy and physiology but have different maps to explain the territory. In the context of medical pluralism, the incorporation of Asian Knowledges has to be considered in light of tactile ability and acquaintance with the relevant knowledge systems and bringing them together.

The influence of Asian medicine flowed through to the manuals written posthumously that interpreted Bowen's work, but none of the teachers have abandoned Western anatomy in favour of exclusively focusing on Eastern anatomy. The interest seems clearly driven by forces of globalisation of the 1970s period, and although these forces gave Bowen access to new perspectives, it is hard to argue cultural appropriation when Bowen himself was arriving at synthesis.

From a Posthumous NRM to Pluralist Secular Interpretations

The vehicle for the first early widespread interpretation of Bowen's work was essentially via a New Religious Movement (NRM) buoyed by the wider New Age culture of the 1980s. The romance of Bowen's symbolic archetypal power as the universal human healer with transcendent, transpersonal talent was successfully captured. The Bowtech company-academy maintained NRM fervour by promoting an aspirational culture of enthralment, unity, peace and healing. For the Bowen family, the early mood felt biblical as one relative described how Bowen fans wanted to touch them as if there was some power in their raiment that could be transmitted to them.[110] The Bowtech company brand is infused with evangelical and religious persuasions illustrated with bible quotes and claims of 'lineage' and 'purity' evident in the company magazine and conference speeches, while article titles underscore an assumed supremacy over competitors.[111] As a powerful unifying central figure, Bowen's authority empowered the belief that the soft tissue techniques taught in his name were revolutionary globally among other modalities.[112] Consumers and fans shared success stories and novice practitioners expected the technique to uniquely address complex medical problems. Other accounts tell of altars and votive candles. When long-term friends and former patients of Bowen met the nouveau practitioners born of this culture on their travels, they recalled:

> This lady had done a few little flicks and gave, I'm not sure, she was working on mental stuff or something else or about his presence and some other stuff. That wasn't Tom Bowen, he hurt you. I didn't matter

> that it hurt, it was getting it [the nerves or ligaments] in the right position and coming back to check and sometimes it would take three or four times and him saying, 'Now it's right'.[113]

And another:

> One therapist would do their Bowen religiously and not mix the Bowen with any other modality at all; it was all Bowen-Bowen-Bowen. One guy found out that I knew Tom because he looked at me and he asked, 'Has that body had Tom Bowen's hands on it?' and I said, 'Yes'. He was just elated and never charged me a cent because he had the privilege of putting his hands on the same body Tom had . . . So, I had a lot of experience with Tom. Tom never changed his style at all and the only person I felt was anything like Tom was Romney [Smeeton].[114]

The early Bowtech teachings were incredibly popular, delivered in a simple, easy-to-learn recipe-based format. Bowen left no written records of his work, his legacy was orphaned from osteopathy and specifically the traditional style he practised, so there was no knowledge system to give a solid base to any initial teachings. The NRM culture was forged on the mystique of Bowen's successes and stories of miraculous healings. Popularity created a demand for instructors, increased when ambassadors Milton Albrecht and Julian Baker paved the way for the teachings to reach America and the European Common Market, respectively. Without a knowledge system to buoy the teachings, by the late 1990s, a schism led to the formation of offshoot schools that developed teachings variously drawn from formal ideas in the emerging field of fascia science, massage systems, chiropractic theory, trigger point therapy and Eastern systems such as acupoints and energy meridians. The critical mass of those trained started a secular direction and the need for professional associations to be established in Australia and overseas. Under Australian Nationally Recognised Training, Registered Training Organisations (RTOs) delivered teachings and courses compliant with the national competency unit standards of vocational training. Until the Natural Therapies Review outcome of 2019, these standards were accepted by Health Fund Insurers allowing rebates for Bowen treatments. In Britain, the Complementary and Health Care Council oversees training acceptable for service provision in the National Health Service (NHS) and in America, the majority of individual State Regulatory Boards control massage with therapeutic touch. An issue for US Bowen practitioners is the likelihood their state will include them under the definition of massage for licensure.

There is a subtheme of pluralism among the various posthumous interpretations too. Since a unifying knowledge system is lacking, schools pursue individual interpretations and the growing field of fascia science is widely embraced to explain how the techniques bring about therapeutic effects. Website descriptions by associations and official bodies tend to focus on 'the

Bowen move', waits or pauses between sets of moves and minimalist application to specific areas of the body. Some refer to knowledge from fascia science; the beneficial influence on the nervous system, the modality's gentleness and allowing the body to reset.[115] Behind this are numerous studies on the benefits of treatments and these have been submitted to Australian Government Natural Therapies Reviews in 2014 and 2019–2020. One author-instructor has written books on the neurological processes of the therapeutic pause and the effect of touch on sensory fibres and another article discusses nerves.[116] Smeeton DC has worked for nearly five decades with Bowen's methods drawing on the knowledge-systems of chiropractic and his self-education in osteopathy during his Roberts' college training in the 1970s. On professional development beyond entry-level training, he says, 'My advice to anybody who is wanting to further their understanding and knowledge is "know your neurology" because everything Tom did was started from a spinal perspective'.[117]

Adversaries of CAM Including Bowen Therapy/Technique

Bowen did not call what he did Bowen Therapy or Bowen Technique. As claimed in this book, he was practising osteopathy with the technical component derived principally from neuropathy within that field. Posthumously as a CAM modality, it has gained accreditation and a level of legitimation in Australia and internationally in various jurisdictions, but like other CAM therapies suffers attack from internationally organised sceptics' organisations who hold all CAM therapies up to the RCT standards of biomedicine. The crux of the fight around legitimation is centred around contested ideas about evidence-based medicine. Advocates and champions of biomedicine criticise CAM as not evidence-based, but they do so on the basis of the RCT being the only acceptable standard. A growing body of literature articulates why the RCT approach is not always suitable for CAM research. For instance, researchers recognising the significant uptake of CAM in oncology treatments conducted the first robust analysis of CAM trials involving comparisons against a large pool of non-CAM studies. This involved 764 trials representing 462,449 patients (including 5,330 patients enrolled in twenty-five CAM RCTs). Instead of simply sweeping CAM aside, the researchers showed the need for improved study design.[118] Medical writers in orthopaedics and physical therapy who uphold the RCT acknowledge that the RCT is a form of research design not always suitable for all research needs and state, 'Yet few things annoy us more than the ***deification*** that clinicians and selected researchers have given to randomize controlled trials'.[119] Five limitations of RCT research are identified with a call to understand them before applying them to clinical practice as well as acknowledging the costly nature of RCTs. They conclude, 'Other research designs are needed to understand the diagnosis, validity of outcomes, and other important research issues'.[120] Chatterjee looked at the widespread popularity of CAM in the USA and the barriers to effective utilisation in integrative care. Financial costs were identified as CAM does not attract insurance and scepticism and discouragement from doctors and the public and the difficulty in understanding efficacy and benefits against cost are issues. As a result, access is enjoyed by demographics unrestricted by income and education.[121]

Today, the shared standards of biomedical sciences in education underpin the allied health system in Australia with a biomedical hierarchy diversified to include physiotherapists, osteopaths and chiropractors who share status with doctors, formalised with the creation in 2010 of APHRA. Medicare resources are uniquely within the remit of those APHRA-registered. Doctors can create Medicare-funded care plans and make referrals to other allied health services. It is interesting to observe patterns that can be interpreted as the consequence of relationships and cultural attitudes forged early last century between biomedicine and other systems of healing that became state-recognised in the medical landscape. A 2022 report by the Australian Institute for Health and Welfare shows nearly 11 million referrals by doctors went to physiotherapy, about 9 million to chiropractic and only 1 million to osteopathy.[122]

Historically, the status of physiotherapy evolved from the groundwork of massage which established medical credibility through registered masseurs operating from the beginning under the oversight of medical doctors in hospital settings. Massage was regulated in Australia early last century and in Victoria from 1922. The story of the Saunders' father and son duo in Chapter 4 is an example of the government setting aside biomedicine's constituency to allow their registration based on ability and not credentials. Qualifications of masseurs expanded mid-century towards university degrees founded on biomedical sciences that strengthened their connection with doctors; the Massage Association in Victoria became the Massage and Physiotherapy Association, then ultimately federally, the Australian Physiotherapy Association. The heritage of the close relationship of physiotherapists (formerly masseurs) with medical doctors is undoubtedly reflected in the dominant pattern of referrals under Australian Medicare today. Similarly, the lower quantum of referrals for osteopathy compared to chiropractic may be seen to reflect the difficult journey of osteopathy following the outcome of the Western Australian Commission 1958–1964 and the national strategy (described in Chapters 1 and 6) to achieve registration under the chiropractic umbrella. Consequently, developments in the medical landscape of last century have a long reach into the twenty-first century and influence cultural attitudes and behaviours among doctors in today's landscape of medical pluralism and diversity of medical systems.

Posthumous Bowen Therapy schools and practitioners are represented as part of natural therapies in CAM. There is a misperception that biomedicine is evidence-based and CAM is not. The key issue is that biomedicine and adversaries of CAM have redefined evidence to strictly mean evidence that follows the RCT gold standard of biomedicine. Campaigns by groups such as the Friends of Medicine (FoM-Australia), Good Thinking Society (GTS-UK), the European Council of Sceptical Organisations (ECSO) and Science-Based Medicine (SBM-USA) are vocal activists against CAM and vigilant about attacking claims about benefits to consumers. The CAM detractors portray themselves as protecting consumers but the agenda is more complex. Consumer protections are valid and claims that sit outside of the scope of practice or remedial benefit should not be made. However, an entire international industry of critics exists to protect the flanks of biomedicine and ignores the right of consumers to look for and invest in therapies of their choosing in a landscape of medical pluralism and diversity.

Biomedicine allows the concept of dignity of risk which honours the right of people to make decisions that support personal growth, self-esteem and quality of life even the choices carry a risk in the worldview of mainstream medical care. Dignity of risk is a crucial part of person-centred care but this seems implicitly ignored in the media efforts of these organisations to denigrate CAM. Their media influence was to the fore during the First Australian government-led Natural Therapies Review in 2014 set up to assess the efficacy, effectiveness, efficiency and safety of CAM therapies, including Bowen, which by then attracted health fund rebates for those with private health insurance extras. The underlying political agenda was to divert government funding to support Health Funds' policies instead to the Medical Fund and biomedical research. The first scientific committee appointed to make recommendations to the federal Chief Health Officer did not represent the CAM sector and some members were affiliated with anti-CAM organisations and declared no conflict of interest. The benchmark for keeping a therapy was the systematic review and gold standard RCT and limited to very recent research which eliminated worthy older studies. As a result, despite a large volume of research describing benefits, efficiencies and effectiveness expressed as consumer satisfaction and therapeutic benefits, seventeen modalities were removed from the rebates schedule, including Bowen Therapy, due to research not being considered compliant with the standards set by the review. In Australia, FoS enjoyed a high profile in the media with academics denouncing CAM and even critical of CAM education being available at the university level. The international collaboration between CAM detractors was clear when a Sydney newspaper poll aimed at Australian consumers was gamed by overseas participants stacking the negative response while Australia was asleep. Since then, another review was conducted under a Liberal government with a more representative committee and the sector awaits results from the current Labor government. The challenge of maintaining its place as a relative newcomer in CAM and building a credible evidence base for therapeutic benefit that stands up to critical scrutiny of biomedicine and its sceptic allies is a challenge, but a growing body of studies has been submitted to the Australian Natural Therapies Reviews.

Bowen Therapy in the UK has received ongoing critical attention from members of the Good Thinking Society formed in 2012 whose members include former sceptic society academics. In 2009, Edzard Ernst started by singling out chiropractic and complementary medicine for attack.[123] More recently, Ernst targeted Bowen Technique.[124] Together with sceptic Simon Sing, Ernst included Bowen among questionable massage techniques.[125]

Likewise, other UK sceptics such as Richard Rawlins incorporated Bowen Technique in his overall critique of CAM therapies as quackery.[126] This serves to illustrate that alongside Bowen's historical legacy impacted by biomedicine's role in the legitimation of chiropractic and osteopathy, its posthumous trajectory is now caught up in the battle of legitimation of CAM against a well-organised and articulate industry of CAM detractors, including in academia. Part of the problem is that some CAM practitioners have minimal qualifications and strong cultural opinions distrusting the pharmaceutical industry and biomedicine, and also for some Bowen therapists, this extends to the critique of the legitimated professions of osteopathy and chiropractic. They can be categorised as belonging to what Uibo and Koppel synthesise from other researchers seeing in recent decades, 'increasingly diverse health-related opinions and expert positions in the mass media. Among them are lay experts who belong to organised online groups creating 'healthcare knowledge cultures that by nature challenge the authority allopathic medicine and allied health generally'. However, Uibo and Koppel are referring to the community, Bowen Therapy is shaped and controlled by practitioners in the pluralist medical landscape and are the arbiters of meaning.

There are practitioners who appropriate and integrate diverse practices into the presentation and practice of Bowen Therapy and this is an area of contention among those who wish Bowen's legacy to be authentically portrayed as a musculoskeletal medicine. As a CAM therapy in the medical landscape, official control of how Bowen is presented to consumers are the official government, professional association and practitioners' websites. However, some practitioners stray from the formal descriptions of the modality and for example, treat Bowen Therapy as an energy therapy that can be transmitted through distant healing. There are British and American practitioners' websites openly promoting this service and the COVID-19 pandemic provided leverage. Consumers millions of miles away from Australia have been introduced to Bowen Therapy through practitioners offering fee-based distance healing services – and they choose to seek out this service regardless of the fact it is not authentic to Bowen's name and clinical practice. Practitioners overseas have made Bowen's legacy their own and assert authority over college-trained observers with first-hand acquaintance over what Bowen's work was and what Bowen stood for personally. This diversified reality supervenes on the real man and his work and is inherited from the introduction of the early popularised interpretations of Bowen's work occurring in the New Age Movement (NAM) of the 1980s. Paul Healas offered an in-depth analysis of the movement that helps to explain these attitudes and describes the trait of 'unmediated individualism: I am my own authority'.[127] Healas stated the NAM as 'an appeal against uncertainties of modernity and identifies from the work of others the spiritual aspirations and characteristics of the movement'.[128] The practitioner-only Bowen Therapy Worldwide Facebook group specifically disallows discussion of Bowen Therapy in the context of energy healing and the position strongly kept is that Bowen is a physical hands-on musculoskeletal therapy. Practitioners concerned about the future of Bowen as a modality are opposed to Bowen's legacy and practice being presented in a manner that sets it up for ridicule and at risk of further attack in renewed opprobrium as quackery.

Distinguishing Bowen Therapy Within CAM

There are several themes and tensions in the positioning and legitimation of Bowen Therapy/Technique in the landscape of medical pluralism and beyond that are worthy of further analysis and monitoring as its future unfolds. Legitimation of osteopathy and chiropractic last century was determined by standards of science in education. Bowen Therapy/Technique has achieved government recognition in Australia and Europe including Britain. In Australia, entry-level training towards a professional career is available at Certificate IV and Diploma level through a Registered Training Organization under the National Qualifications Framework.[129] Therapeutic skills are based on assessment and technical delivery, supported by specific competency units required under the standardised National Health Training Package. These include anatomy and physiology, medical terminology, infection control and working effectively in the health system.[130] In the UK, the Complementary and Natural Health Care Council (CNHC) sets requirements under National Occupational Standards for service provision in the NHS. The approach is similar to the Australian system and requires a level-3 diploma in anatomy and physiology, a certificate of Bowen proficiency from a recognised tutor, an Anatomy and Physiology certificate and a current first-aid certificate.[131] These qualifications allow practitioners to practise identifying as Bowen therapists. Similarly in Canada, training is available accredited with the Canadian Examining Board of Healthcare Practitioners and the Bowen Therapists Professional Association (BTPA-UK).[132] Despite the need for curriculum content to government standards – the key mechanism of legitimation of chiropractic and osteopathy last century, sceptics maintain the attack which suggests the issues are no longer about educational standards as they, at a minimum have established legal competencies to practice.

In America, the situation is more complex and threatens the unique identity of Bowen as a modality. American Bowenwork has two categories of training, certificated and non-certificated.[133] The academy is not board-certified and individuals with Bowen qualifications may not necessarily be allowed to practise as Bowen therapists. In America, the legal definition of massage is broad and subsumes a wide range of therapeutic systems involving touch. To practise massage, the majority of states require a license to touch, involving credentials in massage and Bowen therapists can be caught with these requirements.[134] American Bowenwork objects to Bowen being categorised under massage and encourages would-be Bowen therapists to check with their state licensing board whether they also need massage qualifications.[135] Information online suggests Bills have been prepared in Utah, Arkansas and California to legally exempt Bowen from the business of massage. The Californian bill is interesting as it sets out a legal definition of Bowen that attempts to set it apart from massage on the basis of minimal touch, Bowenwork being largely hands off and the client is fully clothed.[136] However, in the meantime, the National Massage and Bodywork University whose courses are Board-certified offers Bowen training in various states and qualified massage therapists are able to use the techniques as part of their massage repertoire.

Similar objections around preserving the identity of the modality erupted in Australia after the Natural Therapies Review removed Bowen Therapy from the list of modalities that could attract health fund rebates. Remedial Massage was retained and remained eligible. Neil Skilbeck, who operated an Australian RTO in Bowen Therapy, endeavoured to expand offerings and create a massage package that incorporated Bowen Techniques that conformed with nationally recognised training definitions and standards. Skilbeck explained that the techniques of Bowen fell under the definition of remedial massage and included the same basic techniques such as friction, passive soft tissue movements, muscle energy, neuromuscular, press and release and trigger point therapy. Skilbeck was strongly attacked and accused of attempting to defraud the government.[137] His aim was to practise the technique without need to use the 'Bowen' label. The overall key objection was the loss of identity. The sector struggles to differentiate Bowen from massage and a recent attempt focused solely on technique delivery and attributes such as minimalism, non-continuous contact with the body, waits between moves and gentleness.[138] Some would argue these differences are insufficient to distinguish Bowen from massage and massage therapists in the USA have challenged the attempt to differentiate on the touch aspect. An underlying issue is that both draw on the same knowledge systems such as fascia science and claim to be holistic with similar wellbeing benefits. There is a need to distinguish Bowen based on the distinct cognitive framework and knowledge system with a philosophy drawn from traditional neuropathy/naturopathic osteopathy.

Bowen was known to practise craniosacral therapy (CST). Although CST is not generally taught as part of Bowen Training and it is taken up separately by those interested, CST has been subject of strong criticism for those that would. It is not accepted by advocates of osteopathic education based on the biomedical sciences which has underpinned modern trajectory of osteopathy.[139] In 2006, Hartman called for a ban on teaching CST altogether and for insurance companies to cease supporting the practice.[140] Others including Edzard Ernst found no therapeutic benefit in CST.[141]

In Victoria, Australia, especially in the western region, Bowen was well known. He touched the lives of many and survives in living memory but this is rapidly waning. Of the nearly sixty participants who took part in the 2016 centennial celebratory *Healing Hands, Unsung Voices* Anthology, nearly 12 per cent are now deceased. They include clinic associate Kevin Neave DC; patients John Garner, James Barr, Trevor Cole and Bernie Molloy; Bowen's sister Agnes Shaw; Don Mathieson OAM, past president of the Geelong Football League; and Pat Allen, protégé of Bert Donald. Clinic helper and lay masseur Doug Sells contributed accounts after and is now also deceased.

Summary

The Bowen story historically illustrates several themes that fall under medical pluralism and beyond. Bowen stands out as representative of a regulatory process that was draconian, especially when his treatment is compared to that of Kirsté Martinovich under the *Chiropractors Act 1964* (WA) covered in Chapter 1, the registration of the Saunders' father and son duo described in Chapter 4 and the treatment of much less qualified counterparts in NSW described in Chapter 7. Posthumously, Bowen's work was orphaned from osteopathy and although it has been accepted as a standalone therapy in some jurisdictions, its standing is under threat in America where ability to practise can be subsumed under massage. The descriptions flowing from the interpretations of his work lack a distinct knowledge system and philosophical framework that Bowen worked within to consolidate that claim. Osteopaths use massage techniques but osteopathy itself is not classified as massage because the cognitive framework, knowledge system and philosophy that guides the therapist in the use of their hands-on-techniques are distinct from massage.

Notes

1 Venera Khalikova, "Medical Pluralism," in *The Open Encyclopedia of Anthropology*, ed. Felix Stein (2023 [2021]). Facsimile of the first edition in *The Cambridge Encyclopedia of Anthropology*. Accessed November 17, 2024. http://doi.org/10.29164/21medplural
2 S. Cant, "Medical Pluralism, Mainstream Marginality or Subaltern Therapeutics? Globalisation and the Integration of 'Asian' Medicines and Biomedicine in the UK," *Society and Culture in South Asia* 6, no. 1 (2020): 31–51.
3 An overview of the history of the biopsychosocial model is presented by Micah R. Sadigh, "Development of the Biopsychosocial Model of Medicine," *History of Medicine, American Medical Association Journal of Ethics* 15, no. 4 (2013): 362–66.
4 Marko Uibu and Katre Koppel, "Beyond Medical Pluralism, Communicative Positioning of Biomedicine and CAM in Estonia," *European Journal of Health Communication*, 2, no. 3 (2021): 85–109.
5 Uibu and Koppel, "Beyond Medical Pluralism, Communicative Positioning of Biomedicine and CAM in Estonia."
6 Danuta Penkala-Gawęcka and Małgorzata Rajtar, "Introduction to the Special Issue 'Medical Pluralism and beyond," *Anthropology & Medicine* 23, no. 2 (2016): 129–34.
7 Penkala-Gawęcka and Rajtar, "Introduction to the Special Issue 'Medical Pluralism and beyond."
8 Hans Baer, "The Australian Dominative Medical System: A Reflection of Social Relations in the Larger Society," *The Australian Journal of Anthropology* 19, no. 3 (2010): 252–71.
9 Hans Baer, "Osteopathy in Australasia: From Marginality to a Fully Professionalised System of Health Care," *International Journal of Osteopathic Medicine* 12 (2009): 25–31; "The Drive for Legitimation by Osteopathy and Chiropractic in Australia: Between Heterodoxy and Orthodoxy," *Journal of Evidence Based Integrative Medicine* (April 1, 2006): 77–94.
10 S. P. Bolton, "A Retrospective View of Historical Periods in Australian Chiropractic History," *Chiropractic Journal of Australia* 36, no. 1 (2006): 9–16.

11 R. Blaich, A. Steel, D. Clark, and J. Adams, "Challenges and Opportunities for Australian Osteopathy: A Qualitative Study of the Perceptions of Registered Osteopaths," *International Journal of Osteopathic Medicine* 30 (2018): 18–24.
12 Ward Inquiry Report, 3, 1.24.
13 "Former Recipient Gives to Herald Blanket Fund," *Herald (Melbourne)*, May 20, 1938.
14 "A Pageant Organiser," *Journal (Adelaide)*, May 26, 1914.
15 "Register of Masseurs as at 31 December 1927," *Victoria Government Gazette*, No. 19, January 31, 1928.
16 "Life Governors," *Sporting Globe (Melbourne)*, September 10, 1932: 6.
17 "League Trainers," *Age (Melbourne)*, February 9, 1938: 16.
18 " 'Up There, Casaly!' – the Cry Lives on," *Sporting Globe (Melbourne)*, May 20, 1953: 5.
19 Col Hutchinson, *Cat's Tales, The Geelong Football Club 1897–1983* (Geelong: Geelong Advertiser, 1984), 25.
20 "Charity Match," *Age (Melbourne)*, August 22, 1931: 14; "Veteran Athletes Rally to the Globe's Charity Carnival," *Sporting Globe (Melbourne)*, September 2, 1933: 6.
21 "V Leveson's Tour," *Sporting Globe (Melbourne)*, December 22, 1928: 6; "Swimmers and Water Polo Players Ready for Busy Season," *Sporting Globe (Melbourne)*, December 22, 1928: 6.
22 "Mostly Personal," *Western Mail (Perth)*, March 12, 1931: 5.
23 "Trainers to Aid Crippled Children," *Sporting Globe (Melbourne)*, December 2, 1933: 6.
24 Pleass receives no mention in Peter Yule, *The Royal Childrens Hospital a History of Faith, Science and Love* (Broadway, Australia: Halstead Press, 1999).
25 Ron Phelan interview of Rene Horwood in Shirley Strachan, *Healing Hands, Unsung Voices, Thomas Ambrose Osteopath (1916–1982)* (United Kingdom: Cloister House Press, 2016), 25.
26 Ron Phelan personal communication November 18, 2024.
27 Agnes Shaw, video interview by Ron Phelan, excerpt in Strachan *Healing Hands*, 59.
28 Oral history accounts are provided in interviews by author in Strachan, *Healing Hands* of Bettye le Marquand, 94–97, Greg Hutchins, 172–77 and Maryann Cosic, 178–84.
29 Leonie Appelt to Shirley Strachan personal communication, August 23, 2017. Appelt was treated by Mitchell as a teenager.
30 "Family Notices," *Argus (Melbourne)*, February 21, 1951: 17.
31 "Masonic Installation," *Record (Emerald Hill)*, October 3, 1885: 5.
32 "Friendly Society Meetings," *Record (Emerald Hill)*, July 23, 1904: 3.
33 VIC, Parliamentary Debates, Legislative Assembly, May 14, 1996: 7–12: 7.
34 Heather Hay personal communication to author February 18, 2019.
35 "He Loved His Fellow Man," *Sporting Globe (Melbourne)*, February 24, 1951: 9.
36 "He Loved His Fellow Man."
37 Rene Horwood interview by Ron Phelan, in *Healing Hands*, 27.
38 Rene Horwood personal communication to Ron Phelan, nd.
39 "Stephen Grellet 1773–1855 French Quaker and Missionary," Oxford Reference; An image in Smeeton's possession of Bowen's last calendar with this saying appears in Strachan, *Healing Hands*, 276.
40 PROV, Report and evidence Osteopathy Committee (Pt.1–4), 27/11/975 (Pt. 2) 2261, VPRS 3253/P1/, Unit 47. Original papers tabled in the Legislative Assembly, transcripts of proceedings, Bowen transcript: 672.
41 PROV, VPRS 3253/P1/, Unit 47, Bowen transcript: 672.

42 PROV, VPRS 3253/P1/, Unit 47, Bowen transcript: 676.
43 PROV, Osteopathy, Chiropractic and Naturopathy Committee, VPRS 16439/P1, Unit 12, Committee Records, Jens transcript: 964–65.
44 PROV, Osteopathy, Chiropractic and Naturopathy Committee, VPRS 16439/P1, Unit 12, Committee Records, Jens transcript: 964–65.
45 PROV, VPRS 3253/P1/, Unit 47, Bowen transcript, 675 (note the transcript misspelled Shiels as Shields).
46 PROV, Report and Evidence Osteopathy Committee (Pt 1–4), 27/11/975 (Pt. 2) 2261 VPRS 3253/P1, Unit 50, Original Papers Table in the Legislative Assembly, Allchin transcript: 2882.
47 Susan Kruss, *After the Game, Geelong Past Players and Officials Club, 80 Years 1933–2013, Geelong Past Players and Officials Club* (Geelong Print Solutions, 2013), 106; Col Hutchinson, *Cat's Tales, The Geelong Football Club 1897–1983* (Belmont, Victoria: Geelong Advertiser, West Web Printers, 1984).
48 Jim Rose personal communication to author August 21, 2017.
49 "He Loved His Fellow Man."
50 Frank Harrison interview by author, March 19, 2015, transcript in Strachan, *Healing Hands*, 169.
51 Sue Bell, "Great Healers Are Born Healers," October 2014, accessed July 25, 2017, http://midlifexpress.com/great-healers-born-healers/. Reprinted with permission. This blog has now migrated to "Great Healers are Born Healers" and requires a subscription.
52 Mark Whittacker, "Time Capsule," *Weekend Australian Magazine*, May 3, 2003.
53 Julietta Jameson, *Cliffy, the Cliff Young Story* (Melbourne: Text Publishing Company, 2013), 67.
54 Jameson, *Cliffy, the Cliff Young Story.*
55 Betty Boyd (patient of Williams) personal communication to author, April 28, 2017.
56 Boyd (patient of Williams) personal communication to author, April 28, 2017.
57 Lisa Casanelia and David Stelfox, *Foundations of Massage* (Sydney: Churchill Elsevier, 2010), 16–17.
58 "The Age Landmarks, Lake Oval," Wednesday, April 13, 2005, Austadiums, Australian Stadiums and Sport.
59 John Murtagh telephone interview and email messages to author November 8, 2016.
60 Murtagh telephone interview and email messages to author November 8, 2016.
61 Michael Quinlivan personal communication to author; Ron Phelan personal communication to the author
62 Keith Davis, in *In Search*, 123. 165; Smeeton personal communication to author.
63 Bell, "Great Healers Are Born Not Made."
64 Bell, "Great Healers Are Born Not Made."
65 Leonie Appelt email to the author August, 22 2017.
66 PROV, VPRS 6345/P/, Unit 545 Letter and report dated April 14, 1978, Jacka Federal President of ANTA to Digby Crozier forwarded to Houghton, Minister for Health, May 4, 1978.
67 Gregory Munro personal communication to the author, March 15, 2019.
68 Munro personal communication to the author, March 15, 2019.
69 John Garner, interview June 22, 2015, by author in *Healing Hands.*
70 Numerous entries, *Geelong Advertiser* and other newspapers; Image courtesy of Ron Phelan from Rene Horwood Collection.
71 Garner interview in Strachan, *Healing Hands*, 41.
72 Garner interview in Strachan, *Healing Hands*, 41.
73 Garner interview in Strachan, *Healing Hands*, 37.
74 Kevin Ryan comment made in question time at end of "Working alongside Tom Bowen," not included in the transcript.

75 Graham Martin email message to author in Strachan, *Healing Hands*, 106.
76 Phil Dower, Interview by author, in Strachan, *Healing Hands*, 212.
77 Phil Dower, interview by author, in Shirley Strachan, Healing Hands.
78 Kevin Neave, interview by author, *Healing Hands*, 219.
79 Doug Griffiths video interview by Robert Ryder Geelong October n.d., 2003, transcribed by author June 24, 2018.
80 Zachary Comeaux, *Robert Fulford DO and the Philosopher Physician* (Seattle, WA: Eastland Press, 2002).
81 "Helping Hands," *Donald Birchip Times*, December 2, 1983: 6; Barbara Hewitt (daughter) interview by author September 17 2016.
82 "He Loved His Fellow Man."
83 Doug Griffiths video interview by Robert Ryder.
84 Neave record of meeting by Mechner.
85 Lockwood, "The Hands That Have Helped Thousands," 8.
86 VIC, Parliament Legislative Assembly Session 1935, Vol. 197, August 20, 1935, 2042.
87 Fay, *Scientific Massage for Athletes*, 22.
88 Heather Edmonds interview by author April 25, 2015, transcript in Strachan, *Healing Hands*, 62–63.
89 Murray, *In Search*, 184.
90 Diane Perhill, interview by Robert Ryder, Geelong, October, n.d., 2003 transcribed by author.
91 Garner, *Healing Hands*, 37.
92 Garner, *Healing Hands*, 37.
93 Smeeton personal communication to author.
94 Skilbeck, "A Typical Day Working with Tom Bowen," 3.
95 Heather Hay personal communication to author, July 29, 2017.
96 Kevin Norbury, "Bert Gives the Sick a Hand," *Sunday Press*, September 14, 1986: 16.
97 Romney Smeeton personal communication to author, December 5, 2017.
98 Nicholas Comino personal communication to author, 2016.
99 Zachary Coumeaux, *Robert Fulford DO, and the Philosopher Physician* (Seattle, WA: Eastland Press, 2002), Chapter on Adjunctive Modalities, 129–43.
100 Ward Report, "Undesirable Aspects of Fringe Practitioners," 59; PROV VPRS 16439/P0001/000012, Mik transcript, Ward Inquiry, 2942.
101 S. Cant, "Medical Pluralism, Mainstream Marginality or Subaltern Therapeutics? Globalisation and the Integration of 'Asian' Medicines and Biomedicine in the UK," *Society and Culture in South Asia* 6, no. 1 (2020): 32.
102 Cant, "Medical Pluralism, Mainstream Marginality or Subaltern Therapeutics?" 33.
103 Cant, "Medical Pluralism, Mainstream Marginality or Subaltern Therapeutics?" 34, 37.
104 T. Tegiacchi, "Manual Palpation Could Be a Useful Tool to Guide Traditional Acupuncture Point Selection," *Acupuncture in Medicine* 39, no. 5 (2021): 560.
105 A. C. Ahn and O. G. Martinsen, "Electrical Characterization of Acupuncture Points: Technical Issues and Challenges," *Journal Alternative and Complement Medicine* 13, no. 8 (2007): 817–24.
106 John C. Longhurst, "Defining Meridians: A Modern Basis of Understanding," *Journal of Acupuncture and Meridian Studies* 3, no. 2 (2010): 67–74.
107 Longhurst, "Defining Meridians."
108 Longhurst, "Defining Meridians."
109 Frijov Capra, *The Tao of Physics, An exploration of the Parallels between Modern Physics and Eastern Mysticism* (Great Britain: Wildwood House, 1975), 36.

110 Identity withheld, personal communication to author.
111 'Ossie' (O. Rentsch), "The Challenge, the Choice, the Change." *Bowen Hands, the Official Journal of the Bowen Therapy Academy of Australia* 9 (2), no. 33 (June 2000): 5–6; Ossie, (O. Rentsch), "Bowen Chose Me!" *Bowen Hands, the Official Journal of the Bowen Therapy Academy of Australia* 21 (4), no. 83 (December 2012): 1.
112 A banner to this effect appeared on the back of *Bowens Hands* till 1996 and continues in the corporate lexicon.
113 Trevor Cole interview by author, transcript in Strachan, *Healing Hands*, 14.
114 Barry Tattersall interview author, transcript in Strachan, *Healing Hands*, 8.
115 "Bowen Therapy," Better Health Channel; "Welcome to the American Bowen Academy," American Bowen Academy; "Bowen Therapy Core Curriculum', Complementary and Natural Healthcare Council, UK.
116 Louise Tremblay, *The Therapeutic Pause in Osteopathy and Manual Therapy* (Edinburgh: Handsprings Publishing, 2015); Louise Tremblay, *Physiological Pillars of Manual Therapy, Volume 1, Interoceptive Afferent Fibres* (Canada: AIMTC, 2022); Joh Wilks, "The Bowen Technique – Mechanisms for Action," *Journal of the Australian Traditional Medicine Society* 19, no. 1 (2013): 33–35, accessed November 17, 2024.
117 Romney Smeeton, Interview in Shirley Strachan, *Healing Hands Unsung Voices, Thomas Ambrose Bowen Osteopath (1916–1982)* (United Kingdom: Cloister House Press, 2016), 229.
118 Ethan B. Ludmir et al., "The Trials (and Tribulations) of Complementary and Alternative Medicine in Oncology," *Journal of the National Cancer Institute* 111, no. 12 (2019): 1358–60.
119 Chad E. Cook and Charles A. Thigpen, "Five Good Reasons to Be Disappointed with Randomized Trials," *The Journal of Manual & Manipulative Therapy* 27, no. 2 (2019): 63–65.
120 Cook and Thigpen, "Five Good Reasons to Be Disappointed with Randomized Trials."
121 Anwesa Chatterjee, "Evaluating the Barriers to the Utilization of Complementary and Alternative Medicine (CAM) in the United States: An Exploratory Study," *Advances in Integrative Medicine* 10, no. 4 (2023): 167–71, ISSN: 2212-9588.
122 "Use of Chronic Disease Management and Allied Health Medicare Services," Australian Institute of Health and Welfare, December 15, 2002.
123 Edzard Ernst, "Complementary /Alternative Medicine: Engulfed by Post Modernism, Anti-science and Regressive Thinking," *British Journal of Medical Practice* (April 2009): 298–300.
124 Edzard Ernst, "Is the Royal College of Nursing Promoting Quackery?" May 10, 2017 accessed September 7, 2018.
125 Simon Sing and Edzard Ernst, *Trick or Treatment Alternative Medicine on Trial* (London: Bantam Press, 2008), 316.
126 Richard Rawlins, *Real Secrets of Alternative Medicine an Exposé* (Dartmouth, Devon, UK: Placedo Publishing, 2016), Kindle edition, 225.
127 Paul Healas, *The New Age Movement: The Celebration of the Self and the Sacralisation of Modernity* Reprint (Oxford: Blackwell Publishers, 1997), 21.
128 Healas, *The New Age Movement*, 181, 225.
129 "Building a Career in Bowen Therapy," *Bowen Training Australia.*
130 "Building a Career in Bowen Therapy."
131 "Regulation," Bowen Therapy Professional Organisation UK; "Core Curriculum Bowen Therapy." Complementary and Natural Healthcare Council.
132 "Learn Bowen," Bowen College.
133 "Learn Bowenwork," American Bowen Academy.

134 "Massage Therapy State Licensing Requirements," Associated Bodywork and Massage Professionals.
135 "Licensing", American Bowen Academy.
136 AB 2793 Assembly Bill – Bill Analysis.
137 Dialogue took place on Bowen Therapy Worldwide Facebook Group in late 2017 -early 2018.
138 "Is Bowen Therapy Massage?" Bowen Training Australia.
139 Steve E. Hartman, "Cranial Osteopathy: Its Fate Seems Clear," *Chiropractic & Osteopathy* 14, no. 1 (2006): 10.
140 Hartman, "Cranial Osteopathy: Its Fate Seems Clear."
141 Luis Ceballos-Laita et al., "Is Craniosacral Therapy Effective? A Systematic Review and Meta-Analysis," *Healthcare (Basel, Switzerland)* 12, no. 6 (March 18, 2024): 679.

References

Newspapers

"A Pageant Organiser." *Journal (Adelaide)*, May 26, 1914. Accessed November 11, 2024. http://nla.gov.au/nla.news-article204669195.

"Advertising." "Shops, Factories &c, To Let." *Argus*, February 11, 1937: 2 (col.7). Accessed November 17, 2024. http://nla.gov.au/nla.news-article11967941.

"Charity Match." *Age (Melbourne),* August 22, 1931: 14 (col.2). Accessed November 17, 2024. http://nla.gov.au/nla.news-article203030622.

"Family Notices." *Argus (Melbourne)*, February 21, 1951: 17 (col.3). Accessed November 17, 2024. http://nla.gov.au/nla.news-article23035305.

"Former Recipient Gives to Herald Blanket Fund." *Herald (Melbourne),* May 20, 1938: 9. Accessed November 17, 2024. http://nla.gov.au/nla.news-article243158691.

"Friendly Society Meetings." *Record (Emerald Hill),* July 23, 1904: 3. Accessed November 17, 2024. http://nla.gov.au/nla.news-article165172893.

"He Loved his Fellow Man." *Sporting Globe (Melbourne)*, February 24, 1951: 9. Accessed November 17, 2024. http://nla.gov.au/nla.news-article193636732.

"Helping Hands." *Donald Birchip Times*, December 2, 1983: 6.

"League Trainers." *Age (Melbourne),* February 9, 1938: 16. Accessed November 17, 2024. http://nla.gov.au/nla.news-article206747989.

"Life Governors." *Sporting Globe (Melbourne),* September 10, 1932: 6. Accessed November 17, 2024. http://nla.gov.au/nla.news-article189114584.

Lockwood, Keith. "The Hands That Have Helped Thousands." *Mail-Times*, November 13, 1981.

"Masonic Installation." *Record (Emerald Hill*), October 3, 1885: 5. Accessed November 17, 2024. http://nla.gov.au/nla.news-article113011237.

"Mostly Personal." *Western Mail (Perth*), March 12, 1931: 5 (col.3). Accessed November 17, 2024. http://nla.gov.au/nla.news-article38896825.

Norbury, Kevin. "Bert Gives the Sick a Hand." *Sunday Press*, September 14, 1986.

"Swimmers and Water Polo Players Ready for Busy Season." *Sporting Globe (Melbourne),* December 22, 1928: 6, Accessed November 17, 2024. http://nla.gov.au/nla.news-article183971260.

"Trainers to Aid Crippled Children." *Sporting Globe (Melbourne),* December 2, 1933: 6. Accessed November 17, 2024.http://nla.gov.au/nla.news-article181748862.

"Up there, Casaly!" – the Cry Lives on." *Sporting Globe (Melbourne*), May 20, 1953: 5. Accessed November 17, 2024. http://nla.gov.au/nla.news-article178187662.

"V. Leveson's Tour." *Sporting Globe (Melbourne),* December 22, 1928: 6. Accessed November 17, 2024. http://nla.gov.au/nla.news-article183971277.

"Veteran Athletes Rally to the Globe's Charity Carnival." *Sporting Globe (Melbourne)*, September 2, 1933: 6. Accessed November 17, 2024, http://nla.gov.au/nla.news-article181741315.

Whittacker, Mark. "Time Capsule." *Weekend Australian Magazine*, May 3, 2003.

Primary Sources

Chiropractors and Osteopaths (Amendment) Act (VIC). 1992. Accessed November 17, 2024. https://classic.austlii.edu.au/au/legis/vic/hist_act/caoa1992395/.

Cole, Trevor. Interview by author. Transcript in Strachan, Shirley. *Healing Hands, Unsung Voices, Thomas Ambrose Bowen Osteopath (1916–1982)*. United Kingdom: Cloister House Press, 2016.

Cosic, Maryann. Interview by author. Transcript in Strachan, Shirley. *Healing Hands, Unsung Voices, Thomas Ambrose Bowen Osteopath (1916–1982)*. United Kingdom: Cloister House Press, 2016.

Dower, Phil. Interview by author. Transcript in Strachan, Shirley. *Healing Hands, Unsung Voices, Thomas Ambrose Bowen 1916–1982, Osteopath*. United Kingdom: Cloister House Press, 2016.

Edmonds, Heather. Interview by author. Transcript in Strachan, Shirley. *Healing Hands, Unsung Voices, Thomas Ambrose Bowen 1916–1982, Osteopath*. United Kingdom: Cloister House Press, 2016.

Garner, John. Interview by author. Transcript in Strachan, Shirley. *Healing Hands, Unsung Voices, Thomas Ambrose Bowen 1916–1982 Osteopath*. United Kingdom: Cloister House Press, 2016.

Griffiths, Doug. Interview by Robert Ryder n.d., 2003. Transcribed by author.

Harrison, Frank. Interview by author, March 19, 2015. Transcript in Strachan, Shirley. *Healing Hands. Unsung Voices, Thomas Ambrose Bowen 1916–1982 Osteopath*. United Kingdom: Cloister House Press, 2016.

Hewitt, Barbara. Interview by author. In Strachan, Shirley. *Healing Hands, Unsung Voices, Thomas Ambrose Bowen 1916–1982, Osteopath*. United Kingdom: Cloister House Press, 2016.

Horwood, Rene. Ron Phelan interview. Transcript in Strachan, Shirley. *Healing Hands, Unsung Voices, Thomas Ambrose Bowen 1916–1982, Osteopath*. United Kingdom: Cloister House Press, 2016.

Hutchins, Greg. Interview by author. Transcript in Strachan, Shirley. *Healing Hands, Unsung Voices, Thomas Ambrose Bowen 1916–1982, Osteopath*. United Kingdom: Cloister House Press, 2016.

Le Marquand, Bettye. Interview by author. Transcript in Strachan, Shirley. *Healing Hands, Unsung Voices, Thomas Ambrose Bowen 1916–1982, Osteopath*. United Kingdom: Cloister House Press, 2016.

Neave, Kevin. Interview by Vicki Mechner. March 14, 2003. Transcript in possession of author.

Neave, Kevin. Interview by author, February 27, 2015. Transcript in Strachan, Shirley. *Healing Hands, Unsung Voices, Thomas Ambrose Bowen 1916–1982, Osteopath*. United Kingdom: Cloister House Press, 2016.

Osteopaths Registration Act 1996, Act No. 75/1996. Accessed November 17, 2024. https://www.legislation.vic.gov.au/as-made/acts/osteopaths-registration-act-1996

Perhill, Diane, and Beverley Smith. Interview by Robert Ryder Geelong, October n.d., 2003. Transcribed by author, 2018.

PROV. Osteopathy, Chiropractic and Naturopathy Committee, VPRS 16439/P1 Committee Records, Goldby transcript: 447–54.

PROV. Osteopathy, Chiropractic and Naturopathy Committee, VPRS 16439/P1/, Unit 12. Committee Records, Jens transcript: 953–65.

PROV. Osteopathy, Chiropractic and Naturopathy Committee, VPRS 16439/P1, Unit 12. Committee Records, Mik transcript: 2941–56.
PROV. Osteopathy, Chiropractic and Naturopathy Committee, VPRS 16439/P1, Unit 13, Committee Records, Cogan transcript: 428–35.
PROV. Registration of Chiropractors and Oestopaths [*sic*]– New Act VPRS 6345/P/, Unit 545. General Correspondence, Jacka ANTA report April 14, 1978 to Digby Crozier, Member for Western Province April 19, 1978 forwarded to Houghton, Minister for Health, May 4, 1978.
PROV. Report and Evidence Osteopathy Committee (Pt 1–4) VPRS 3253/P1 27/11/975 (Pt. 2) 2261, Unit 50, Original Papers Table in the Legislative Assembly, Allchin transcript 2881–95.
PROV. Report and Evidence Osteopathy Committee (Pt.1–4), 27/11/975 (Pt. 2) 2261, VPRS 3253/P1/, Unit 47. Original papers tabled in the Legislative Assembly, transcripts of proceedings, Bowen transcript: 672–78.
"Register of Masseurs as at 31 December 1927." *Victoria Government Gazette*, No. 19, January 31, 1928: 493–96. Accessed November 17, 2024. http://gazette.slv.vic.gov.au/images/1928/V/general/19.pdf.
Ryan, Kevin. "Working alongside Tom Bowen." Presentation to National Conference of Bowen Interest Groups, August 21, 1999. Transcript in Strachan, Shirley. *Healing Hands, Unsung Voices, Thomas Ambrose Bowen 1916–1982, Osteopath.* United Kingdom: Cloister House Press, 2016.
Shaw, Agnes. Interview by Ron Phelan. Transcript in Strachan, Shirley, *Healing Hands, Unsung Voices, Thomas Ambrose Bowen 1916–1982 Osteopath.* United Kingdom: Cloister House Press, 2016.
Skilbeck, Neil. "Typical Day Working with Tom Bowen." *Vic Bowen News* 1, no. 2 (May 1998): 3.
Smeeton, Romney. "The Bowen Approach to Manipulative Therapy." 1992.
Smeeton, Romney. Interview in Shirley Strachan, *Healing Hands Unsung Voices, Thomas Ambrose Bowen Osteopath (1916–1982).* United Kingdom: Cloister House Press, 2016.
Tattersall, Barry. Interview by author, January 9, 2015. Transcript in Strachan, Shirley. *Healing Hands, Unsung Voices, Thomas Ambrose Bowen 1916–1982, Osteopath.* United Kingdom: Cloister House Press, 2016.
VIC. Parliamentary Debates. Legislative Assembly. Volume 197, August 20, 1935.
VIC, Parliamentary Debates, Legislative Assembly, May 14, 1996: 7–12: 7.
Ward Inquiry Report – full title – Victoria Parliament, Osteopathy, Chiropractic and Naturopathy Committee, et al. *Report from the Osteopathy, Chiropractic and Naturopathy Committee: Together with Appendices.* Melbourne: C. H. Rixon, Government Printer, 1975. Accessed November 17, 2024. http://www6.austlii.edu.au/au/other/vic/VicLASelCPubInq/1975/1.pdf.

Secondary Sources

Ahn, A. C., and O. G. Martinsen. "Electrical Characterization of Acupuncture Points: Technical Issues and Challenges." *Journal Alternative and Complementary* Medicine 13, no. 8 (2007): 817–24. Accessed November 17, 2024. https://doi.org/10.1089/acm.2007.7193.
Baer, Hans A. "The Drive for Legitimation by Osteopathy and Chiropractic in Australia: Between Heterodoxy and Orthodoxy." *Journal of Evidence Based Integrative Medicine* (April 1, 2006): 77–94. Accessed November 17, 2024. https://journals.sagepub.com/doi/pdf/10.1177/1533210106292467.
Baer, Hans A. "Osteopathy in Australasia: From Marginality to a Fully Professionalised System of Health Care." *International Journal of Osteopathic Medicine* 12,

no. 1 (2009): 25–31. Accessed November 18, 2024. https://doi.org/10.1016/j.ijosm.2008.05.002.

Baer, Hans A. "The Australian Dominative Medical System: A Reflection of Social Relations in the Larger Society." *The Australian Journal of Anthropology* 19, no. 3 (2010): 252–71. Accessed November 18, 2024. https://doi.org/10.1111/j.1835-9310.2008.tb00353.x.

Blaich, R. A. Steel, D. Clark, and J. Adams. "Challenges and Opportunities for Australian Osteopathy: A Qualitative Study of the Perceptions of Registered Osteopaths." *International Journal of Osteopathic Medicine* 30 (2018): 18–24. Accessed November 17, 2024. https://doi.org/10.1016/j.ijosm.2018.10.004.

Bolton, S. P. "A Retrospective View of Historical Periods in Australian Chiropractic History." *Chiropractic Journal of Australia* 36, no. 1 (2006): 9–16. Accessed November 17, 2024. https://search.informit.org/doi/10.3316/informit.530550519029873.

Cant, S. "Medical Pluralism, Mainstream Marginality or Subaltern Therapeutics? Globalisation and the Integration of 'Asian' Medicines and Biomedicine in the UK." *Society and Culture in South Asia* 6, no. 1 (2020): 31–51, page 32. Accessed November 17, 2024. https://doi.org/10.1177/2393861719883064.

Capra, Frijov. *The Tao of Physics, an Exploration of the Parallels between Modern Physics and Eastern Mysticism*. Great Britain: Wildwood House, 1975.

Casanelia, Lisa, and David Stelfox. *Foundations of Massage*. 3rd ed. Sydney: Churchill Elsevier, 2010.

Ceballos-Laita, Luis et al. "Is Craniosacral Therapy Effective? A Systematic Review and Meta-Analysis." *Healthcare (Basel, Switzerland)* 12, no. 6 (18 March 2024): 679. Accessed November 17, 2024. https://doi.org/10.3390/healthcare12060679.

Chatterjee, Anwesa. "Evaluating the Barriers to the Utilization of Complementary and Alternative Medicine (CAM) in the United States: An Exploratory Study." *Advances in Integrative Medicine* 10, no. 4 (2023): 167–71. Accessed November 17, 2024. https://doi.org/10.1016/j.aimed.2023.10.002.

Comeaux, Zachary. *Robert Fulford DO and the Philosopher Physician*. Seattle, WA: Eastland Press, 2002.

Cook, Chad E., and Charles A. Thigpen. "Five Good Reasons to Be Disappointed with Randomized Trials." *The Journal of manual & manipulative therapy* 27, no. 2 (2019): 63–65. Accessed November 17, 2024. https://doi.org/10.1080/10669817.2019.1589697.

Ernst, Edzard. "Complementary /Alternative Medicine: Engulfed by Post Modernism, Anti-Science and Regressive Thinking." *British Journal of General Practice* 59, no. 561 (2009): 298–301. Accessed November 17, 2024. https://doi.org/10.3399/bjgp09X420482.

Ernst, Edzard. "Is the Royal College of Nursing promoting Quackery?" May 10, 2017. Accessed November 17, 2024. http://edsardernst.com/2017/05/is-the-royal-college-of-nursing-promoting-quackery/.

Fay, Joseph H. *Scientific Massage for Athletes*. London: Athletic Publications, n.d.

Hartman, Steve E. "Cranial Osteopathy: Its Fate Seems Clear." *Chiropractic & Osteopathy* 14, no. 1 (2006): 10. Accessed November 17, 2024. https://doi.org/10.1186/1746-1340-14-10.

Healas, Paul. *The New Age Movement: the Celebration of the Self and the Sacralisation of Modernity*. Reprint. Oxford: Blackwell Publishers, 1997.

Hutchinson, Col. *Cats' Tales the Geelong Football Club 1897–1983*. Geelong: Geelong Advertiser, 1984.

Jameson, Julietta. *Cliffy, the Cliff Young Story*. Melbourne: Text Publishing Company, 2013, 67.

Khalikova, Venera. "Medical Pluralism." In *The Open Encyclopedia of Anthropology*, edited by Felix Stein. Facsimile of the first edition in *The Cambridge*

Encyclopedia of Anthropology (2021) 2023. Accessed November 17, 2024. http://doi.org/10.29164/21medplural.

Kruss, Susan. *After the Game, Geelong Past Players and Officials Club, 80 Years 1933–2013, Geelong Past Players and Officials Club.* Geelong Print Solutions, 2013.

Longhurst, John C. "Defining Meridians: A Modern Basis of Understanding." *Journal of Acupuncture and Meridian Studies* 3, no. 2 (2010): 67–74.

Ludmir, Ethan B. et al. "The Trials (and Tribulations) of Complementary and Alternative Medicine in Oncology." *Journal of the National Cancer Institute* 111, no. 12 (2019): 1358–60. Accessed November 17, 2024. https://doi.org/10.1093/jnci/djz117.

Murray, Col. *In Search of Tom Bowen and the Therapy he Inspired and Lots of Other Stuff.* Armadale: Palmer Higgs, Booksonline, 2010.

Penkala-Gawęcka, Danuta, and Małgorzata Rajtar. "Introduction to the Special Issue 'Medical Pluralism and Beyond'." *Anthropology & Medicine* 23, no. 2 (2016): 129–34. Accessed November 17, 2024. https://doi.org/10.1080/13648470.2016.1180584.

Rawlins, Richard. *Real Secrets of Alternative Medicine and Exposé.* Dartmouth, Devon, UK: Placedo Publishing, 2016, Kindle edition, 225.

Sadigh, Micah R. "Development of the Biopsychosocial Model of Medicine." *History of Medicine, American Medical Association Journal of Ethics* (April 2013). Published in *Virtual Mentor* 15, no. 4 (2013): 362–66. Accessed November 17, 2024. https://doi.org/10.1001/virtualmentor.2013.15.4.mhst2-1304.

Sing, Simon, and Edzard Ernst. *Trick or Treatment Alternative Medicine on Trial.* London: Bantam Press, 2008, 316.

Tegiacchi, T. "Manual Palpation Could Be a Useful Tool to Guide Traditional Acupuncture Point Selection." *Acupuncture in Medicine* 39, no. 5 (2021). Accessed November 17, 2024. https://doi.org/10.1177/0964528420987568.

Tremblay, Louise. *The Therapeutic Pause in Osteopathy and Manual Therapy.* Edinburgh: Handsprings Publishing, 2015.

Tremblay, Louise. *Physiological Pillars of Manual Therapy, Volume 1, Interoceptive Afferent Fibres.* Canada: AIMTC, 2022.

Uibu, Marko, and Katre Koppel. "Beyond Medical Pluralism, Communicative Positioning of Biomedicine and CAM in Estonia." *European Journal of Health Communication* 2, no. 3 (2021): 85–109. Accessed November 17, 2024. https://doi.org/10.47368/ejhc.2021.305.

Wilks, John. "The Bowen Technique – Mechanisms for Action." *Journal of the Australian Traditional Medicine Society* 19, no. 1 (2013): 33–35. Accessed November 17, 2024. https://search.ebscohost.com/login.aspx?direct=true&db=ccm&AN=107997148&site=ehost-live.

Yule, Peter. *The Royal Childrens Hospital a History of Faith, Science and Love.* Broadway Australia: Halstead Press, 1999.

Websites

"AB 2793 Assembly Bill – Bill Analysis." Accessed November 17, 2024. http://www.leginfo.ca.gov/pub/15-16/bill/asm/ab_2751-2800/ab_2793_cfa_20160425_093928_asm_comm.html

American Bowen Academy. "Learn Bowenwork." Accessed November 17, 2024. https://americanbowen.academy/why-learn-bowenwork/.

American Bowen Academy. "Licensing." Accessed November 17, 2024. https://americanbowen.academy/licensing/.

Associated Bodywork and Massage Professionals. "Massage Therapy State Licensing Requirements." Accessed November 17, 2024. https://www.abmp.com/practitioners/state-requirements.

Austadiums, Australian Stadiums and Sport. "The Age Landmarks, Lake Oval." Wednesday, April 13, 2005. Accessed November 17, 2024. http://www.austadiums.com.au/forum/viewtopic.php?t=1118.

Australian Institute of Health and Welfare. "Use of Chronic Disease Management and Allied Health Medicare Services." Accessed November 17, 2024. https://www.aihw.gov.au/reports/chronic-disease/medicare-chronic-disease-allied-health-items/contents/allied-health-services.

Bowen College. "Learn Bowen." Accessed November 17, 2024. https://www.bowencollege.com/learn-bowen/.

"Bowen Therapy." *Better Health Channel.* Accessed November 17, 2024, https://www.betterhealth.vic.gov.au/health/conditionsandtreatments/bowen-therapy.

Bowen Therapy Professional Organisation UK. "Regulation," Accessed November 17, 2024. https://www.bowentherapy.org.uk/regulation.php

Bowen Training Australia. "Building a Career in Bowen Therapy." *Bowen Training Australia.* Accessed November 17, 2024. https://bowentraining.com.au/build-a-career-in-bowen-therapy.

Bowen Training Australia. "Is Bowen Therapy Massage?" Accessed November 17, 2024. https://bowentraining.com.au/is-bowen-therapy-massage/.

Complementary and Natural Healthcare Council, UK. "Core Curriculum Bowen Therapy." Accessed November 17, 2024. https://www.bowentherapy.org.uk/docs/standards/CoreCurriculum_Nov20.pdf.

Oxford Reference. "Stephen Grellet 1773–1855, French Quaker and Missionary." Accessed November 17, 2024. https://www.oxfordreference.com/display/10.1093/acref/9780191826719.001.0001/q-oro-ed4-00005064.

Conclusion

> When you start this college, what system is to be used. Are you going to use the chiropractic theory or are you going to use another theory? There are many branches of this profession.
>
> Thomas Ambrose Bowen, 1973[1]

Bowen left no memoirs or writings to explain his work and posthumously, this led to the popularised interpretations of his work being orphaned from the knowledge system he embraced, he presumed the inventor of his approach and the focus directed to his techniques rather than what can be deduced about his cognitive framework.

This book has placed the Bowen story in the context of the larger forces of the last century that propelled chiropractic and osteopathy towards legitimation, rafting on biomedical standards of education that had its roots in Flexner's educational reform in America. This reform cast aside Dr Still MD, DO's college and the naturopathic colleges alike and set in train a medicalised pathway for osteopathy in America and a modernised mainstream scientific pathway for legitimated osteopathy as it evolved away from the original sometimes eclectic osteopathic philosophy. Bowen's work represents a long-forgotten practice that came to Australia via the separate naturopathic route. There is evidence of uncompleted formal studies at a British College with Stanley Lief's British College of Naturopathy and Osteopathy most likely – a college connected to others influential in Bowen's world and to Thomas Dummer dean of the European School of Osteopathy (ESO) who played a role in accrediting Australian colleges controlled by the professional organisation Bowen was a member of before regulation.

Oral histories captured how Bowen communicated about and practised his work. These in conjunction with documentary evidence from the Ward Government Inquiry and his comments to the press have been set in historical context and allowed his methods and ideas to be traced to neuropathy and early traditional osteopathy that came to Australia from America and Britain via Australia's naturopathic pioneers. Bowen's genius was in using his unusual tactile sensitivity and giftedness to pioneer these cosmopolitan influences and

DOI: 10.4324/9781003602125-10

their origins into a treatment system that was uniquely Australian and exquisitely minimalist according to Dr Still MD, DO's dictum of, 'Find it, Fix it and leave it Alone'; sometimes extended to 'Nature will do the Rest.'

Bowen's work was all about nerves: the resonances in symbolic interaction associated with neuropathy and lifting pressure off nerves are strong in accounts of his practice, along with Bowen's own words and those of his contemporaries in addressing the Ward Inquiry, especially those educated as osteopaths in the early Roberts' College period in the 1930s. The work of Dr Still MD, DO was principally soft tissue work; Bowen practised like a neuropath and within the tenets of Still's traditional osteopathy as articulated by his disciples who convened the 1924 Roundtable and generated the sequential Universal or General Natural Treatment Tonic (U/GNTT). The system could be creatively adapted and used to deliver techniques tailored to a patient's complaint and Bowen's approach strongly resonates with its concurrent diagnostic and therapeutic aspects.

Rather than the quiet lone wolf, Bowen emerges as culturally fluid in the political landscape of the 1970s and contemplated deeply about how to resolve his patient's problems. Figure 9.1 captures him in contemplation.[2]

He responded to the Victorian Government's Ward Inquiry, was commented on by leading medical figures in positive terms and recorded as a leading osteopath in the Ward Inquiry Report. He networked with other professionals, influenced directors of ACONPAL/South Pacific who adopted his ideas in their teachings and he was invited into the politically elite world of the United Chiropractors Association of Australasia (UCAA) to attend their conferences and demonstrate his techniques at the Sydney College of Chiropractic at

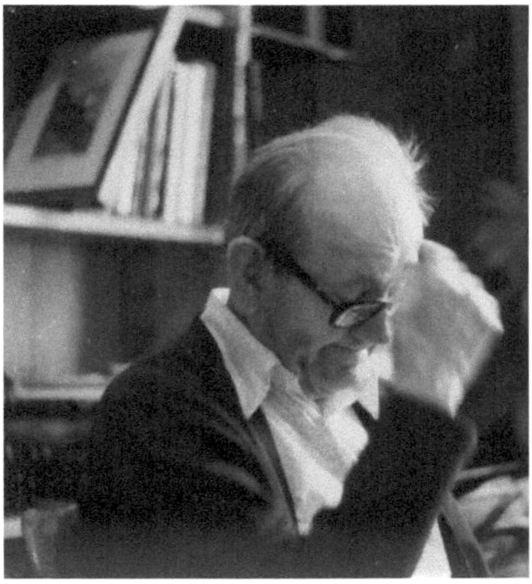

Figure 9.1 Tom Bowen captured in contemplation, taken at Smeeton Residence, Colac, late 1970s.

Source: Image courtesy Romney Smeeton DC.

workshops aimed at professional advancement. He was in demand by lay and professional practitioners alike. Bowen emerges fluid in indulging his intrigue about Eastern medicine and acupoints and demonstrates the ability to integrate the Western and Eastern systems on a sensory level. Bowen's fluid worldview was humanistic; people from all walks of life were welcomed into his practice where he treated factory workers, farmers, general public, individuals in sport, politicians and doctors and would often treat for free. He was devoted to helping those crippled by neurological conditions (see Figure 9.2).[3]

Despite his enormous, acclaimed talent, Bowen's treatment before the Victorian Registration Board was unjust and he became a victim of both the biomedical powerbase and the new powerbase of the legitimated professions working together to regulate professional practitioner registration. Practitioners like Bowen were supposed to have been grandfathered into registration in the same way their counterparts with lesser experience were in New South Wales. With a professional career of nineteen years standing and a lay career dating to the war period, his track record exceeded by far the legislative requirements of five years in Victoria. It is inconceivable to consider that not only was he not given a real living case to work on, but also he was denied the opportunity to demonstrate his skills in-clinic. Bowen suffered his first leg amputation shortly after the Act was introduced; he lost his second in hospital shortly after the Registration Board's verdict and died soon after and this conveys a symbolism of its own. He did not live to witness Marcus Try's successful Supreme Court case against the Registration Board, which if he had survived, would have established a legal precedent to have the Board's decision against him invalidated and overturned.

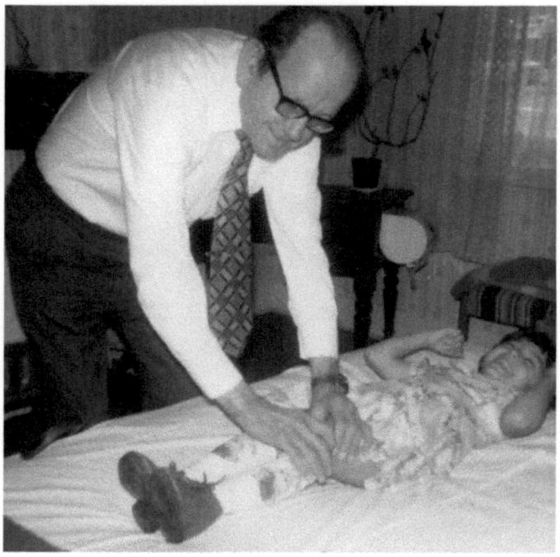

Figure 9.2 Bowen treating Maryann Cosic as a child at a Villamanta Street Clinic between 1978 and 1982.

Source: Image by Maryanne's mother and courtesy Romney Smeeton DC and Maryann Cosic.

We can never access Bowen's inner world to understand how he as a self-titled osteopath worked with his higher intelligence of a gifted healer. All we can appreciate is that Bowen found a home in osteopathy to channel his sensory giftedness and exceptionally intuitive way of addressing issues. The sensitivity trait also cursed Bowen with the relentless compulsion to tend to living things in pain and took its toll on his health. He died aged sixty-six suffering severe atherosclerosis that affected the circulation to his legs. His death was tragic but his legacy has survived and been impactful in two different domains – close to home in the hands of clinicians who have treated thousands of Australians, many of who still recall Bowen in living memory: in teachings by the clinicians to professional colleagues, final-year osteopaths and those adept in TCM and able to combine Bowen's physical techniques with that system.

Through the teachings of Bowen Schools nationally and internationally, Bowen Therapy or Technique has become a formal part of the global medical landscape of complementary and alternative medicine (CAM). It is undergoing transformation by growing its research base. Orphaned from the osteopathic wellsprings that provided a knowledge system for Bowen, the modality relies on differentiating on the basis of minimalist moves and waits and suffers from a lack of a distinct cognitive framework to clearly separate it from massage. The significance of Bowen's legacy nationally and internationally lies in the global reach of his methods. Historically, Bowen is uniquely representative of early cosmopolitan naturopathic osteopathy – including neuropathy – brought from American colleges inspired by Dr Still MD, DO and spread across the world via British Colleges to the antipodes by Australia's naturopathic pioneers FG Roberts and Maurice Blackmore who promoted and practised these forms until mid-century when likely due to chiropractic politics, neuropathy fell away from view.

As Bowen asked the Ward Inquiry, 'Are you going to use the chiropractic theory or are you going to use another theory? There are many branches of this profession'. History has brought to the fore a forgotten knowledge system that resonates with Bowen's work, allows his genius to shine in having evolved and pioneered it to a higher level of sophistication and calls for the title 'A History of Australia's Early Cosmopolitan Naturopathic Osteopathy: The Pioneering Practice and Global Symbolism of Thomas Ambrose Bowen'.

Notes

1 PROV. Report and evidence Osteopathy Committee (Pt.1–4), 27/11/975 (Pt. 2) 2261, VPRS 3253/P1/, Unit 47. Original papers tabled in the Legislative Assembly, transcripts of proceedings, Bowen transcript: 676.
2 Tom Bowen Captured in Contemplation. Image courtesy Romney Smeeton, DC.
3 Bowen treating MaryAnne Cosic as child at Villamanta Street Clinics between 1978 and 1982. Image by Mrs Cauchi (Mother) and courtesy Maryann Cosic and Romney Smeeton DC.

Abbreviations

AAC&O	Australian Association of Chiropractors and Osteopaths
ACA	Australian Chiropractors Association (represented those overseas trained)
ACN	Australian College of Naturopathy
ACONPAL	Australian Chiropractors Osteopaths and Naturopathic Physicians Association Limited
AFL	Australian Football League
AHPRA	Australian Health Practitioner Regulation Agency
AIF	Australian Infantry Force
AMA	Australian Massage Association
ANPA	Australian Naturopathic Practitioners Association
ANTA	Australian Natural Therapists Association
AOA	Australian Osteopathy Association (represented those overseas trained)
ASIC	Australian Securities and Investment Commission
ASO	American School of Osteopathy
ATMS	Australian Traditional Medicine Society
ATSU	Andrew Taylor Still University
BAIN	British and Australian Institute for Naturopathy
BCN/O	British College of Naturopathy and Osteopathy (see BCOM)
BCOM	British College of Osteopathic Medicine
BSO	British School of Osteopathy
BTPA-UK	Bowen Therapists Professional Association UK
CAM	Complementary and Alternative Medicine
CCA	Chiropractic College of Australia/Australasia
CMA	Complementary Medicine Association
CMF	Civil Militia Force
CNHC	Complementary and Natural Health Care Council
COCA	Chiropractic and Osteopathic College of Australasia
COCSA	College of Chiropractic and Osteopathy South Australia
COSS	College of Somatic Studies
CRTS	Commonwealth Reconstruction Training Scheme
CSF	Cerebrospinal Fluid
CST	Craniosacral Technique
DC	Doctor of Chiropractic
DO	Doctor of Osteopathy

ESO	European School of Osteopathy
EBSCo	Elton B Stephens Co Information Services
FBRA	Fellow British Reflexology Association
IFPNT	International Federation of Practitioners of Natural Therapeutics
IPM	Immediate Past Master
GNTT	General Naturopathic Treatment Tonic (see Universal Naturopathic Treatment Tonic)
KCOM	Kirksville College of Osteopathic Medicine
LCSP	London and County Society of Physiologists
LSNT	London School of Natural Therapeutics
LSO	London School of Osteopathy
MET	Muscle Energy Technique
MSNT	Manchester School of Natural Therapeutics
NAA	National Archives of Australia
NAM	New Age Movement
NAN/NANC/NANOC	National Association of Naturopaths (NAN), later including Chiropractors (NANC) and Osteopaths (NANOC)
ND	Naturopathic Doctor
NHMRC	National Health and Medical Research Council
NHS	National Health Service
NLA	National Library of Australia
NMT	Neuromuscular Therapy/Technique
NPH	*Natures Path to Health* Magazine
NRM	New Religious Movement
NST	Neurostructural Integration Technique
NSW	New South Wales
OAM	Order of Australia Medal
POW	Prisoner of War
PROV	Public Records Office of Victoria
QLD	Queensland
RCT	Randomised Controlled Trial
RMIT	Royal Melbourne Institute of Technology
RTO	Registered Training Organisation
SA	South Australia
SACA	South Australian Chiropractors Association
SACO	South Australian College of Chiropractic and Osteopathy
SCC	Sydney College of Chiropractic
SCO	Sydney College of Osteopathy (see SCOC and SCC)
SCOC	Sydney College of Osteopathy and Chiropractic (see SCC)
SOT	Sacro Occipital Technique
SPFNT	South Pacific Federation of Natural Therapeutics
SPCNT	South Pacific Council of Natural Therapeutics
SSNT	Southern School of Natural Therapies
TBT	Tom Bowen Therapy
TCM	Traditional Chinese Medicine
UCA [A]	United Chiropractors Association [later titled of Australasia] (represented those Australia trained)
UNTT	Universal Naturopathic Treatment Tonic (see GNTT)
UOPG	United Osteopathic Practitioners Guild
UPAA	United Practitioners Association of Australasia
VCA	Victorian Chiropractic Association

VFL	Victorian Football League
VIC	Victoria
VPRS	Victorian Public Records Series
VSSO	Victorian Society of Specialist Osteopaths
WA	Western Australia
YMCA	Young Men's Christian Association

Index

Note: locators in *italics* and **bold** refer to *figures* and **tables**.